RUSSIAN/SOVIET AND WESTERN PSYCHIATRY

A Contemporary Comparative Study

Paul Calloway

A WILEY-INTERSCIENCE PUBLICATION

JOHN WILEY & SONS, INC.

New York   •   Chichester   •   Brisbane   •   Toronto   •   Singapore

Copyright © 1992 by S. P. Calloway.
Copyright © 1993 by John Wiley & Sons, Inc.

All rights reserved. Published simultaneously in Canada.

Reproduction or translation of any part of this work
beyond that permitted by Section 107 or 108 of the
1976 United States Copyright Act without the permission
of the copyright owner is unlawful. Requests for
permission or further information should be addressed to
the Permissions Department, John Wiley & Sons, Inc.

This publication is designed to provide accurate and
authoritative information in regard to the subject
matter covered. It is sold with the understanding that
the publisher is not engaged in rendering legal, accounting,
or other professional services. If legal advice or other
expert assistance is required, the services of a competent
professional person should be sought. *From a Declaration
of Principles jointly adopted by a Committee of the
American Bar Association and a Committee of Publishers.*

Library of Congress Cataloging-in-Publication Data:

Calloway, Paul.
    Russian/Soviet and Western psychiatry : a contemporary comparative
study / Paul Calloway.
        p.   cm.
    Includes bibliographical references and index.
    ISBN 0-471-59574-8 (cloth : alk. paper)
    1. Psychiatry—Soviet Union. I. Title.
    [DNLM: 1. Mental Disorders. 2. Cross-Cultural Comparison.
    3. Mental Health Services—Russia.   WM 100 C163r 1993]
    RC451.S65C35   1993
    616.89′00947—dc20
    DNLM/DLC
    for Library of Congress   93-19938

Printed in the United States of America

10 9 8 7 6 5 4 3 2 1

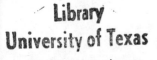

In Memory of my Father
Vernon Calloway

FOREWORD

Joseph Wortis, Emeritus Professor of Psychiatry at the State University of New York, has had a long and distinguished career in psychiatry. In the 1930s he had psychoanalysis with Sigmund Freud in Vienna. He is currently the editor of "Biological Psychiatry". In 1950 he wrote the book "Soviet Psychiatry".

A foreword usually focusses on the book it introduces, but because certain issues are involved I shall take the liberty of first reviewing some relevant history. At the close of World War II when a publisher proposed that I write a book about Soviet psychiatry, I asked the late Bob Felix, then head of the National Institute of Mental Health, if he would write a foreword for it. He responded cordially, writing, "We might learn something from the Russian experience," but he soon afterwards telephoned to say his public relations people advised against it because it could embarrass his dealings with Congress, "... and I depend on those guys for my appropriations," he explained. My friend Horsley Gantt, Pavlov's pupil, also backed off because his departmental chairman opposed the idea. They had reason to be cautious. I soon learned that anybody who enters that area is likely to be drawn into a mirky Byzantine complex of intrigue, hostility and suspicion. The John Hopkins Office of Strategic Services wrote to say they heard of my project and were "much interested in learning of the psychological weaknesses of the Communist states." Meanwhile Senator McCarthy was flourishing. The only foreword that the book finally had was an apologetic one by the publisher explaining and justifying the printing of such a book. Soon afterwards he was delighted to let me know that a batch of copies was sold to the US Department of Defense.

Though I was critical of some aspects of Soviet psychiatry, I credited Soviet psychiatrists with serious scientific interests and humane concern for their patients. In spite of the prevailing atmosphere, the book was surprisingly well received, had mostly good reviews, sold pretty well, was chosen for distribution by a small book club, and enjoyed a couple of foreign translations. But it caused me no end of trouble, and I was harried and harassed for years thereafter. Soon after the book's publication I was subpoenaed by Senator Jenner's Congressional committee on subversive infiltration into education.

Who was this Senator Jenner who presumed to monitor a scientific report on psychiatry? He was a small-town lawyer from Shoals (pop.1022), Indiana, who had managed to arrange his discharge from the armed forces during the war just in time to be elected Senator. He then promoted his political career by following the rabid anticommunistic line that was fashionable at the time, calling the highly respected General Marshall "a front man for traitors," and charging in 1951 on the Senate floor "... that this country today is in the hands of a secret inner coterie which is directed by agents of the Soviet Government. Our only choice is to impeach President Truman and find out who is the secret invisible government," It was at this unfortunate juncture that I entered the scene. The committee tried to establish that I was the gullible dupe of Soviet propaganda. When they badgered me with political questions and innuendoes, I quipped that my mother taught me it was impolite to ask people questions about their politics, and it was this that hit the newspapers, sparing me the ignominy of adverse publicity. Besides, my appearance coincided with the coronation of Queen Elizabeth, which commandeered all the headlines. One week later the committee brought up a refugee Russian psychiatrist who attested that everything in my book was false.

This bit of history should serve to show that nothing about the late Soviet Union can be separated from politics. Though times have changed, Dr. Calloway's excellent book is also likely to encounter similar politically charged evaluations. One foreign observer not long ago remarked that in the USA any opinion, however absurd, obnoxious, venal, false or malicious could be regarded as unobjectionable if paraded under the banner of anticommunism. In spite of the elation over the recent successes of the free market, any slouching towards socialism would be regarded by many as a no-no. What this book is all about is a description of a particular kind of psychiatry that developed in a socialist setting with a philosophically materialistic outlook, and with certain long-standing traditions. The picture that Dr. Calloway describes will not be duplicated in any other country, and will undoubtedly change in the new east European republics in the years ahead. It is practically certain, however, that in all these countries some form of national health service will remain. The USA and South Africa are the only two remaining industrialized countries with no national health program in place, and the time is not far distant when the USA will recognize its necessity, as the American public already does. In Britain even the Thatcher government could not divest itself of its National Health Service.

This book by Dr. Calloway updates and supersedes my own, which was put together in the midst of the cold war. The Berlin Crisis made it impossible for me to gain entry into the Soviet Union, and my account was drawn entirely from secondary sources. Moreover, my Russian was very elementary: I could always get a laugh by saying, "Ya ponyamayu Russki yazik tolko kogda ya goveryu," which means, "I understand only when I am talking." When I first visited the Soviet Union ten years after my book appeared I was curious to discover if what I wrote was true. Essentially it was, but it lacked the breath of life. This lack is corrected by Dr. Calloway, who not only knows the language well, but had ample opportunities to explore the scene. With the transmutation of the former USSR, the animosities have abated, and people may be more willing to learn about the Russian way; but the antipathy to socialism remains, and much that is in the public interest is denigrated as socialist. This book should satisfy Bob Felix's early hope that "we might learn something from the Russian experience."

JOSEPH WORTIS
January 1992

APPRECIATION

Maurice R. Green, series editor of the Wiley Series in General and Clinical Psychiatry, is clinical professor of psychiatry at the New York University School of Medicine and project director for brain research at the Nathan Klein Research Institute. He has made several observational trips to Russia and has been invited to consult with colleagues at the Russian Institute of Mental Health and the Bekhterev Institute.

As Joseph Wortis quotes from Bob Felix in the Foreword—"We might learn something from the Russian experience." In these brief pages I will try to summarize what might be valuable to learn from the Russian experience detailed in this fine book, which describes psychiatry among the former Soviet republics prior to the rise of Yeltsin and the separation of the republics to separate nationhoods. My recent trips to Russia and the other newly independent republics indicate that although the political system has changed, psychiatric practice has not. Aside from the elimination of its political uses in the interests of the Soviet state, the practice of psychiatry functions in much the same way as it did before the dissolution of the USSR. It is possible that, in the new climate, changes will occur, but they are not yet apparent and not likely to happen quickly.

What is striking about Russian psychiatry is not only the variety of views represented but also the continuity of the behavioral and psychophysiologic mainstream of psychiatric theory from the mid-nineteenth century to the present. But then if we take a hard look, isn't there a similar continuity between the work of Kraepelin, 100 years ago, and today's *Diagnostic and Statistical Manual of Mental Disorders (DSM-III-R)* of the American Psychiatric Association?

With the amazing growth of neuroscience in the Western world, we have become very mindful of navigating between the Scylla of biologic reductionism and the Charybdis of psychologic reductionism. One can even look now at the effects of psychologic and interpersonal interventions on neurotransmittors in the brain. Adolf Meyer, a German immigrant to the United States at the beginning of the century, is often acknowledged to be the father of American psychiatry; he fought hard and eloquently against mind-body dualism with his psychobiology. Nevertheless, psychiatry in the United States has tended to be dualistic in practice, with its apprehension of organic factors emphasized only in the past two decades in much psychopathology—psychoses, phobias, obsessive-compulsive disorders, anxiety disorders, and even adjustment disorders.

By contrast, in the monolithic dictatorship of the old Soviet Union, the materialistic view presided, with Pavlovian theory receiving official support. Even so, there is still great emphasis on harmful environmental factors interacting with genetic vulnerability—not an unfamiliar or uncommon perspective in Western psychiatry today.

One must not forget Ivan Petrovich Pavlov when speaking of Russian psychiatry, as he was the official theorist of the Soviet Communist party, who even after his death in 1936 had the full approval and endorsement of the infamous Joseph Stalin. In spite of this, the value of his experimental work has been recognized worldwide. In 1928, Pavlov began to apply his conditioning theory and account of cerebral activity to psychiatric problems. He was less successful in this endeavor and is no longer cited much in psychiatric work. However, his emphasis on objective experiment and his rejection of mind-body dualism clearly show their influence even today. This influence is not limited to Russia and Eastern Europe but can be seen throughout the Western world wherever laboratories of experimental psychology and neurophysiology extend the earlier experimental work. The application of animal models to human behavior is most conspicuous in the preliminary phases of testing new drugs designed to help psychiatric patients.

In Soviet psychiatry, as in all of Soviet medicine, the social dimension is given great weight in all diagnoses and treatments "with no distinction between mental illness and physical illness in this respect." (Calloway, p. 17) Soviet psychiatry follows a longitudinal as opposed to the cross-sectional approach of Western psychiatry. This is reflected in the Western literature on Soviet psychiatry that praises their system of community care, day facilities, partial hospitalization, rehabilitation, work therapy, and restricted use of hospital beds.

Soviet psychiatry, as epitomized by Snezhnevsky, pays much more attention to the variety of changes that occur over a period of years in the presenting phenomenology of the particular psychiatric disorders—tending to become more complex with age. This is becoming more and more appreciated in the West, as longitudinal studies comprising the same set of individuals over a course of twenty or more years are undertaken.

Mental health care has been provided to Soviet citizens through "psychoneurologic" outpatient clinics over the past 70 years. These clinics developed intensively and provided valuable research data from their statistical files. They also offered social as well as medical care to the mentally ill—offering job training and placement, legal services, help with housing, child care, and other social services.

The Russians, who have been interested in providing care outside of hospitals since the nineteenth century, established their first Day Hospital in 1932. Later, a network was developed of outpatient clinics, farm work colonies, and home care. Since the mid-1950s, there has been a decrease in the reported incidence of catatonic states, stuporous conditions, and other forms of severe psychopathology. By the early 1980s, 90 percent of psychiatric patients did not require hospitalization. Also, by this time, the use of psychiatric dispositions for political dissidents had begun to fade as Mr. Gorbachev took power.

This emphasis on caring for patients in their own community, as mentioned earlier, is part of the heavy investment in the rehabilitation of the mentally ill that is rooted in nineteenth century Russian psychiatry. The V. M. Bekhterev Psychoneurological Institute in St. Petersburg has been a leader in laying the scientific foundation for the rehabilitation of the mentally ill, enhancing medical evaluation of the work capacity of the disabled and coordinating scientific research on these problems. The director of the institute, M. M. Kabanov, has been an outstanding leader, worldwide, in the field of rehabilitation psychiatry. This approach involves not only traditional work therapy supported by medication, but also various forms of group therapy, relaxation training, family education, therapeutic physical training, and active use of therapeutic leaves of absence to discourage dependency on hospitals and to encourage resumption of normal work and normal social life.

In line with this emphasis on the social aspect of psychiatry is newly developing research into preventative psychiatry—taking account of age-related characteristics, nature of the patient's activities and interests, problems of school regimens, working conditions on the job, changes in occupational status, and changes in the life-style and family life of the elderly. This should lead to the delineation of high-risk groups and to prophylactic measures of preventing or minimizing illnesses in these groups.

With the cessation of the Cold War, the Russian peoples have become free and open to the exchange of ideas from the West. Its end has also freed Americans to be more open to Russian contributions without the old fear of being labeled a Communist sympathizer. Given the possibililities inherent in this new era of acceptance and accessibility, we each can learn much from the other.

MAURICE R. GREEN
February 1993

PREFACE

There is an established tradition of psychiatry, dating back to pre-Revolutionary Russia, in the former Soviet Union. This, however, is largely unfamiliar in the West. There are few translations from the Soviet psychiatric literature and, although there have been articles and books about specific aspects of Soviet psychiatry, most recent material has focussed on political issues. The primary aim of this book is to introduce Western readers to the theory and practice of Soviet psychiatry. To some extent the book is a comparative account, and, in addition to examining Soviet psychiatry through Western eyes, it includes Soviet criticism of Western psychiatry.

During four years as a research fellow reading articles and monographs from around the world it became apparent to me that a large body of work was not easily available to Western readers. This comprised the research from the many institutes and hospitals in the Soviet Union. Articles which appeared to be relevant were available only in the form of short abstracts which conveyed little useful information. The terminology seemed to be obscure and different. The difficulty in obtaining translations, together with a long-standing interest in the country and the language, prompted me to study Russian and this eventually led to the idea of writing this book. I attempted to establish a link with Soviet psychiatrists but had no response from the Soviet embassy or the various departments within the Soviet Union (this was just after the Soviet Union withdrew from the World Psychiatric Association in 1983). My only reply was from Professor Yuri Nuller in Leningrad with whom I had already corresponded about research. I therefore arranged a trip to Leningrad and made contact with him. This was my starting point. I tried to arrange a formal attachment through the Ministry of Health in Moscow but was unable to do so on the grounds that there were no bilateral agreements. It was made clear that the lack of cooperation was partly the result of the bitterness felt by Soviet psychiatrists, especially with regard to the role of the Royal College of Psychiatrists in what they saw as a politically motivated campaign.

Despite this, or perhaps because of it, I managed to visit and observe clinical practice in many different psychiatric institutes, hospitals and day facilities in three cities: Moscow, Leningrad and Smolensk. I was able to arrange attachments through official local channels and also make unofficial visits through other contacts. In all I made six separate visits to the Soviet Union, spending a total of four months in the country. The theoretical material is derived from the books and journals listed in the bibliography.

It is clearly not possible to provide a comprehensive account of Soviet psychiatry in one book, and I have tried to present an overall picture, giving more detail on certain topics. There was a tendency for Western observers to use the Soviet Union as a gigantic Rorschach ink-blot on which to project their own ideas and beliefs. To counter this I tried to present the material, read, seen or heard, as it came to me, avoiding, where possible, interpretation or comment. The opening chapters examine the concept of mental illness and aspects of diagnosis and classification. There are chapters on the delivery of service, aetiology, treatment and specific disorders. Mental health legislation and forensic psychiatry are described and there is a discussion of political issues, both general and those relating to the question of psychiatric abuse.

Some of the issues discussed are as much to do with different approaches within psychiatry in general as with the differences between Soviet and Western psychiatry. There is no single "Soviet" view of psychiatry and even before the era of glasnost there was a heterogeneity of views, some influenced by the West. There are different schools of psychiatry, and, more obviously, wide individual differences in philosophy and practice. This especially applies to treatment where there is probably greater diversity than in the West. Clearly there are likely to be greater differences in theory and practice in future. The material in this book reflects the prevailing tradition of Soviet psychiatry up to the 1990s, in particular the important influence of Snezhnevsky, who died in 1988.

Psychiatry is concerned with how people think and behave. It inevitably touches upon social, cultural, religious and political issues. It is therefore neither surprising nor unreasonable that psychiatry should be subject to wide interest and public scrutiny and that it should provoke controversy.

Note on recent developments and terminology

Although current developments will affect the scope of this book, many theoretical aspects of Soviet psychiatry will remain the same in that they are not simply the product of a particular social or economic system. With the dissolution of the Soviet Union the main changes are likely to be in the pattern of health care and service delivery. What is described here is the basic Soviet system which will presumably be modified to different degrees in the different republics. Some general terms and names have changed and in others there is uncertainty about their usage, but I have retained the names of various institutes and the city of Leningrad and also the general term Soviet. The term West is used loosely to describe psychiatry in the English-speaking world, although there is also discussion of psychiatry in Europe and Japan in this context.

ACKNOWLEDGMENTS

It would be impossible to acknowledge everyone who has contributed to this work over the course of ten years. A full list would include all those who have taught me Russian, the many people who have helped me during my visits to the Soviet Union and the USA, and colleagues, Soviet, American and European, with whom I have discussed aspects of psychiatry. I am especially grateful to my friends and colleagues at the Royal Free Hospital in London and Fulbourn Hospital, Cambridge and to Joyce Rolph, Mike Todd-Jones, Natasha Franklin, Joseph Elgar, Gordon Hyde, Stewart Britten, German Berrios. In the Soviet Union Yuri Nuller, Evgeny Zubkov, Yuri Popov and Modest Kabanov were particularly helpful. Carol Brayne, Ray Dolan and Eric Chen were all kind enough to read the book at various stages and the following read particular sections: German Berrios, Tony Daniels, Richard Latcham, Peter McKenna, Jim Birley, Eugene Paykel, Mervyn London, Geoff Shepherd, Adrian Grounds, James Rafferty, John Hodges, Ian Goodyer. I am most indebted to the financial support that I received from the Jannsen Research Foundation, and to Stephen Burton, then of Jannsen, and Gerry Hammond.

BIBLIOGRAPHY

The main sources are two multi-author texts, the "Handbook of Psychiatry" (1983) and the "Manual of Psychiatry" (1985), both under the editorship of Snezhnevsky. Two publications from the Ukraine are also referred to. These are "Clinical Psychiatry" (1989) edited by Bacherikov and colleagues and "Manual for psychiatrists" (1990) edited by Voronkov and colleagues. There are monographs and books on more specific topics including "Neuroses" (1980) by Karvasarsky, "The Affective Psychoses" (1988) by Nuller and Mikhalenko and "The treatment of mentally ill patients" (1981) by Avrutsky and Neduva. There are also references to other monographs and multi-author books, most of which have small print-runs. The main Soviet psychiatry journal is the "Journal of Neuropathology and Psychiatry" (the "Korsakoff Journal"), first published in 1901. There are also references to articles in a variety of journals such as the Journal of Higher Nervous Activity, Clinical Medicine, Feldtscher and Midwife. I have scanned the medical newspaper *Meditsinskaya Gazeta* for material on psychiatric topics over a period of ten years. There are a few references to other Soviet newspapers and magazines, including *Pravda, Komsomolskaya Pravda, Izvestia, Trud, Literaturnaya Gazeta* and *Moscow News*.

English language bibliography
There have been many accounts of Soviet medicine, fewer of Soviet psychiatry. Many are rather subjective, often based on a single visit to the Soviet Union. One of the first comprehensive accounts of Soviet Medicine was that of Sigerist, a Professor of the History of Medicine at Johns Hopkins in his "Socialised Medicine in the Soviet Union", (1937). This is an account of the health care system, with much on its history and development. There is, however, little on psychiatry, although he describes the emphasis on care in the community, commenting that patients are only admitted as a last resort. Field's "Soviet Socialized Medicine" (1967) concentrates on the structure and organization of health care, and there are numerous sets of statistical data. There is a brief section on psychiatry. More recent accounts of the health care system include Lisitsin and Batygin (1978) and Kaser (1976). Hyde (1973, 1974 and 1988) and Ryan (1982, 1985, 1989) discuss various aspects of the Soviet Health Service including mental health issues.

    "Soviet Psychiatry" by Wortis (1950) is a comprehensive and learned account of theoretical issues in Soviet psychiatry, although it is limited by the fact that he was not able to visit the Soviet Union at the time. The book gives excellent summaries of the material available to the author and is interesting on theory, concepts, historical aspects and psychology. Accounts in the psychiatric literature of the 1960s and 1970s, especially by American psychiatrists, tended to concentrate on the service and delivery of care (Auster, 1967; Hein, 1968; Sirotkin, 1968; Visotsky, 1968; Fuller Torrey, 1971; Allen, 1973; Holland, 1975). On the whole there were favourable reports on the system of community care, day facilities, partial hospitalization, rehabilitation, the emphasis on work, restricted use of beds, although most described conditions as fairly basic. Kiev (1968) describes some features of psychiatry in various Eastern European countries, but is mainly concerned with service aspects and is limited on other issues. Holland (1975, 1976 and 1977), an American psychiatrist, describes her experiences of eight months working in Moscow 1972, a visit arranged by the NIMH. Babayan (1985) gives a patchy account of the system and structure of Soviet Psychiatry. Cohen (1989) gives a entertaining, journalistic account based on a brief visit to the Soviet Union in order to make a film. The book is mainly about political issues although there are brief descriptions of the dispensary system and conditions within hospitals.

There are several books on specific topics, for instance Morozov and Kalashnik (1970) on forensic psychiatry and Rollin (1972) on child psychiatry. Corson (1976) concentrates on psychology and Umansky (1989) discusses the work of a neuropathologist, covering some aspects of psychiatry, especially with regard to the organic disorders. Aspects of schizophrenia are given in papers by Snezhnevsky (1968), Shakhmatova-Pavlova et al (1975), Holland (1977) and Holland and Shakhmatova-Pavlova (1977). Kazanetz (1979 and 1989) discusses the concept of sluggish (slow-flow) schizophrenia. In Schizophrenia Bulletin (1989) volume 15, number 4, pages 515-571 there is a section on American and Soviet concepts of dangerousness, also an account in English on sluggish (slow-flow) schizophrenia by Smulevitch and a comparison of American and Soviet concepts of schizophrenia by Andreasen. There is a collection of papers by Soviet authors edited by Masserman (1986). "Soviet Neurology and Psychiatry", published by M.E.Sharpe, Armonk, New York, is a quarterly journal of translations, mainly from the Korsakoff journal.

Much of the Western material on Soviet psychiatry is confusing, partly because of difficulties in translation, but also because the material is hard to understand without a background knowledge of basic concepts and terminology. Many Western articles and books also contain frank inaccuracies, especially when quoting authors such as Snezhnevsky.

Psychotherapy

There are a number of the books and articles in English about psychotherapy in the Soviet Union. These include Wynn (1962), Salzman (1963), Ziferstein (1966), Rollin (1972), Segal (1975), Lauterbach (1984) and Ponomareff (1986, 1988). In an interesting historical document, Wynn (1962) gives a selection of papers read at the conference on psychotherapy in Moscow in 1956. Ziferstein (1968) spent a year at the Bekhterev Institute in Leningrad and describes wide availability of treatment. In his book "Soviet Psychotherapy" (1984) Lauterbach gives a fairly comprehensive account of psychotherapy in the Soviet Union based on his time at the Bekhterev Institute in Leningrad. Ponomareff (1988) includes extracts from Karvasarsky's book "Psychotherapy" (1985) published by Meditsina, Moscow.

Political aspects

The main works are Bloch and Reddaway (1977 and 1984) and Wynn (1987). Lader (1977) is mainly concerned with political issues, although he does attempt a somewhat broader approach, describing aspects of mental health legislation and forensic psychiatry. There are the personal accounts of Tarsis (1967), Medvedev and Medvedev (1971), Bukovsky (1978) and Podrabinek (1980). There are letters and articles in newspapers and medical journals, some of which are quoted in this text or in the above sources. The main primary source was the Samizdat publication "A chronicle of current events", produced in the West by Reddaway. Amnesty International relies upon secondary sources, mainly the Samizdat publications. The main Amnesty International publication was their booklet "Prisoners of Conscience in the USSR" (1975). Stone (1984) by gives an interesting analysis of some important theoretical issues.

CONTENTS

Chapter One

THE CONCEPT OF MENTAL ILLNESS

Towards the end of the nineteenth century it first seemed possible that mental illness could be explained in terms of what was happening in the brain. However, the notion that mental illness was more or less synonymous with brain disease was only just gaining credence when alternative, psychological, concepts of mental illness, influenced by psychoanalysis and phenomenology, were introduced. Their impact on Western psychiatry remains to this day and has fuelled the controversy about the nature of mental illness. Both the terms "mental" and "illness" are disputed and at the core of the debate are issues to do with the mind-body question and the concept of disease.

Concept of mind in Soviet psychiatry
The mind-brain or mind-body problem refers to the nature of mind and how it relates to the material substance of the body. Is the mind separate from matter (broadly the dualist position) or can it be explained in terms of the workings of the nervous system (the materialist position)? If the mind is something that is separate from matter, how does it interact with the brain?

Historical aspects
Materialist views about the nature of man were popular with sections of the intelligentsia in nineteenth century Russia [1]. A number of explanations have been suggested for this, among them the strong tradition of natural sciences with the prominent status of physiology. The physiologist Sechenov (1829-1905) had a profound impact with his book "Reflexes of the Brain", published in 1863 and subsequently banned. Sechenov had a materialist stance and argued that it needed an external sensory stimulus for even the slightest mental activity, writing that "the initial cause of any human action lies outside the person." He is considered to have discarded philosophical theories of the mind or soul and opened up the way for the direct investigation of the materialist substrate of mental phenomena. The publication of the book is described by some Soviet writers as the dawn of the science of the brain, providing the foundation for the materialist psychology and

---

1. Bazarov in Turgenev's novel "Father and Sons" which was first published in 1862 is a good exemplar of this. "Nourished on biology and physics, Bazarov would cast away religious and metaphysical conceptions in order to reorganise society on strictly scientific and utilitarian principles" (Edmonds, 1965).

psychiatry of the twentieth century. Sechenov's important successors were Bekhterev (1857-1927) and Pavlov (1849-1936) who considered mental activity (higher nervous function) to be the elaboration of multiple conditioned reflexes. Early "Soviet" views of mind largely arose from this pre-Revolutionary tradition of materialist physiology.

The early years of Soviet government also saw the development of a parallel view of mind which emphasized the importance of social processes and was partly based on Marxist philosophy but also incorporated some psychoanalytic concepts. This was associated with the psychology of Vygotsky, Luria and, later, Rubinstein. Rubinstein (1942) considered that the mind, although a function of matter, had its own dialectical development and he put forward the theory of the unity of consciousness and activity which related consciousness to the external environment and rejected the notion of a repressed layer of unconscious ideas.

After the Second World War there was a shift back to the physiological, Pavlovian, position at the expense of social concepts. Pavlov's view of the higher nervous system was seen as consistent with Marxist-Leninist philosophy and declared to be the logical scientific foundation of psychiatry in contrast to "idealistic and mechanistic theories" in Western psychiatry. More recently Pavlovian concepts have been less prominent. Mental activity is still considered to be firmly based on psychophysiology, but there has been more emphasis on social and interpersonal processes in explanatory models of the mind.

Current position

Although there are divergent views in the Soviet Union about the nature of mind and the interaction between mind and brain, the psychiatric literature generally presents an unambiguous view about the nature of mind and mental processes. The Soviet concept of mind, especially from a psychiatric perspective, is not simply an assimilation of the theories of Marx and Engels. It would be truer to say that some of the philosophy of dialectical materialism or Marxist-Leninism has been grafted on to an earlier materialist view of the mind and brain.

The dialectical materialist concept regards mental phenomena as a function of matter ie the mind is a product of the working brain. Thus, a particular individual's mind (and "spirit") cease to exist when that human brain no longer works. The mind, however, cannot be explained simply by considering the physiology of an individual brain, and to stop at this point would be regarded as crude materialism. There is a social and cultural dimension which cannot be reduced to the summed experiences of one individual brain. Thus, the brain is necessary but not sufficient to explain the mind in that mental processes are the product of environmental influences ie the experiences that the individual has had. Moreover, these mental processes in turn will affect an individual's experiences. Mind is thus the product of the interaction between an individual and the environment, the most important component of which is other people. This interaction means that an individual mind can incorporate the experiences of other people and explains the continuation of culture. Thus, although the mind is a product of the physiological processes of the individual brain, and cannot happen without them, it is actually created by social experiences. Ideas are determined by social factors, including economic factors and man's consciousness comes from the people around him.

2

Dialectical materialism rejects the idealist or dualist view that mental processes may be independent of the world of matter. This is closely linked to the whole question of religion. Mchedlov (1982) writes: "Consider, for instance, one of the central concepts of religion - that of the immortality of the soul. Data supplied by physiology, medicine and psychology have proved convincingly enough that there is no isolated spiritual substance independent of the human body and continuing to live after man's death, and that consciousness is a property of the brain." Although most printed material tends to reflect this position, a much broader range of views is expounded in discussion. People hold a wide range of philosophical, religious and political views, and some psychiatrists, especially those with religious beliefs, do hold alternative models and believe in the existence of a mind which is not the product of the nervous system.

The contribution of psychology
Soviet psychology has had an important influence upon the development of psychiatry and many of the current concepts have been moulded by the neurophysiology of Pavlov and Bekhterev and the neuropsychology of Luria. I will not attempt to discuss this in any detail, and there are many English texts on Soviet psychology. The section below is drawn from Soviet psychiatric texts and also Wortis (1950), Corson (1976), Gray (1979), Mangan (1982), Levitan (1982), Kozulin (1984) and Lauterbach (1984).

There was a school of materialist psychology, based on the physiology of Sechenov and Pavlov, in pre-Revolutionary Russia, although the "idealist" school led by Chelpanov at the Institute of Experimental psychology in Moscow was dominant. Chelpanov continued to work after the Revolution, but in the 1920s there was a move away from what was seen as the "mentalism" of the psychology of the time. Materialist psychology then developed along two lines: the physiological and the social.

The physiological trend, which was essentially concerned with mechanisms, dominated up to the 1930s and was based on the work of Pavlov and Bekhterev's reflexology. The theories were developed to explain personality, neurotic disorders and even psychoses. This was based upon investigating the balance between excitation and inhibition (which is an active process, not just absence of excitation) of the reflex system. In the 1930s and 1940s social psychology, essentially based upon dialectical materialist philosophy, came to the fore with the work of Rubinstein, whose influential book "Foundations of General Psychology" (1942) was awarded the then prestigious Stalin prize. In the late 1940s and 1950s there was a swing back to a psychology based upon Pavlovian physiology, and it was not until the mid 1960s that these polarized views were replaced by attempts to integrate social and physiological aspects. This was facilitated by the acceptance of concepts of functional systems and feedback [2].

This is, of course, an over-simplified version of the history of Soviet psychology, and several important workers were developing their ideas in parallel to this. Vygotsky (whose work influenced the film-maker Eisenstein) attempted to

2. Developments in cybernetics were slow to be accepted in the Soviet Union, partly because of ideology. The ideas were actually introduced in the 1930s and 1940s by Bernstein and Anokhin. Anokhin, a student of Pavlov and Bekhterev, described the nervous system as the *functional* link between the organism and the outer environment and considered the functional system as the basic unit of neurological activity.

3

explain various phenomena, especially consciousness, by the relationship between thought and speech. He argued that social interactions and activity generated consciousness, but that the external things were transformed into psychological functions by signs. Leontiev and the so-called Kharkov school, mainly former students of Vygotsky, developed the idea further into the psychology of activity, placing more emphasis on the importance of the direct link between physical activity and thought. Luria, who owed much to Vygotsky, has made an important contribution to neuropsychology which is familiar to Western psychologists.

The historical trends in psychology were mirrored by changes in the concept of personality. Thus, in the 1930s and 1940s personality was seen as the sum of acquired knowledge, abilities and habits - that is essentially experience [3]. With the switch to Pavlovian psychology in the 1950s, personality theory was seen in terms of the expression of a particular type of nervous system (although it was emphasized that this could be modified by the environment). Certain parameters of higher nervous system function, for instance stability and the balance between excitation and inhibition, were considered to be the neurophysiological basis for individual psychological differences.

According to Pavlov there were three levels at which the human organism reacts to the environment. The basic level, the unconditioned reflex, is laid down in evolution. The next layer is the first signalling system, the conditioned reflex (which reflects sub-cortical processes). The third level is the second signalling system, the level of language and symbolic representation (which reflects cortical processes). More recently, other properties of the nervous system have been investigated. These include "dynamism" (similar to reaction time), lability and concentration.

Personality theory based upon the theory of *otnoshenia* was developed by Miasishchev (1960). *Otnoshenia* are the attitudes and relationships that link an individual to his environment. The theory is discussed further in chapters 7 and 10.

The individual and the collective
According to Marxist-Leninism what differentiates man from other living things is the social dimension which develops out of his interaction with other human beings and his participation in human society. It is this dimension which is said to distinguish dialectical materialism from the reductionism of crude materialism, which fails to account for the significance of social and cultural life. Human consciousness is not just the result of the workings of the nervous system of one individual. The consciousness of the collective is fundamental, so that society and social history determine consciousness and there is some social/cultural expression of the individual that continues after his death. Ultimately, of course, this consciousness depends upon the workings of the different nervous systems of each living human being. If there were no more people then there would be no human consciousness [4].

However, the Soviet attitude to collective life has not developed simply as a result of this doctrine. There are pragmatic and historical reasons, including the

---

3. A reflection of how these theories were transformed into dogma was the banning of IQ testing in 1936.
4. The dialectical materialist concept of mind does have some features in common, albeit without recourse to any mystical element, with the Jungian view of the collective unconscious. It might be thought of as the Jungian collective unconscious, but with brains. There are also features in common with some of the notions of Teilhard de Chardin and his "omega" state and even some of the newer, Californian theories of consciousness. There is, of course, a fundamental difference. Many of these views imply a consciousness free of the material of the nervous system, so that consciousness would continue even if there were no matter left.

traditions of the village community or *mir* [5]. Aronson (1968) writes about the importance of the "collective" in the Soviet Union and suggests that this explains some of the differences between Soviet and American psychiatry. He writes that in the USA "the dominant orientation is individualistic; the individual is seen as independent and responsible for himself. In the Soviet Union the individual is seen as being secondary to the group." He considers that this tradition is rooted in the Russian village which was ruled by the commune or *mir* in which discussions continued until a unanimous decision was reached.

Comparative aspects

Although the mind-brain problem is perhaps the central philosophical question that concerns psychiatry, it is not easy to give a coherent account of current "Western" views about this. It is rare for the issue to be discussed in depth in the psychiatric literature. The paucity of material might indicate confusion or disagreement, but as much as anything seems to reflect unease about the subject. There may be a number of reasons for this, some related to the fact that psychiatrists work within a culture which, broadly speaking, still holds a dualist philosophy of mind and body. Sims (1988), for instance, writes: "The whole discipline of psychiatry tacitly accepts a dualistic background for its very existence." This tacit dualism has had a considerable impact on the theory and practice of psychiatry, particularly in the USA. It has led to the idea that there are two separate fields of endeavour, one concerned with the world of brain and the other with that of the mind, or soul. The split goes right down the line into diagnosis. The psychoses are seen as brain disorders whereas the neuroses and personality disorders are considered to lie within the sphere of mind. The reasons are partly historical. Jaspers attempted to apply Husserl's philosophy of phenomenology to psychiatry, introducing "verstehen" psychology, the process of understanding the connections between a person's life and his mental state by using empathic understanding. He essentially gives psychological explanations for psychiatric symptoms, and he believed that these things happen in the realm of mind, separate from matter or brain. He is clear about his orientation, arguing that it is necessary to have a dualist position with regard to mind and body. He argues that the materialist position leads one to "impossible consequences", although he does not say what these are. Although Freud considered that eventually a neural substrate would be found for the processes which he wrote about, most psychoanalytic writing has been dualist in orientation and has been concerned with things happening in the realm of mind.

Most Western definitions of neurosis incorporate the absence of an organic component. For instance, Cawley (1983), in the Handbook of Psychiatry, defines neuroses as being mental disorders with no known or even suspected basis in organic pathology. The split also leads to a dichotomy with regard to aetiology. It is assumed that genetically determined abnormalities, for instance in neurotransmitter systems, are important in the aetiology of "biological" disorders whereas psychosocial factors are of little relevance. Neurotic disorders on the other hand are equated with "problems of living", with psychosocial factors having an aetiological role.

---

5. The word *mir* has two other meanings: peace and the world.

5

In a chapter on "Mind and Body", Granville-Grossman (1983), also in the Handbook of Psychiatry, writes that there is "considerable doubt that any approach - scientific or otherwise - will resolve the problem of the way in which physical and mental events appear to co-exist and interrelate." He himself, however, comes down on the side of some variation of Cartesian dualism, quoting such possibilities as the existence of the mind (or soul) after death, and notions of "one person's mind, entire and intact, becoming intimately related to a new body." He considers that dualism is a "common-sense point of view" that might be held by the "man in the street who knows little of philosophy" but also by influential philosophers like Karl Popper and scientists like John Eccles [6]. He concludes, however, that "the mind-body problem may never be finally solved."

The main American textbooks do not address the issue although it is raised in a number of articles in major journals. Cooper (1985) attempts to refine the dualist position and maintains that advances in neurobiology will redefine the boundaries between mind and body. He argues that there is no bridge from neurobiology to the unconscious or, indeed, to consciousness and states that there is "no danger that the mind will disappear". Other authors also want to preserve the world of "mind", without firmly committing themselves to just what they mean by it (Reiser, 1988; Wallace, 1988). Pollock (1988), in his retiring address as President of the American Psychiatric Association, discusses the "problems of mind versus body". He poses the familiar dualist dilemma, writing that there is a major difficulty in reconciling what he calls two cultures: that of science and molecules and that of meaning and aesthetics. He does not suggest a solution and seems to imply that there is no solution. However, he concludes: "Ultimately, I believe we will not have dualism."

By contrast, materialists, Soviet or Western, reject the view that the mind is some kind of unfathomable mystery that can never be solved. Bekhtereva (1984), for instance, quoting some of the writing of Eccles and Penfield, criticizes their "paradoxical conclusions in various verbal disguises" that man does not think through the working of his brain. She argues that advances in neurosciences and more sophisticated understanding of social factors will eventually be able to explain all mental processes. Scientific progress is seen as eroding away the dualist position as the physiological basis for mental processes (both normal and abnormal) becomes apparent. Although some dualists might argue that these findings are not relevant to the question, they are still left with the task of explaining the interaction of mind and body. The main difficulty for dualists is not so much that the boundaries keep changing (with more disorders being incorporated into the biological realm) but that the boundaries keep getting crossed. Biological changes are found in disorders which have traditionally been reserved for the "mind" category and psychosocial factors are shown to be significant in the aetiology and outcome of somatic disorders. The dualist position is not always easy to reconcile with developments in medicine and biology or with observations made in clinical practice.

The mind-body problem is inevitably of particular concern to those with religious beliefs [7]. In general, people with religious beliefs, especially if they

6. Popper and Eccles (1977) suggest that the cortex is the place where mind and body interact (with Descartes it was the pineal). Their view seems to be that neurones in a particular layer of the cerebral cortex send messages backwards and forwards from the non-material, self-conscious mind.

involve a belief in some kind of spiritual existence after death, are most likely to hold to a dualist notion of mind and brain. A separate world of mind, unencumbered by the material brain, is seen as the necessary place for spiritual life. The general approach is to emphasize the split between mind and brain and to reinforce the dualist position by establishing clear brain-based disease entities as opposed to mental or spiritual problems or "problems of living". In practice, most psychiatrists keep their personal philosophy out of their work, which, at a practical level, rarely has need for religious speculation. Occasionally, however, the association between religious ideation and psychiatric disorder does raise this issue. The possibility of altering an apparently religious experience by pharmacological means does require a clear distinction to be made between "mad" religious experiences and "proper" ones. An exchange of views in the British Journal of Psychiatry illustrates this. Signer (1988) reports the case of a 26 year old man who was described as having had "a life-long interest in mystical and religious philosophy" and joined a Cistercian monastery. During the course of meditation he had developed a prolonged ecstatic state with increased awareness. He reports that it "was initially pleasant and thought to be derived from spirituality and the contemplation of God." Unfortunately, however, this ecstatic state became a permanent feature which he was not able to control and led to symptoms of anxiety, panic and depression. There was some question as to whether the man wanted to give up the "mystical ecstasy" to gain relief from the severe symptoms. He was treated with phenelzine which did indeed prevent the ecstatic states and associated panic as well as leading to normalization in his mood.

This approach is questioned by Pelosi (1988) who writes that he "feels obliged to place on record my view that religious phenomena such as these are not the legitimate concern of psychiatrists." He argues that mysticism is a part of the Christian tradition and feels that the patient might be considered privileged to have undergone the experiences. He makes the point that the "greatest ever Cistercian", a Bernard of Clairvaux, was also a mystic. He suggests that a religious supervisor might have been more appropriate and urges Signer to stop the drug and advise the patient to get help from a "spiritual mentor."

It is worth bearing in mind that the original report by Signer makes it clear that the patient had a strong family history of psychiatric disorder (with a father who was a chronic alcoholic and a brother and sister with depression). The patient also had evidence of frontal lobe damage and there were various abnormal neurological signs. It is unlikely that the appropriateness or otherwise of treating severe symptoms with a drug (which worked) would be questioned if the associated experiences had not been of a religious nature.

In current practice these issues have little impact on the day-to-day work of psychiatrists, and most psychiatrists would claim to be 'eclectic' in their philosophy as well as their psychiatry. I asked several American psychiatrists about their philosophical orientation and their views on the mind-body question. Most said that they used different systems for different purposes, which, when argued through, generally seemed to imply some kind of dualist philosophy. Others said

---

7. According to Galanter (1991), of 192 "born-again" Christian psychiatrists most considered that bible reading or prayer was more effective than drugs for suicidal patients, alcoholics, sociopaths and those suffering from grief reactions.

that the idea of the psyche as a separate entity was fading rapidly and that materialist views were becoming predominant [8], although two American psychiatrists told me that it was unusual for people to declare themselves as being out-and-out materialists, partly because of the implications with regard to religious and political beliefs. This kind of circumspection would be rare in Europe.

Many of these issues are not really to do with the differences between Soviet and Western psychiatry. They are more to do with the clash of two different orientations, and the fires of debate are fuelled by the implications for religion, culture and art. The scientist, claiming that he is simply trying to understand the natural world, of which man is a part, is accused of trying to reduce interesting and meaningful phenomena to neuronal discharges or describe interesting people in terms of their brain processes. This debate crosses cultures, systems and countries.

The concept of disease

The difficulty in defining health and disease is not confined to psychiatry, but it is perhaps only within psychiatry that it has generated such fierce controversy. There are two fundamentally different concepts of disease. The realist view (sometimes referred to as essentialist or "Platonic") holds that a disease has an independent existence of its own. Put crudely this is the notion that there are such things as pneumonia or schizophrenia out there waiting to get you. The nominalist view (also referred to as empirical, physiological or "Hippocratic") regards disease as an arbitrary concept, a convenient name for a group of phenomena, and classifies diseases on the basis of groups of patients that resemble one other.

There is also a controversy about the medical model as opposed to the social concept of mental illness. This is related to the question of whether or not mental illness should be considered in the same way as other illnesses [9]. Several polarized positions have been taken up. What might be called the extreme biological position is to consider mental illnesses as clear-cut disease entities which are biologically determined and have no social component. The "anti-psychiatry" view denies the existence of mental illness altogether, maintaining that the so-called diseases are no more than labels that society applies to people with socially deviant behaviour.

The Soviet concept of mental illness

There is no single concept of mental illness in the Soviet Union, and, as in the West, individual psychiatrists hold their own views which vary considerably. There is, however, probably more of a consensus about the main concepts than is found amongst Western psychiatrists. This is partly because, until recently, there

---

8. Wortis (1950) wrote: "Stripped of the forbidding terminology and its sometimes pedantic or dogmatic tone, many principles of Marxist theory will be found to coincide with the common sense and scientific judgement of American scientists, who may be surprised, if not embarrassed to discover, like Moliere's character, that they were talking materialism all their lives."

9. Much of the writing in this area does not appear to challenge traditional disease concepts as applied to physical medicine. Sedgewick (1982), however, argues that there is no distinction between mental and physical illness, claiming that social criteria define physical as much as mental illness. All diseases, mental and physical, are 'social constructions'. Diseases and attitudes to them vary with time and place. He argues that there are no diseases in nature, but that disease is a human notion, determined by "anthropocentric self-interest". Potato blight is only a blight because we want chips. Cholera in humans is like the souring of milk by bacteria. A fractured femur in a seventy-year-old is like the 'snapping of an autumn twig'. He does not imply that these disorders should not be treated.

8

were relatively few psychiatric textbooks and hand-books [10]. Features of the Soviet concept of mental illness are:

1. The materialist basis. Psychiatric disorders have a neural substrate, that is they are brain-based.
2. The "Hippocratic" tradition. This is patient-oriented rather than disease-oriented.
3. The longitudinal and syndromal approach. This emphasizes the importance of considering the changes in the syndromes over time.
4. The dimensional approach. This postulates the existence of a continuum of disease, or intermediate forms, rather than distinct, discrete entities.
5. The role of environmental or exogenous factors, both physical and psychosocial.

1. The materialist basis.

The Soviet concept of disease is based on a natural sciences view of man, regarding man as an organism which interacts with the environment like other living things. Environmental factors, which may be physical or social, act upon the host organism to produce changes which result in either adaptive or pathological responses. When these pathological responses fall into recognizable clinical patterns they are considered to be syndromes or diseases. These have a basis in matter in that there is a material substrate for mental processes, and thus for mental illness. Psychological and social factors are considered to be of importance, but these act upon the material substrate, the nervous system.

One manifestation of the materialist view of mental illness has been the association between psychiatry and neurology in the Soviet Union, although this in fact dates back to the nineteenth century. There has been a single association of psychiatrists and neurologists as well as a common journal. However, at the Eighth Congress of Psychiatrists and Neurologists, held in 1988, it was decided that separate associations of neurologists and psychiatrists should be formed, although the Korsakoff Journal of Neuropathology and Psychiatry will continue in its present form.

It has been claimed that the Second World War helped to consolidate a more "organic" view of mental illness. According to Zilboorg (1944) the massive casualties sustained by the Red Army led to a considerable experience in the field of neuropsychiatry and confirmed the view that there was an organic factor in apparently psychogenic disorders and also that social factors played a part in all organic disorders. Soviet psychiatrists like Yudin noted that hysterical disorders (usually considered to be functional) were common in patients after brain injury, especially when there was damage to the frontal lobes.

Soviet psychiatry has concentrated on the investigation of the functioning of the central nervous system in psychiatric disorders in order to try and establish a pathophysiological basis for mental illness. Up until recently this was closely

---

10. According to Snezhnevsky (1983), there were two double volume handbooks over the previous century: Korsakoff (1893) and Osipov (1923, 1927 and 1931). There were also two single volume handbooks: Serbsky (1906) and Giliarovsky (1931, 1935, 1938 and 1954). He writes that these books had an important influence in the development of psychiatric thinking in Russia and then the Soviet Union. Korsakoff took the first steps in developing a nosology which was further established in Osipov's book. Since the 1950s the influence of Giliarovsky has been prevalent, and, partly because of the Handbook (1983), partly because of his position, Snezhnevsky's concepts have moulded current psychiatric thinking.

bound to Pavlovian theory. The result was a considerable amount of work in the field of psychophysiology, not always with fruitful results, possibly because it was so bound to theory. More recently there has been less emphasis on Pavlovian theory although psychophysiological research is still directed towards the investigation of the neural substrate of mental illness.

2. The Hippocratic tradition.

The Soviet concept of disease is nominalist and rejects the notion that diseases are independent entities that exist in their own right. Thus, a disease is considered to be an arbitrary concept, a convenient name for a group of phenomena. The approach has its roots in the pre-Revolutionary tradition of Russian medicine [11] and is described in the Soviet psychiatric literature as "Hippocratic" or patient-oriented. This is said to contrast with the "Platonic" or disease-oriented tradition which is considered to be rife in the West. However, the historical importance and pragmatic usefulness of the "Platonic" approach is recognized. Snezhnevsky (1985) writes that the two different trends have run through the history of medicine. The Platonic tradition led to an emphasis on classification and diagnosis, whereas the Hippocratic tradition was more concerned about prognosis than diagnosis. He argues that the clinical-descriptive approach, which takes account of the patient's personality and life history, is descended from the Hippocratic school, and is empirical rather than speculative.

Snezhnevsky (1985) writes that the era of scientific medicine began with the Platonic tradition and the systematization of disease. Thus, the Kraepelinian classification, in which each individual illness was seen as a nosological entity with its own distinctive presentation, cause and outcome, was influenced by the work of Koch and Pasteur and the germ theory, the notion of one cause for one disease. In dialectical fashion, however, running alongside these continuing attempts to systematize illness, there was a resurgence of the Hippocratic tradition towards the end of the eighteenth and beginning of the nineteenth century. He quotes the English psychiatrist, Henry Maudsley as writing that temperament was more important in defining the form of an illness than the cause of the illness. The struggle to make sense of the picture continued into the twentieth century. According to Snezhnevsky the two approaches are not mutually exclusive. Medical students learn about illnesses in a disease-oriented way and then, during their clinical training, should see their manifestations in the patient and move on to the Hippocratic approach.

3. The longitudinal and syndromal approach.

The clinical-descriptive approach emphasizes the importance of observation over time. The course that an illness takes is considered to be crucial to understanding aetiology and outcome [12]. It is, in fact, its essence in that the illness is the interaction between the individual (the host) and the basic pathological process [13]. Diagnosis, therefore, is based on the syndromes and the way they change over

11. Botkin, one of the leading physicians of the nineteenth century, considered that an illness was an interaction between the individual and the basic pathological process. Another nineteenth century Russian physician, Mudrov, is often quoted as saying that there were no illnesses, only patients.

12. This again has pre-revolutionary roots. Botkin considered that syndromes were transient stages in the overall development of an illness.

time. This contrasts with the "Platonic" cross-sectional approach where diagnosis depends upon what symptoms are present at a particular point in time.

This approach explains one of the major differences between Western and Soviet systems of classification. In the Soviet system each of the main "forms" of schizophrenia is defined on the basis of the course of the disorder over time rather than on the cross-sectional syndromal picture. There are, for example, continuous, episodic-progressive and slowly-flowing forms. The different syndromes, the clusters of symptoms, can occur at different points in time in the basic forms. This has important implications for research, particularly for epidemiological studies.

4. The dimensional approach.

One implication of the distinction between the realist and nominalist concepts of disease concerns the difference between the categorical and dimensional approach to diagnosis. The realist view of disease is generally associated with the categorical approach in that you either have the disease or you don't. The dimensional approach, on the other hand, fits better with the nominalist or natural sciences view. The dimensional approach in this context has no implications about social as opposed to medical models in that any continuum would be seen as biologically based. Thus, just as there are varying degrees of hypertension in the population so there might be varying degrees of depression or intermediate forms of schizophrenia.

This view clearly has implications for diagnosis and treatment. Treatment is not simply a question of prescribing a particular treatment when a particular disease is present. It leads instead to a syndromal approach, the treatment of particular syndromes, even symptoms, when they arise during the course of an illness.

5. The role of environmental factors.

From a Western perspective Soviet psychiatry appears to put a disproportionate emphasis on environmental rather than genetic factors in mental illness. This is partly accounted for by historical and political reasons. The role of heredity was more or less ignored during the years in which neo-Larmarckianism dominated Soviet science [14] and it is still relatively neglected. The current view would be to accept that there is a relationship between heredity and harmful environmental factors, but to stress that the way in which they interact is unclear and that it is not diseases as such that are inherited. The view is that some form of vulnerability is inherited but that it is still necessary to identify the external (environmental) factors which are involved. There have been two practical manifestations of this. Firstly, it has led to various aetiological theories to do with environmental (usually physical) factors. A second result has been the tendency to whittle down the numbers of patients within the diagnostic categories by attributing their pathology to various external causes.

---

13. The notion that an illness is defined by its course (essentially that the course of the illness is the illness) fits comfortably with dialectical materialism. However, once again pre-Revolutionary psychiatry is cited, and Snezhnevsky (1985) quotes the psychiatrist Orshansky, author of a textbook of psychiatry published in Kharkov in 1910, as saying: "only the course of an illness provides the material for explaining aetiology, pathogenesis and outcome".

14. A modification of Lamarckianism, the doctrine that acquired characteristics or traits can be genetically transmitted to the next generation, was promoted by the influential Soviet geneticist, Lysenko. For some time Mendelian genetics was ignored. For a geneticist's account of this period see "Acquired Traits" (1988) by Raissa Berg. Also "The Rise and Fall of T. D. Lysenko" (1971) by Zhores Medvedev.

This led to the concept of the exogenous psychoses linked to specific aetiological agents. It still influences the classification in that the vascular disorders in the "exogenous-organic" rubric represents a sub-group which in the West would be divided up amongst dementia, depression and schizophrenia. Also from this perspective the various organic disorders such as diencephalitis (discussed on page 191) would explain some Western cases of neurosis and depression.

"Leningrad" and "Moscow" schools.

Although the search for external factors in the aetiology of mental illness is a feature of Soviet psychiatry as a whole it has generally been more associated with the so-called "Leningrad" school of psychiatry. The Moscow school is said to be more concerned with endogenous processes and psychopathology in contrast to the Leningrad school with its emphasis on environmental factors, both physical and psychosocial. The concept of exogenous psychoses led to extensive investigation for aetiological agents, and it was thought that infectious diseases such as typhus, malaria or brucellosis were the cause of specific psychoses. This approach led to the view that schizophrenia should be a last resort diagnosis, that it should only be diagnosed when all other aetiological factors have been ruled out [15]. There has been a wide debate about this, and it is related to the question of the unitary psychosis. It can be argued that when infectious diseases such as malaria and typhus were common, as they were in the early years of Soviet rule, one would have expected to see many cases in which there was a coincidental occurrence of an infectious disease and psychosis in the same person.

There is less interest in this approach at the present time partly because the results have been limited [16]. The search for environmental factors now tends to take place within the context of the established nosology, leading, for instance, to the search for a viral aetiology of schizophrenia. One legacy of this trend may be the greater emphasis placed by Leningrad psychiatrists in distinguishing between schizophrenia and manic-depression, putting them closer to the traditional British position.

The second feature which is said to distinguish the Leningrad from the Moscow school is the emphasis on the psychosocial aspects of mental illness. The importance of psychosocial factors, both in relation to aetiology and outcome, is part of the theoretical framework of all Soviet psychiatry, as is the strong tradition of rehabilitation. However, the Bekhterev Institute in Leningrad has been more active, both in terms of research and practical applications, in the fields of psychotherapy and rehabilitation. The Moscow school has tended to concentrate on areas concerning diagnosis, classification, psychopathology, and the underlying biological abnormalities.

---

15. Isaev (1974), a child psychiatrist in Leningrad, writes that schizophrenia in childhood and adolescence is rare. The differential diagnosis includes oligophrenia, the results of trauma, the autistic disorders, inflammatory and infectious diseases such as encephalitis, the affective disorders and the "recurrent psychoses". He considers the post-infectious psychoses due to infections such as brucellosis were common in the past.

16. Some of the results are of interest. Golant of the Bekhterev Institute, in Leningrad, considered that some atypical affective disorders were due to diencephalitis, infection or inflammation of certain deep structures within the fore-brain, the thalamus and hypothalamus. She suggested that this presented with some features of depression, but that there tended to be shorter episodes which were rapidly cycling. There were atypical features and, in particular, vegetative reactions (disorders of the autonomic nervous system, resulting in abnormalities of cardiovascular function, sweating and temperature control).

12

Comparative aspects

The date of the Russian revolution was significant for the development of psychiatry within the Soviet Union and perhaps accounts for the relatively limited impact of psychoanalysis and phenomenology upon diagnosis and classification. Psychoanalysis has had an important influence upon the Western concept of mental illness, especially in Northern America. The traditional psychoanalytic approach is to eschew nosology, so that symptoms of psychiatric disorder are seen as manifestations of conflicts and/or defence mechanisms. Essentially this model produces its own system of classification, based upon psychodynamic processes. However, psychoanalytic concepts have also been incorporated into the general psychiatric nosology, for instance into Bleuler's concept of schizophrenia. More recently this position has been modified to allow for some 'biological' processes, particularly in disorders such as manic-depressive disorder. Jaspers phenomenology also had a profound influence upon Western concepts of mental illness. Jaspers writes about a psychopathology which is "not enslaved to neurology and medicine", arguing against the notion of mental disorder being cerebral disorder [17]. This model sets up a parallel "medical model" for the psychiatric disorders. Broadly the idea is that the psyche can have its own diseases, defined in similar kinds of ways to bodily diseases.

There have obviously been considerable difficulties in trying to integrate these concepts with more naturalistic and biological views about the nature of mental illness. The concepts have been taken up by the "anti-psychiatry" movement which continues to influence Western psychiatry and Western psychiatrists.

Psychiatric diagnosis and "anti-psychiatry"

The more radical critics of psychiatry have argued either that mental illness does not exist or that it should not be regarded in the same way as other types of illness. The "anti-psychiatry" movement [18] eschewed the process of diagnosis and classification and condemned most forms of treatment. Essentially it sought to dismember the body of psychiatry altogether. Laing (1965), whose early ideas were based on existential philosophy, saw insanity as the product of "ontological insecurity", the lack of a real sense of being-in-the-world. This was an appealing idea, mainly because many people could identify with it, but its weakness was that it was never shown to have anything to do with psychiatric illness. "Ontological insecurity" was undoubtedly felt by many people with mental illness, especially those with certain types of personality disorder, but it was also experienced by people who were never seen by psychiatrists, and, of course, by some psychiatrists.

Laing's early ideas were about people being driven mad by a mad world, but in his later writing, along with his colleagues Esterson and Cooper, he questioned the concept of mental illness in a more fundamental way. He drew upon labelling theory (for instance the views of Thomas Scheff who argued that mental illness was a response to being labelled as mad) and introduced the notion of the

17. He drew a clear distinction between man and the natural world and even maintained that Kant was logically correct in stating that expert opinions about mental states should be given by philosophers.

18. "Anti-psychiatry" is a broad church which includes those who deny the existence of mental illness altogether as well as those who promote their own concepts of mental illness. The movement was most influential in the late 1960s and early 1970s, but the arguments are still put forcibly by various professional and lay groups. The Church of Scientology is perhaps the most vociferous body currently active in the West.

scapegoated ("labelled") child in a mad family. The theme eventually broadened to suggest that it was in fact the mentally ill who were sane whereas society and the family were mad. These views did not gain wide acceptance. Interestingly, however, they are echoed in the "anti-psychiatry" movement in the Soviet Union. In a passage which could be taken out of the writings of the Western anti-psychiatry movement, Podrabinek (1980) writes: "Thank God the 'abnormal' people still exist in our country. They are not only mentally but also ethically healthy people who bring to our spiritually ill society a culture of freedom and democracy. For this reason alone they are condemned to incarceration in psychiatric hospitals."

Much of the controversy about the nature of mental illness was focussed on schizophrenia. It was with regards to this diagnosis, above all, that psychiatrists were subjected to the wrath of labelling theorists, accused of tidying up the streets for an authoritarian state and labelling those who did not conform to the dictates of society. Szasz in "Schizophrenia: The sacred symbol of Psychiatry" attacks the whole concept of schizophrenia as a medical condition. He argues that the paradigm of general paresis had an unduly strong influence upon psychiatry. Szasz claims that schizophrenia and other mental illnesses are not illnesses in the sense of "real" illnesses such as brain tumours. He argues from a dualist position, maintaining that mental illness lies within the moral-social realm, dealing with so-called "problems of living" rather than being medical disorders. His widely quoted analogy is of the inappropriateness of calling in the television repairman because you do not like the television programme [19]. As is apparent from the criticisms made by Roth (1986), Szasz generally appears to be vague about psychopathology, although he can justify himself to some extent in that the psychoanalytic tradition in the USA has meant that form and content are sometimes confused. Szasz is, however, more cogent when he gets on to his main theme, which is political. He is a strong advocate of individual liberty and "freedom from constraint". He sees psychiatrists as enemies of liberty because they look to the interests of society over and above those of the individual and that they seek to impose collectivist values. Szasz's view is that the psychiatrist should not be working in "public hygiene" but that his only responsibility should be to the patient, as laid out in a contract made in the open market [20].

Current views in the West
An effort has been made to describe the anti-psychiatry movement, because,

19. This analogy does not hold up when one considers his basic premise which is that diagnosis is based upon the content of the programme. As discussed in Chapter 2, diagnosis in psychiatry is based on *form* not *content*. Using his analogy, the diagnosis would actually be based on the fact that the screen was flickering (hallucinations?) or that the picture was badly faded (depressed mood?), not that the dialogue was boring.

20. Sedgewick (1982) points out that psychiatry is not alone in facing such criticisms. Advocates of the laissez-faire society and the free market make similar criticisms of social workers, health visitors and inspectors of more or less any kind (tax, factory or parking). He argues that much anti-psychiatry thinking is linked to the ideas of Herbert Spencer and 19th century Social Darwinism. Misapplied theories of natural selection, advocating open competition and the weak going to the wall, lead to opposition to any form of "interference" such as taxation, factory legislation or trade union bargaining. Sedgewick is particularly fierce in his condemnation of the anti-collectivism and individualism of the new right. He accepts that mental illness is a social construction, but claims that this applies to all illness. He argues, however, that it is useful to have a concept of mental illness, not least to be able to make demands of society on behalf of the disadvantaged. He condemns the passivity of anti-psychiatrists who play into the hands of the new right with their "psychiatric monetarism", justifying economic stringency on the grounds that mental illness does not exist. Like Szasz, Sedgewick is mainly concerned about the political issues, and puts up the collectivist case against Szasz's dream of a laissez-faire society with psychiatry practised solely on a contractual basis.

although much of the polemic has gone, there is no doubt that its influence remains [21]. The movement was to some extent a reaction to a confident period in the history of psychiatry, the 1950s and early 1960s, when there was optimism about real and potential sucesses in treatment, deinstitutionalization and the removal of stigma. There was a notion that psychiatry might have a wider role in solving social problems and improving the lot of mankind in general (perhaps it is no coincidence that this was also the high point of the cold war). It lined up with other scientific disciplines to challenge old beliefs and systems. In this context the reaction against psychiatry took many psychiatrists unawares. Some reacted with bewilderment or resentment. Many, however, perhaps alarmed by the possible implications of their discipline, were happy to retreat from the science and emphasize the humanitarian and caring aspects. To some extent this produced an atmosphere of scientific stagnation which remains to this day, with dogma taking the place of enquiry [22]. This is not to say that the tenets of anti-psychiatry have been accepted. What does seem to have happened is that the movement has acted as kind of militant wing for more conventional psychological and social approaches. Psychological concepts of mental illness have been shored up at a time when they could have come under threat because of the developments in biological psychiatry. Many psychiatrists influenced by the ideas have been left with a somewhat nihilistic view of mental illness and a tendency to view biological research findings with scepticism. It has also resulted in other psychiatrists retreating from anything psychosocial into a biological world of genetically-determined diseases waiting to be established by further advances in molecular biology.

Mainstream psychiatry, however, is still trying to make sense of both the biological and the psychosocial. Ginsberg (1985), writing in the Comprehensive Textbook of Psychiatry, makes the point that American psychiatry is still trying to integrate two themes. The first is that psychiatric diseases exist, and that patients either have them or do not, the approach adopted by DSM-III. The second is the psychoanalytic tradition which is concerned with content and meaning rather than form. The psychoanalytic tradition is still powerful within mainstream American psychiatry and it does influence the concept of mental illness. The Comprehensive Textbook of Psychiatry (1985) states that the importance of psychoanalysis for the student of general psychiatry should not be underestimated and that psychoanalysis is a fundamental discipline in psychiatry which is the basis for understanding the neuroses. Psychoanalytic theories are given much space. Reflecting the different trends, Grinker (1982) states that the psychoses are genetic-environmental diatheses whereas the neuroses are psychological processes, the product of defences against anxiety. Personality disorders have an uncertain position. Some modification of this view does appear to be held by many American psychiatrists. Indeed, despite the criticisms made by Ginsberg, the DSM-III definition of mental

---

21. There was no open anti-psychiatry movement within the Soviet union. Indeed, it has been argued that the accusations of psychiatric abuse are partly the result of a suppressed, externally fostered anti-psychiatry movement. The opening up of the press has meant that Soviet psychiatrists are now subject to the same pressures that Western psychiatrists experienced three decades earlier.

22. It could be argued that the anti-psychiatry movement was part of a more general reaction against science. Wolpert (1987) discusses the tradition of hostility to science in the broader context of art and religion, suggesting links with vitalism, which he defines as "an idea that gives man and life a special quality outside science".

illness does allow room for the dualist position [23].

The British position is harder to come by. Lewis (1953) argued in favour of the medical model, writing that the "traditional" medical criteria for disease are that a person feels ill or that the functioning of some part of him is disordered or that he has symptoms which conform to a recognizable clinical pattern. He argues that these apply to mental illness and that there is essentially no distinction between mental and physical health. He does, however, caution the reader that the second criterion, a disturbance of part-function, is not always a sufficient criterion on its own. Thus someone might have abnormal perceptions, including hallucinations, without necessarily being ill. His way round this is to suggest that to fulfil this criterion the abnormality should be statistically deviant and also have a basis in some kind of psychopathological process ie it is a maladaptive rather than an adaptive mechanism. He writes that "the concept of disease, then - and of health - has physiological and psychological components, but no essential social ones." This line has been criticized for taking too narrow a view of social. The point at which a disorder of part-function is considered pathological is often determined by social factors for physical as well as mental illness. Indeed, there are social components to the other criteria - whether a patient feels ill and when symptoms are recognized as falling into a clinical pattern. Kendell (1975) attempts to define mental illness by invoking Scadding's criterion of biological disadvantage [24]. In doing so he narrows down his list of psychiatric diseases to schizophrenia, manic-depressive psychosis, some forms of drug dependency and certain sexual disorders, including homosexuality. He writes that these disorders "carry with them an intrinsic biological disadvantage, and on these grounds are justifiably regarded as illness." The place of psychopathy and the neuroses is uncertain.

Clare (1986), in keeping with the Maudsley tradition, tends to be sceptical about most approaches. One has to deduce a position by taking the least criticized approach. Laing and Szasz, as might be expected, are attacked. The Lewis notion of disorder of part-function is criticized on the grounds that it does not let in some personality disorders and alcoholism. A vaguely medical model which makes no assumptions about the brain seems to come out best. The important criteria for psychiatric disorders are considered to be statistical deviation from the norm with some adverse consequences and, possibly, help-seeking behaviour. This allows for the possibility of diseases occurring in the realm of mind, and would seem to be a compromise stance to satisfy those with a psychological understanding of mental illness. Both dimensional (the theory of a continuum of disease) and categorical (discrete disease entities) approaches are criticized, the categorical less so. Clare concludes that there is a broad consensus within psychiatry favouring the disease approach and "the present rudimentary classification".

The social model
The Soviet view is that there is no dichotomy between the biological and social

23. The DSM-III definition of mental disorder is: "a clinically significant behavioural or psychological syndrome or pattern that occurs in an individual and that is typically associated with either a painful symptom (distress) or impairment in one or more important areas of functioning (disability)." This definition allows for most concepts of mental illness.

24. Scadding (1967) defined disease in the following way: "A disease is the sum of the abnormal phenomena displayed by a group of living organisms in association with a specified common characteristic or set of characteristics by which they differ from the norm for their species in such a way as to place them at a biological disadvantage."

models of illness. The social dimension is considered important in all diagnosis, with no distinction between mental illness and physical illness in this respect. The split between the disease model and the social model can be seen as one of the weak points of Western psychiatry. Psychiatrists with a biological view tend to talk in terms of clear-cut disease entities, defending the established nosology rather than considering the possibility of dimensional approaches or alternative systems of classification. Because the existing nosology fails to account for what is seen in day-to-day practice it is easy, by association, to challenge the biological basis of mental illness ie just because of the (false) affiliation between the disease-entity model and the biological position. The dichotomy has meant that the natural sciences view of man as an organism interacting with his environment has been obscured and with it the importance attached to the effect of environmental factors upon the body.

The result of the two different trends in Western psychiatry has been to produce two separate lines of research. Biological researchers tend to investigate small groups of patients, diagnosed according to strict criteria, ignoring patients with mixed clinical pictures or "atypical" features. The findings of such studies, based on small groups of patients, themselves highly atypical, often appear to confirm the disease model. Social psychiatry, on the other hand, investigates populations but tends to ignore biological findings. As yet there has been relatively little research which combines both the biological and psychosocial, for instance the application of epidemiological methods to biological research. If the current nosology does not reflect what is actually out there in the population it would seem likely that high-technology biological work based upon its categories will only serve to mislead. There are also practical consequences with regards to treatment. There is a tendency to think that patients suffer either from biological disorders which require physical treatments, or, alternatively, that they have problems of living or psychological problems which should respond to psychotherapy or counselling.

The dimensional approach
As with many psychiatric issues, the question has been put most eloquently by a writer of fiction, in this case Herman Melville: "Who in the rainbow can draw the line where the violet tint ends and the orange tint begins? Distinctly we see the difference of the colour, but where exactly does the first one visibly enter into the other? So with sanity and insanity. In pronounced cases there is no question about them. But in some cases, in various degrees supposedly less pronounced, to draw the line of demarcation few will undertake..." [25]

There is little in the Western psychiatric literature to indicate interest in the continuum theory with regard to the psychoses, although the notion that there might be degrees of neurosis and personality disorder are generally accepted. However, the dimensional approach to the psychoses has been mooted by the psychologist Eysenck and, more recently, by Claridge (1987). The latter argues that many of the features characteristic of schizophrenia can also be observed in normal, healthy people and that the disorder should be conceptualized as a

---

25. He goes on, rather unkindly: ". . . though for a fee some professional experts will. There it nothing nameable but that some men will undertake to do for pay."

biologically-based continuum [26]. The fact that there is no clear boundary between psychosis and so-called normality should not be taken to imply that schizophrenia is not a disease. It implies, instead, that schizophrenia should be considered in the same light as conditions like hypertension, in which a continuum exists between normal blood pressure, mild hypertension and severe hypertension. Decisions about what treatment is appropriate are made on the basis of the severity or the point on the continuum. That decision is partly clinical and partly social, just as it is with many somatic disorders. It does not take us away from the medical model; rather, it brings biological concepts to the medical model.

The Soviet concept of schizophrenia fits the continuum model better than the more traditional models of disease or non-disease. Soviet psychiatrists, in particular those of the Moscow school, would argue that the idea that a patient has mild features of the disorder is in keeping with the nominalist or patient-oriented approach. It is argued that there is no evidence to support the disease-oriented notion, that you either have the disease or you don't. The evidence favours the existence of intermediate forms, reflecting an underlying pathological process which manifests itself in different ways. There are various theories as to what the process might be, including those to do with imeir psychiatry. I asked several American psychiatrists about their philosophical orientation and their views on the mind-body quenon-specific. How it affects someone, what symptoms it produces and what the long-term outcome is, depends on many other factors. Important factors will be basic constitutional make-up, for instance the robustness of the nervous system, also factors related to personality and quality of upbringing. The result, therefore, will be a variety of different reactions and therefore a range of clinical manifestations from mild forms to severe forms of the disease. This explanation would also apply to the distinction and overlap between schizophrenia and manic-depression.

It is important, as Soviet psychiatrists themselves emphasize, that the correctness or otherwise of this concept of disease should not be confused with issues to do with the social consequences of receiving a diagnostic label, say of schizophrenia. Social consequences should not be the result of a label, but should reflect the degree of disability, irrespective of what a disease process is called. In reality, of course, there is no doubt that the label schizophrenia does have adverse social consequences, not necessarily sanctioned by the law, and that this applies as much in the Soviet Union as in the West. This might suggest that there is a pragmatic case for keeping the label schizophrenia for people who fall at the severe end of the spectrum, irrespective of whether or not this reflects reality. It means that the social consequences apply to a smaller proportion of people with symptoms. This benefits those with milder forms of the disorder, but the corollary is that it makes things worse for those with more severe forms. There is inevitably more stigma attached to the label of schizophrenia if it applies only to the most severe form of the disorder.

The Soviet view is that many of these difficulties stem from the categorical, disease-entity model in the context of a dualist approach. This has led to a rigid distinction between ill and not ill, with implications for treatment and stigma. The stigma of mental illness is due to the notion that it is distinct from other types of

26. The "new genetics" provides some evidence in favour of the continuum. It suggests that you inherit a predisposition to develop either schizophrenia or a range of other personality disorders and non-psychotic disorders (the borderline disorders in Soviet psychiatry). Thus, the same genotype may produce schizophrenia or a range of disorders running into normality. There is evidence that there may be a schizophrenia-related spectrum and a manic-depression related spectrum (Mullan and Murray, 1989).

illness, and this arises from the dualist position and the various bizarre ideas about aetiology associated with it. It is argued that stigma will remain, and with it the crude notion that someone is either sane or insane, until the biological basis for mental illness is accepted, and with it a dimensional concept.

The longitudinal and syndromal approach

The longitudinal as opposed to cross-sectional approach leads to differences in diagnostic practice although these are not absolute and are less than the theoretical implications might suggest. Western diagnosis attaches relatively more weight to the symptoms present at a particular point in time as compared to the longitudinal picture [27]. The two approaches are not just the result of different theoretical concepts, but also arise out of differences in the psychiatric services. The dispensary system (see page 49), which has produced much of the psychiatric research in the Soviet Union, facilitates investigation of the course of a disorder. There are fewer studies of this nature in the West where research tends to concentrate on cross-sectional population samples. One consequence of the strict use of the cross-sectional approach is that it leads to changes in diagnoses over time as symptoms change. It is not uncommon to see case notes where there have been several different admissions to hospital with a different diagnosis on each occasion. A common sequence might run the nosological gamut: anxiety state, manic-depression, schizophrenia, schizo-affective disorder and personality disorder. This does not happen because several different psychiatrists held different concepts of mental illness (indeed it could be the same psychiatrist who makes all the different diagnoses), but is the result of a changing clinical picture and a cross-sectional approach to diagnosis. Thus, applied to a realist concept of disease, logically leads either to the view that the person did indeed happen to suffer from several different conditions or that some of the earlier diagnoses were incorrect.

The longitudinal approach, which makes a diagnosis on the basis of symptoms and syndromes over time, would not consider that one disease had "gone" and another had developed just because the symptoms had changed. The disorder would be seen as an ongoing process.

There are important practical consequences to these differing concepts of illness. As already discussed, the patient-oriented, longitudinal approach produces a model of service which expects long-term follow-up. The obvious dangers are that this is excessively intrusive, although it is important to distinguish between the clinical significance of a diagnosis and what society does with the information. By contrast the cross-sectional, disease-oriented approach fits in with the contractual model. There is no doubt that the disease-oriented as opposed to the patient-oriented concept of medicine is having a major impact upon current American medicine. Diagnosis-related groups (DRGs) have been introduced to standardize payments for the treatment of similar conditions. The result is the shift away from charging per item of service to charging a fixed amount for a particular hospital admission, essentially for a particular diagnostic or disease grouping. Case management schemes are having a similar impact. It can be argued that these will prop up the "Platonic" disease-entity model in the emphasis on treating diseases rather than patients.

---

27. However, Adolf Meyer, Professor of Psychiatry at Johns Hopkins from 1909-1940, emphasised biography over phenomenology, referring to the "life history" of the patient. His multifactorial approach led him to stress the importance of basic aspects such as nutrition and sleep before going into details of psychopathology.

Chapter Two

DIAGNOSIS AND CLASSIFICATION

A disease or disease process is diagnosed on the basis of the syndromal presentation, preferably accompanied by evidence of a particular aetiological agent or pathological process. Psychiatric diagnoses remains at the syndromal level as there are not, as yet, any "biological" features which have been incorporated into diagnostic criteria. The lack of any obvious external validation means that diagnosis rests upon clinical description and the definition and delimitation of the disorders. In order to do this it is necessary to classify them, and the process of diagnosis is intimately linked to that of classification. This requires consensus, both with regards to what symptoms make up a particular disorder, and, perhaps more importantly, what constitutes a particular symptom.

Diagnosis in Soviet psychiatry
Soviet psychiatry emphasizes the longitudinal course of a disorder, whereby a disease is seen as a dynamic process characterized by the different syndromes that constitute it and the changes in these syndromes over time. This implies that a disease cannot be diagnosed just on the basis of the cross-sectional clinical picture, that is the symptoms at a particular point in time. Clinical diagnosis rests upon the recognition of the dynamic process. Thus, symptoms are necessary, but not sufficient, to make a diagnosis, and a cross-sectional picture allows only a provisional diagnosis.

Snezhnevsky (1983) stresses that a diagnosis cannot be based upon individual symptoms, but that these only become significant when they occur in conjunction with other symptoms to make up recognized syndromes. These in turn make up the independent "forms". These forms, each of which has its own typical pattern in which syndromes change over time, are assumed to represent separate disease processes, although it is recognized that different forms may be variations of the same disease. The syndrome, therefore, does not constitute the form or "disease", and the same syndrome may occur across different independent forms. The hypochondriacal syndrome, for instance, occurs in neurotic disorders but also in the psychoses, organic states and somatic illnesses (Zavilianskaya, 1987).

Individual variation is also critical. Snezhnevsky (1983) writes that the development of the syndromes and the course of an illness will be profoundly modified by factors particular to the individual in whom the process is taking place.

Each patient has individual characteristics which will alter their own manifestations of the syndromes.

Forms and syndromes

A syndrome, which is made up of a combination of interrelated symptoms, is the first order clinical entity and it reflects the underlying pathological process. Snezhnevsky (1983) describes it as a "biological functional formation" which can be considered as a reaction of the brain to a noxious agent. Syndromes are never static in that they reflect impaired activity in particular functional systems of the brain. They develop as symptoms change over the course of an illness. There is usually a consistent pattern to this process in any given disorder. There is emphasis on the connections or *sviasi* [1] between the syndromes. It is these which define the pathological process - they are fundamental to the disease. Diagnosis of an independent form, or disease, therefore, is not based on the recognition of syndromes, but in recognizing the connections between the syndromes, and the sequence of changes. Each stage is a product of the preceding stages and this, in turn, predicts the future stages. Thus each static cross-sectional picture is, in fact, a "slow dynamic". This process of change is due to a mixture of physiological (adaptive) reactions along with morbid, pathogenetic reactions. This dynamic view of illness is at the heart of the Soviet approach to rehabilitation.

The distinction between the syndrome and the form is less emphasized in Western psychiatry in which the diagnostic process consists of moving directly from symptoms to the disease, essentially cutting out the middle-man (the syndrome). Thus, if anxiety symptoms (enough to make up an anxiety syndrome) are present in a patient with schizophrenia they are subsumed under schizophrenia. The implications for treatment are that the schizophrenia is treated not the subsumed anxiety syndrome. By contrast, the Soviet approach recognizes the anxiety syndrome and assumes a distinct pathological process which might require treatment in its own right as part of the overall treatment.

The symptoms of mental illness

Despite the different approach to diagnosis the list of psychiatric symptoms is similar to that found in Western psychiatry. This chapter cannot hope to provide a comprehensive account of Soviet psychopathology and for more detail it will be necessary to turn to the source texts [2]. Symptoms are classified in various ways. Korkina (1980) lists the symptoms in a similar order to that used in Western textbooks. In the Manual (1985) there is no attempt to order them, but the symptoms are listed in alphabetic order. This is not particularly helpful for those with little psychiatric experience and is surprising in a book intended for doctors in other specialties as well as for psychiatrists. Snezhnevsky (1983) classifies symptoms according to the different parts of the reflex arc, reflecting the theories of Sechenov and Pavlov. However, this is essentially pragmatic rather than truly theory-based. Although a symptom is considered to be the expression of disturbed function in an organ or functional system it is considered to be due to an interaction

1. The term *svias*, which translates as connections or links, is widely used and carries the implication of a causal interconnection.

2. The key ones are the Handbook (1983) and the Manual (1985). In the English language there is a brief list of symptoms in "Forensic Psychiatry" (1970) edited by Morozov and Kalashnik.

rather than due to disturbance in a single system. Thus, a delusion is not just a disorder of thinking, but also involves affect and memory.

1. Symptoms due to disturbance of the receptor arc.
These include various types of distorted perceptions, including hyperthesia, hypothesia, metamorphopsia and senestopathia. Derealisation is put somewhere between a disorder of the receptor arc and of intrapsychic disorders. The symptom of "deja vu" is considered to be similar to this.

2. Symptoms due to disturbance of the intrapsychic region.
These include disorientation, in time, place or person, and depersonalization. Also described are a number of disturbances of self-awareness. Pathological emotions are included in this section. These are hyperthymia (manic affect) and hypothymia. Hypothymia refers to depressed affect or depression. This is distinguished from dysphoria, in which there is gloomy, irritable mood with increased sensitivity to outside stimuli, often associated with feeling embittered, and, possibly, a tendency to sarcasm and fault-finding [3].

The word *strakh* is described as a feeling of inner tension with the expectation of menace. It is akin to the English term anxiety although it is generally translated as fear or terror. There is no separate word for anxiety in Russian. The emotion is the same as fear *or strakh* but concerns the future - to do with something unknown or something that might happen.

Other pathological emotions are apathy, emotional blunting and emotional weakness (referring to a labile and fluctuating quality to the emotions). Parathymia refers to emotions which are inadequate with regard to the stimuli provoking them.

Disturbances of thought processes include speeding up and slowing down of thinking and also mentism, the presence of an involuntary, continuous and uncontrolled flood of ideas and images. There may also be incoherence or circumstantial thinking, reduction in the quantity of thought, perseveration and thought stopping. Much attention is given to the obsessional phenomena (these are discussed on pages 169 and 173). Disorders of memory, including dysmnesia, amnesia, paramnesia, confabulation, are included here. Delusions and over-valued ideas are discussed below.

Hallucinations are included in this section rather than under disorders of the receptor arc because they are defined as perceptions in the absence of a real stimulus. There is emphasis on differentiating between hallucinations, pseudohallucinations, illusions and imagery. Pseudohallucinations were described first by the Russian psychiatrist, Kandinsky, which may partly account for the greater emphasis on these in Soviet psychiatry. The original concept of Kandinsky, elaborated upon by Jaspers, was that the term should be used for hallucinations occurring in inner, subjective space rather than out in objective space. Some authors speculate that they are essentially a form of imagery, the product of thought but experienced "as if" they were perceptions. They differ from ordinary imagery

---

3. This distinction is recognized in the West but the term dysphoria is less widely used, generally being lumped together with depressed mood. Bech (1987) writes that anhedonia (a mood state similar to dysphoria) tends to be included with depression but argues that it has a different quality. In his view it is more akin to a loss of vitality and is often associated with "borderline" patients who have poor relationships with other people. He argues that neuroleptics are more likely to be effective than antidepressants if pharmacological treatment is required.

in that they are not under voluntary control. This is essentially how they are regarded in Soviet Psychiatry [4].

3. Symptoms due to disturbance of the effector arc.

These reflect pathology of motivation and movement. Hypobulia is described as a lack of drive and decreased volitional activity. In abulia there is a complete loss of will and absence of motivation. There may be hyperbulia (increased activity) or parabulia (distorted activity). Catatonic stupor, stupor and various sub-stuporous states are also described. In hypokinesia and akinesia there is reduction or lack of voluntary movements. In hyperkinesia there is motor excitement and the most extreme form of which is raptus, in which there may be periods of frenzied excitement with sudden, explosive actions interrupting a period of stupor. Various impulsive phenomena are also included here as are disorders of speech, which are given a detailed and lengthy classification.

Delusions and over-valued ideas
Snezhnevsky (1983) defines delusions as ideas or beliefs which arise as the result of links and relationships being established between events and people without any basis in reality. Delusional ideas or beliefs do not correspond to reality and they are held firmly in the face of clear contradictory evidence. They are inaccessible to correction and fully occupy consciousness. The development of a delusional idea is often preceded by a period when there is a strong presentiment of some impending catastrophe, a sense of vague unease and danger. A delusional mood state occurs when the surroundings seem to acquire a different meaning and the world is seen in a new light which is only recognized by the patient. The delusional idea develops at the height of this state when there is a sudden sense of understanding of what is going on, often with a sense of relief. This was described as the "crystallization of the delusion" by the Russian psychiatrist Balinsky.

The qualities of a delusion are that they are held with unshakeable conviction, they are held with the strength of an irrefutable truth which it is impossible to argue with despite the fact that they clearly contradict reality. The person holding the delusion ignores logical counterargument or other people's experience or evidence. Snezhnevsky (1983) emphasizes the point that mistakes of cognition (thinking) are common and that conclusions (*umozakluchenie*) which do not correspond to reality are found in healthy people, convinced of their authenticity. Although such mistaken conclusions are often held with stubborn conviction and are based on unshakeable beliefs they cannot be considered delusional. It is not enough that the idea/belief does not correspond to reality, but there must be a pathological basis for the way in which it developed.

---

4. There is confusion in the Western literature about the meaning and significance of pseudohallucinations. As well as the view described in the text, there is also the view that pseudohallucinations are hallucinations in the usual sense, but that the patient has insight into the fact that they are not real. This is unsatisfactory in that it confuses the two modalities of perception and conation. This definition suggests that the nature of the experience might change over the course of a couple of minutes during which time a patient has been persuaded that the experience is not real but is due to an illness. There is also no consensus about their diagnostic significance. Most American texts get round the problem by simply not discussing this. Thus, there is no mention of pseudohallucinations in the Comprehensive Textbook of psychiatry (1985) or in the DSM-III manual. Several European authors discuss the concept but do not commit themselves to a view about their significance whilst others state that they are of no diagnostic significance. On the other hand the PSE, used in many major studies of schizophrenia, considers them to have the same diagnostic significance for schizophrenia as do true hallucinations.

He stresses the importance of distinguishing between delusions and over-valued ideas or judgements. The latter are considered to arise as the result of real circumstances which have achieved extreme significance for an individual and become emotionally loaded. There is often a minor, but real, injustice and a sense of natural grievance. This does not disappear over time but intensifies and occupies a prominent place in the consciousness. Subsequent events strengthen this and the person keeps returning to the theme. People may act on these, even plan revenge and so on, but, despite their prominence, they don't fundamentally change the personality or overall outlook or system of relationships with people. By contrast, delusions *always refer to the patient* and distort the relationships with people around the patient, often tending to isolate him.

Thus, the distinction from a delusion is that the over-valued ideas arises as a pathological transformation, often delayed, of a natural reaction to a real event. In a delusion there is pathological interpretation of reality from the beginning. According to Korkina (1980), over-valued ideas are mainly found in patients with personality disorders.

Snezhnevsky (1983) draws on the ideas of Griesinger and Jaspers and argues that there are two basic types of delusion: the primary (intellectual) and the sensory or imagic. He considers that primary delusions are to do with disturbance of rational, logical thinking. The senses are in order and the outside world is perceived correctly. It is essentially a disturbance of judgement. The content of delusions varies: there are delusions of persecution, delusions of jealousy, delusions of exalted rank or birth, hypochondriacal delusions, litigious delusions and delusions of reform. Patients with delusions of reform ".. develop new principles of classifying human knowledge and develop projects for the good of mankind eg plans to establish an academy of human happiness." Most Soviet psychiatrists are surprised that this particular symptom has attracted attention in the West. They stress that delusions of reform meet the criteria for delusions like other delusions. This issue is discussed further on page 233.

Sensory or imagic delusions are secondary delusions which arise as the result of other symptoms such as hallucinations or abnormal mood states. The content is often more figurative, with much imagery and fantasy. Logic is generally fragmentary and inconsistent and the delusion is not systematized in the way that primary, intellectual, delusions are. They are more often related to real events, but with a fantastic twist. Patients may see things on a grandiose, world scale, for instance in terms of a battle between good and evil with the patient in the middle. There are often extremes of fear and ecstasy. He quotes various authors who refer to Manichaean delusions [5]. Affective delusions are a type of imagic delusion, arising alongside a mood disorder. There are delusions of guilt, judgement, death and nihilistic delusions in depression and delusions of greatness, wealth etc in mania.

Snezhnevsky (1983) makes the point that the content of delusions depends upon social and cultural factors, although he quotes Greisinger's observation that there are remarkable similarities in the themes of delusions. The detailed content, however, reflects the age in which patients live. In the middle ages they were often about devils and witchcraft whereas hypnosis, magnetism and telepathy figured

---

5. Based on the third century religious doctrine in which the world was seen as being in a state of eternal struggle of light against darkness, good against evil.

24

prominently in the nineteenth century. Delusions about radio waves, atomic power and cosmic rays are now common.

The syndromes

The following is a brief summary of some of the more common syndromes described in the Handbook (1983).

The *psychoorganic syndrome* is a condition of general mental enfeeblement with impairment in memory and understanding and incontinence of affect, also referred to as the triad of Walther-Buel. There may be specific features depending upon the site of the lesion. In frontal lobe lesions motivation and initiative are lost (the apathetic-abulic syndrome). In brain stem pathology there are changes, increases or decreases, in affects and *vlechenie* (attractions, inclinations or desires). In mid-brain disorders there is reduced mental energy, tiredness, apathy, somnolence. There may be affective, endocrine and metabolic changes.

Various syndromes to do with impaired consciousness are described under *clouding of consciousness*. A distinction is made between disorders in which there is disturbed or reduced awareness of the outside world and delirium, in which there are more productive symptoms: an abundance of vivid images and memories, hallucinations, illusions. There is an excellent account of the syndrome *oglushenie*, which is hard to translate, but comes from the verb to stun, deafen or muffle [6]. It describes the impoverishment of mental processes. New experiences cannot be integrated into mental life. Mental imagery is scanty and memories are faded. There is general slowing, reduced movement, sleep without dreams. Perplexity, hallucinations or delusions are not features.

Other syndromes described in this section are *amentia* (possibly a sub-type of delirium) and the *twilight states* which are subdivided into fugues, with delusional and hallucinatory variants. The *oneroid states* are characterized by the confusion of reality and imagination with dream-like changes in self-awareness, fantastic imagery and bizarre experiences [7].

Various psychotic syndromes are described in detail, including the *hebephrenic syndrome* and several different catatonic syndromes: *catatonic-hebephrenic excitement, impulsive excitement,* different variants of *catatonic stupor.* The hallucinatory-delusional syndromes include *hallucinosis,* the *paranoiac syndrome*[8] and the p*aranoid or hallucinatory-paranoid syndrome.* The s*yndrome of Kandinsky-Clerambault* or the syndrome of mental automatism consists of an aggregate of various symptoms: pseudohallucinations, delusions of persecution and influence. The chief manifestations are mental passivity phenomena such as thought insertion, thought withdrawal and thought echo. There are other "made" experiences including those of feeling (senestopathic automatism) and movement

6. It has been translated as "stupefaction" but this doesn't fully convey the sense of the syndrome.

7. Western psychiatry places less emphasis on the changes in consciousness in the functional psychoses (referred to as endogenous psychoses in Soviet psychiatry). This perhaps reflects the lingering view, in keeping with the dualist tradition, that these are psychological disorders. Thus, clouded consciousness of the oneroid type is often overlooked or attributed to some other factor, for instance the effects of drugs or of some accompanying organic disorder, rather than as a feature of the functional psychosis itself. Soviet psychiatrists are more ready to seek evidence of brain dysfunction and impairment of consciousness in patients with acute schizophrenia.

8. Translation note: *paranoidnii* and *paranoialnii*. *Paranoidnii* translates as paranoid and is the more familiar term. As in the West it implies the presence of delusional ideation. As an adjective describing schizophrenia it allows for the possibility of other features such as hallucinations being present. *Paranoialnii* will translate as paranoiac, and can refer to a person or an episode. This implies the presence of delusional features only and no hallucinations.

(kinesthetic automatism). *The paraphrenic syndrome* shares many of the above features but in addition there are often fantastically grandiose delusions. Thus, patients may think that they are the God of Gods, that they have the ability to change natural laws and the climate. There are acute and chronic paraphrenic syndromes.

The emotional (affective) syndromes include the *manic syndrome* and *depressive syndrome* and there are various subdivisions of these eg ironic (smiling) depression, tearful depression, whining depression, sullen depression, asthenic depression, adynamic depression, anxious depression, agitated depression. Neurotic syndromes include the *asthenic, obsessional, phobic and hypochondriacal syndromes*, also *neurotic depression* and a number of somatic syndromes, movement disorders and the so-called *vegetative syndromes*. These are described in chapter 10.

"Negative syndromes"
Negative syndromes include reduced level of mental activity, reduced energy, various changes in personality, and partial or total dementia. It is thought rare to have positive symptoms, such as hallucinations or delusions, without there being some negative symptoms. Snezhnevsky's view, similar in this respect to that of Bleuler, is that the negative symptoms reflect the underlying pathological process in a fundamental way and therefore that these are inevitable if positive symptoms are to develop. The nature of the underlying process, which is reflected in the negative symptoms, will determine the nature of the positive symptoms. Thus, delusions in a patient with dementia will be different from delusions in the context of recurrent psychosis or schizophrenia.

The manual (1985) gives a list of negative syndromes, starting with the personality changes. The mildest of these is *impoverishment of mental activity* and comprises some reduction in mental activity along with weakness, irritability and hyperaesthesia. There may be a subjective sense of personality change before anything can be observed objectively. In *disharmony of personality* there is a greater reduction in the level of mental activity and productivity. There are more profound personality changes, essentially resembling acquired schizoid traits with social withdrawal, egocentricity, paradoxical emotions and loss of emotional resonance. In the syndrome of *loss of mental energy potential* there is a more profound change in personality with reduced mental activity and productivity. *Lowered level of personality* is a stage of the development of the negative changes in which the reduction in activity and ability to work is more fixed and there is marked loss of interests, social withdrawal and a narrowing of the circle of interests. This leads on to *regression of the personality*, the most serious stage, in which there may be marked personality changes, possibly with disinhibition, aggression, inappropriate behaviour and a lack of any ability to adapt.

The Manual describes the other negative syndromes as the amnestic disorders (disorders of memory), partial (dysmnestic) dementia, Korsakoff's (amnestic) syndrome, paralytic syndrome due to tertiary syphilis and pseudoparalytic syndromes due to other causes.

The development of syndromes over time
Despite this description of the different syndromes it is stressed that these are not

clearly defined and that syndromes merge into each other. As the illness develops, often over the course of many years, the presenting syndromes tend to become more complex and polymorphic. Thus the manic syndrome transforms into a manic-delusional, manic-catatonic or manic-oneroid syndrome. What might have presented as a clear-cut depressive syndrome may later present as a depressive-oneroid, depressive-paranoid or depressive-stuporose syndrome. Most disorders have an inherent pattern to their development.

Snezhnevsky (1983) writes that studies, including those based in out-patient settings, have shown that in the early stages of progressive psychiatric disorders such as schizophrenia patients may present with asthenic, neurotic or affective syndromes and only later develop delusional or hallucinatory features. Development is gradual, but always moves from simple to complex. Some disorders, such as manic-depressive psychosis, tend to retain a more homogeneous picture, although even here there is a tendency to develop more complex presentations with age. The cross-sectional approach means that this is often ignored or dismissed, with the result that diagnoses change (one cross-sectional diagnosis to another) over time.

Snezhnevsky (1983) emphasizes the close relationship between the positive and negative syndromes. Positive syndromes arise in the context of negative syndromes, even though these are not always readily recognized. Negative syndromes have their own progression, for instance from mental exhaustion through to personality changes, memory problems and finally dementia. The way in which these negative syndromes develop, either with age or as the disorder progresses, changes the way in which positive syndromes manifest. Some combinations are not compatible. One would not, for instance, find the paranoiac syndrome (complex, systematized, intellectual delusions) in the context of someone with the negative syndrome of total dementia. The diagnosis of mental illness is based on the combination of the negative and positive symptoms. Simply taking the positive syndrome is viewed as misleading. Thus, someone presenting with the asthenic syndrome might have a neurotic disorder, arteriosclerosis or schizophrenia. Negative syndromes can only be diagnosed if there is information about previous personality, previous level of functioning and the history of the disorder.

"Functional diagnosis"

Volovik (1986) writes that one does not diagnose a disease but a patient, and that many aspects of the patient's life must be taken into consideration. The disease process must be recognized, but the functional diagnosis relates to the level of adaptive behaviour and social functioning.

Adaptive behaviour is an important aspect of the Soviet concept of personality. There are different types of adaptive behaviour which determine how a person adapts to his illness. They influence remissions or at least the consequences of remissions. Thus, energetic and self-reliant people who are sociocentric show a constructive pattern of adaptive behaviour even if the pathological process has caused a lot of personality damage. Passive, dependent, egocentric patients with poor social integration and regressive personality tendencies show poor adaptive behaviour even if they have had only a mild form of the disease. A patient with constructive adaptive behaviour might respond to a depressive episode by easing up on his work and sitting it out. Someone with poor adaptive behaviour, especially if there are poor social supports, might require admission.

The level of social functioning is determined by the interaction between pathodynamic, psychological and social factors [9]. The three vectors - pathodynamic, psychological and social - are dialectically interrelated and a disease causes changes in all of these. Thus, adequate evaluation must take into account the state of each of these vectors at the point of onset of the disorder. Evaluating only one factor produces a distorted picture. Functional diagnosis is particularly important for the process of rehabilitation in that it identifies the areas to concentrate on. Without it one is left only with intuition. It is argued that there is no point in treating symptoms vigorously if one should really be concentrating on the personality or the family situation.

Tests as an aid to diagnosis
Biological tests:
As might be expected from the greater emphasis on the biological basis of psychiatric disorders, both the Handbook (1983) and the Manual (1985) have long sections on physical, especially neurological, examination, and on investigation. As in the West, tests are carried out to exclude organic disorders. However, these are also done when there is a clear diagnosis of functional disorder, in that various physical indices such as autonomic nervous system function may influence treatment. Investigations are also more widely used in the Soviet Union because psychiatrists treat a wider range of disorders such as epilepsy and the consequences of trauma and infection. There are also a number of organic disorders such as diencephalitis and arachnoiditis (see pages 190-193) which are not generally diagnosed in the West.

Electroencephalography (EEG) is carried out on most psychiatric in-patients and is thought to provide information on functional systems, and thus help in evaluating the potential for adaptation, ability to work and so on. A number of studies have attempted to correlate EEG patterns with psychopathology and even diagnostic groupings [10]. An example of the clinical application is a study by Bochkarev et al (1987). They comment that sub-clinical astheno-depression is the commonest form of psychiatric presentation in a student population and write that the symptoms are often inappropriately considered as laziness or treated as fatigue or the result of intercurrent illnesses. They analysed the EEG patterns in an attempt to demonstrate that many of these conditions are forms of endogenous depression, showing that patients with the sub-clinical astheno-depressive syndromes show some of the abnormalities found in depression. This was based on factor analysis

9. Pathodynamic factors refer to the severity of the disorder and the rate of development of negative symptoms. Psychological factors refer to the development and maturity of the personality, attitudes, skills, concept of self and social perceptions. Social factors concern the relationships within the family and the social milieu. It would include things like sense of duty, altruism, enthusiasm for work.

10. On the whole there is little work in this area in the West, although there are some consistent results, for instance the finding of increased slow wave activity in depression. There have been many individual studies such as that of Howard (1984) who found that 60% of Broadmoor patients had EEG abnormalities. Those with higher psychopathy scores showed posterior temporal slow wave activity and those convicted of violent acts against strangers showed bilateral paroxysmal features. The advent of computer technology led to some interesting though controversial developments. John et al (1988) report on EEG studies with computer-assisted quantification to allow differential classification. Essentially it consists of analysing the four main wave bands, alpha, beta, gamma and delta. Different patterns emerged in dementia, schizophrenia, depression and alcoholism, as well as in cognitive dysfunction in children.

studies of EEG frequency-amplitude characteristics which identified factors distinguishing between psychotic depression and the normal state.

There is an interesting study on computer-assisted EEG diagnosis by Sidorenko and Soroko (1989) who studied 123 patients from the Kashenko Hospital. There were three groups of patients (those with schizophrenia, manic-depressive psychosis and organic psychosis) and a control group. The results look impressive with reasonably discrete groupings of the different diagnostic entities. There is extremely good differentiation between controls and patients with the psychoorganic syndrome. As might be expected, there is most overlap between schizophrenia and manic-depression and between schizophrenia and organic. Accuracy of prediction of controls was 80%, organic 78%, schizophrenia 75% and manic-depression 67%.

Another form of EEG investigation is the measurement of evoked potentials to various stimuli. The intercorrelations of the evoked potentials from various brain areas are thought to reflect the integration of brain function and to correlate with pathology and distinguish between patients and controls. Pneumoencephalography, an air-contrast X-ray technique, was in wide usage, but, as in the West, is now more or less obsolete. Computed Tomography was introduced relatively late into the Soviet Union. There have been a number of studies with relatively non-specific results. Echoencephalography is also in use (eg Lukacher et al, 1989).

Investigations of blood and CSF are widely used, mainly for differential diagnosis. There have been numerous studies of immune function in psychiatric disorders, much of it for research purposes, although it is thought that there are also a number of clinical applications. From the Serbsky Institute, Oskolkova (1985) reports that the development of antibodies to antidepressants drugs might be an indication for switching them.

Nuller and Mikhalenko (1988) report on biological tests in the differential diagnosis of depressive disorders, of which the dexamethasone suppression test and TRH-test are familiar in the West. They also comment that intravenous diazepam (10-30mgm given over a few minutes) is useful in distinguishing endogenous depression with anxiety-depressive syndrome from "endogenous" anxiety combined with depressive mood. In the latter there is a transient but marked improvement in mental state. A test thought to be sometimes helpful in differentiating between depression and dementia is intravenous imipramine. 25mgm is given intravenously over 20 minutes. If the memory for words (eg on the Wechsler sub-test) improves this suggests depression and if it worsens dementia.

Psychological tests:
Psychological testing has little place in routine diagnosis although tests of attention, concentration and cognitive function are carried out as part of the interview process. It is only in recent years that psychologists have had significant input into psychiatry, although specialized centres such as the Bekhterev Institute have been an exception. More sophisticated psychological tests may be used as an aid to diagnosis when psychology services are available. This is considered particularly important in forensic work, especially when there is any question of impairment in cognitive function. Thus, analysis of cognitive processes (memory, thinking, perception) may help in the differential diagnosis of neurosis from

29

schizophrenia and organic states. The neuropsychological battery of tests, especially those devised by Luria and his co-workers, are used in the diagnosis of organic states.

Classification in Soviet psychiatry

Snezhnevsky (1983) writes that there is no universally accepted classificatory system, but that they reflect the prevailing theories of the time [11]. He claims that most systems have used three broad groupings. The first are those disorders which are predominantly endogenous, but in which exogenous factors play a part. The second group are disorders which are mainly exogenous, but in which endogenous factors play a part and the third group consist of conditions due to pathological development, including oligophrenia and psychopathy (personality disorder). The classification used in the Handbook (1983) is based on these groupings and is given in Table l.

Table 1 *The classification of mental illnesses (Handbook of Psychiatry, 1983)*

ENDOGENOUS MENTAL ILLNESSES
    Schizophrenia
    Manic-depressive psychosis
    Functional psychoses of old age

ENDOGENOUS-ORGANIC ILLNESSES
    Epilepsy
    Disorders associated with atrophic changes in the brain: Senile dementia, Alzheimer's disease, Pick's disease, Parkinson's disease, Huntingdon's Chorea.
    Genetically based organic illnesses.

EXOGENOUS-ORGANIC ILLNESSES
    Vascular diseases of the brain.
    Mental disorders associated with trauma.
    Mental disorders associated with tumours.
    Mental disorders associated with infectious diseases.
    Mental disorders associated with endocrine diseases.
    Periodic organic psychoses (a)

EXOGENOUS MENTAL ILLNESSES
    Symptomatic psychoses (b)
    Toxicomania
    Alcoholism and other forms of substance abuse.

PSYCHOGENIC ILLNESSES
    Neuroses
    Reactive psychoses (psychogenic psychoses) (c)

PATHOLOGICAL MENTAL DEVELOPMENT
    Psychopathy (the personality disorders)
    Oligophrenia (mental retardation)

Notes to Table 1

(a) The periodic psychoses are a mixed group of psychoses caused by trauma, infection or toxins, but developing 2-10 years after the exposure (Tiganov, 1983). There is sudden onset and it is often provoked by a minor illness. The concept was described in nineteenth century by, amongst others, Korsakoff and was developed by Golant (1941) and her colleagues in Leningrad. The overlap with affective disorders and other psychoses is not clear.

(b) The symptomatic psychoses are psychotic disorders which arise as a result of a general somatic illness or its treatment. They may be due to cardiovascular disorders, especially myocardial infarction, heart operations, infectious, metabolic and endocrine disorders, also various drugs, nutritional and industrial substances.

(c) These are psychotic reactions to some form of psychogenic trauma or unfavourable situation. They are sub-classified as:

1. Affective-shock reactions
   There is a hyperkinetic type with motor excitement and a hypokinetic type with stupor. They are reactions to such things as natural disasters, catastrophes and military situations.

2. Hysterical psychoses
   These tend to be less dramatic responses to severe, often more prolonged, crises. They include the twilight states, pseudodementia (the Ganser state), puerilism and hysterical stupor.

3. Reactive depression
   Unlike the above two this is not always directly connected to a mental trauma. It is a less clear-cut entity and has more links with affective disorders.

4. Psychogenic paranoid reactions (psychogenic paranoia).

The differences between Soviet and Western systems are most apparent with regard to the classification of schizophrenia, given in table 6 on page 123, which is classified according to the course of the disorder rather than the traditional syndromal presentation.

Use of ICD-9

For official purposes the classificatory system used in the Soviet Union is an adapted version of the ninth revision of the International Classification of diseases (ICD-9). This is the system of classification used in the Manual (1985). It follows the ICD-9 sequence, but attempts to accommodate a number of different features of Soviet psychiatry. This is difficult in the case of schizophrenia in that the Soviet classification, based on the course of the disorder, is particularly hard to accommodate to the syndromal/cross-sectional ICD-9 classification (the principle types being simple, catatonic, hebephrenic and paranoid). Looking at the modified ICD-9 classification (for instance in the Manual) gives a muddled view of the

11. Sartorius (1988), director of the WHO division of mental health, gives a comprehensive account of the issues and difficulties involved in the classification of psychiatric disorders. He writes: "A classification is a way of seeing the world. It is the reification of an ideological position, of an accepted stand of theory and knowledge. Classifying means creating, defining or confirming boundaries of concepts."

system. The syndromes, which are not considered nosological entities, are given the same status as the forms and it appears as if there are about forty different disorders, some based on syndromal presentation and some on course. Academic centres generally use the modified ICD-9 for statistical purposes and keep to the Soviet system for teaching and research. This is thought to be a better representation of what is seen clinically.

There are controversies about classification within the Soviet Union. Snezhnevsky has been accused of excessive lumping, putting too much into the schizophrenia basket. Many psychiatrists hold a narrower concept of schizophrenia, more readily diagnosing affective disorders and using ICD-9 instead of the Snezhnevsky classification. Some psychiatrists at the Bekhterev Institute, for instance, consider all patients with slow-flow (sluggish) schizophrenia to be suffering from cyclothymia and diagnose patients with recurrent schizophrenia as manic-depressives. Other psychiatrists in the same Institute hold more traditional (from the Soviet perspective) views. Western oriented psychiatrists are more likely to be found in places like Leningrad and the Baltic republics.

The other Soviet way of narrowing down schizophrenia is to adopt what has been called the traditional nosological approach. Kazanetz (1979), writing in an American psychiatric journal, maintained that there were two schools of Soviet psychiatry. The "nosologists", he claims, represent the traditional Russian school of psychiatry, and hold the view that there are different psychoses with their own aetiologies (what has been referred loosely above as the Leningrad school). The "syndromologists" emphasize the similarity between the psychoses and consider that the different psychotic syndromes represent variations on common underlying pathological processes. He acknowledges that this second view, that of the Moscow school, predominates, but argues for the former position. He argues that the Soviet variant of the ICD, which differentiates exogenous psychoses from schizophrenia, should be more widely used. He reports that in a ten year follow-up of patients with a diagnosis of schizophrenia it was possible to make a diagnosis of exogenous psychosis (reactive, infectious or traumatic) in one third of cases. These patients had a much better outcome in terms of social adaptation and work.

Comparative aspects
Diagnosis
Many of the criticisms directed against Soviet psychiatry have been about diagnostic practice. This is not really surprising in that the process of diagnosis has been a particular target for critics of psychiatry in general. Diagnosis is condemned as being invalid, unreliable and dehumanizing, and for extending into areas where it ought not. Rosenhan (1973) writes that there are no tests for schizophrenia and claims that "medical" diagnoses are well validated whereas psychiatric diagnoses are "...maintained by consensus alone." Laing (1965) challenges the whole process of diagnosis, mainly on the basis that people behave differently towards different people, particularly towards psychiatrists. Similar criticism of diagnostic practice in the Soviet Union is made by Bukovsky and Gluzman in their "Manual on Psychiatry for Dissenters", written in 1974 in a Samizdat publication. This document, which is widely quoted, for instance by Bloch and Reddaway (1977), makes many of the criticisms of psychiatry made by Western anti-psychiatry groups.

There is no doubt that the process of diagnosis can be made to look fatuous if symptoms are taken in isolation, out of context of the diagnostic process. Critics of psychiatry tend to quote descriptive phrases as if they determined diagnosis. The weakness of these criticisms is that they ignore the reality that diagnosis often does not rest upon what people say to psychiatrists. Diagnosis, admission and changes in civil status usually result from disturbances in behaviour, relationships and social functioning. Tacitly or otherwise these tend to carry more diagnostic weight than details of psychopathology. However, these factors are given less prominence as diagnostic criteria than psychopathology, generally based on an interview at a particular moment, giving a cross-sectional picture. This is particularly striking in disorders which rest on the presence of only one symptom.

Soviet psychiatrists claim that their own diagnostic practice is less open to error because of the emphasis on the course of the disorder, personality change and social functioning. They argue that this multidimensional approach ensures that a complete picture of the illness is available. Thus, Volovik (1986) criticizes DSM-III on the grounds that the psychosocial variables are dealt with on a separate axis or "in isolation". He argues that this means they are not incorporated into the diagnostic process which still relies upon a cross-sectional, syndromal picture. This is considered to be unreliable because of the undue influence of Jaspers phenomenology and the impact of psychoanalysis.

Similar criticisms are made of psychiatry in the English-speaking world, especially in the USA ie that the influence of psychoanalysis has led to poor diagnostic practice because dynamic psychopathology is concerned with content rather than form. It is certainly true that descriptive psychopathology has lagged behind classification. Fish (1967) made one of the first comprehensive attempts to introduce systematized psychopathology to the English-speaking psychiatric world[12]. He maintained that American and British psychiatrists tended to confuse form with content and claimed that the careful description of psychiatric signs and symptoms was "conspicuous by its absence". However, since his contribution there has been considerable progress in the field of descriptive psychopathology. A measure of consensus has been achieved about definitions of symptoms and syndromes, and several sets of diagnostic criteria have been introduced. Standardized interview schedules which include definitions of symptoms have gradually come into use, both in Europe and America.

In the USA the influence of psychoanalysis was partly responsible for a broad, even vague, concept of schizophrenia. According to Kendell (1981) this was the result of diagnosis based on psychological attributes and defence mechanisms [13]. It is inevitable to some extent that a psychoanalytic concept of illness is broad in that to be healthy from the psychoanalytic perspective it is necessary to be fully adjusted to the world and other people, to function optimally and, preferably, to be happy as well. Psychoanalytically conceptualised psychotic symptoms are still present in

12. "Clinical psychopathology" by Fish (1967) was the backbone of British psychopathology for two decades. The book was unpopular in some quarters, partly because of his rather strident style of writing. He had a number of targets, the favourite being religion. Fish was tamed in later editions edited by Max Hamilton with some of the more exotic clinical material edited out. It seems likely that Sims' "Symptoms in the Mind" (1988), which is heavily influenced by Jaspers' phenomenology, will become a mainstay of psychopathology.

13. Kendell et al (1971) showed that British and American psychiatrists who saw the same patients would regularly come up with different diagnoses. The main trend was for Americans to diagnose schizophrenia where British psychiatrists diagnosed manic-depression or personality disorder.

American psychiatry, although with DSM-III they are no longer part of the official criteria for the major disorders. However, Lipkowitz and Iduputanti (1985) write that even after DSM-III many psychiatrists still diagnose schizophrenia in an "individualistic, unsystematic way". In the emphasis on the "feel" of schizophrenia and the importance of clinical judgement there does perhaps remain the lingering influence of the eminent American psychiatrist, Nolan Lewis, who remarked that "even a whiff of schizophrenia is schizophrenia". The broadening of the concept of mental illness and the vague diagnostic practices inevitably led to criticisms, the most influential of which was Rosenhan's "thud" study [14].

In mainland Europe, especially Scandinavia and France, the schizophrenia or manic-depression debate is less acute because of a greater readiness to use other categories of psychosis such as schizoaffective disorder and acute reactive psychosis. Saugstadt and Odegard (1985) make the point that third category of psychosis was included into ICD-8 because of this, but that it was not used in Britain because of the wider concept of manic-depression nor in the USA or USSR because of the wider concept of schizophrenia. They report that in Norway only 10% of admissions to a psychiatric hospital are for manic-depression or schizophrenia! Most British or American psychiatrists find that well over half the patients on their wards would carry one or other of these diagnostic labels.

One practical result of the differences between the realist and nominalist approaches to diagnosis is apparent in the different content of Soviet and Western case conferences. From a nominalist perspective the actual name (diagnosis) is less important than understanding the underlying process and deciding upon treatment and prognosis. My impression of case conferences in the Soviet Union is that the theoretical nominalist stance does in fact translate into practice. The emphasis is on the different features, including psychosocial factors, that make up the total picture. The actual label is considered to be fairly arbitrary, with no particular significance attached to one or other term. Western case conferences, on the other hand, are often taken up with debate about diagnosis. Strong views are expressed about what does or does not constitute, say, schizophrenia. In practice, diagnosis often has little relevance to the treatment of a particular patient. As discussed on page 158 patients with a DSM-III diagnosis of personality disorder might receive exactly the same treatment, the same drugs and compulsory admission, as a patient with a DSM-III diagnosis of schizophrenia.

At a case conference at a London hospital there was discussion about a twenty-six year-old woman who was threatening harm to her baby. She had a history of bizarre episodes of deliberate self-harm as a child and a disturbed adolescence. She then married and had two sons, during which period she seemed to be well. She then gave birth to a daughter, having a traumatic delivery, and it was when the girl was nine months old that she again became disturbed and developed hostile

---

14. Rosenhan (1973) described an experiment in which a number of "pseudopatients", including Rosenhan, managed to get themselves admitted to 12 different American psychiatric hospitals by complaining that they were hearing voices. When asked to elaborate they said that these were vague, but seemed to consist of the words "thud" or "hollow". They gave no other symptoms and once admitted to hospital behaved normally. They all acquired and retained a diagnosis of schizophrenia. This study irritated many psychiatrists. Spitzer (1976) condemns the study on scientific grounds and argues that it demonstrates that it is possible to make psychiatrists look foolish but that this is irrelevant to the problems of diagnosis in psychiatry. The study did highlight the problems of using analytic criteria. For instance, the genuine life histories and relationships of these "normal" pseudopatients were thought to demonstrate certain conflicts and relationships characteristic of schizophrenia.

feelings towards the baby. She tried to harm her, saying that the child was a powerful force for evil and that she could control both her and the world. There were a number of other symptoms. At the conference there was much speculation about underlying psychodynamic factors, mainly related to the fact that her troubles began with the arrival of a daughter rather than a son, but, despite this, the majority view was that the correct diagnosis was schizophrenia, or, possibly, an atypical puerperal psychosis, the presentation being rather late. However, the psychiatrist under whose care the patient was argued vehemently against this diagnosis but for one of hysterical personality disorder, giving much greater weight to the psychodynamic factors. Despite this, he had admitted the patient to hospital against her will and his treatment to date had included neuroleptics and a course of ECT.

There may be important social consequences to diagnosis. In forensic psychiatry a label can make the difference between prison or hospital, even death or hospital. There are less dramatic consequences, for instance those arising as a result of the familiar old debate, conducted on psychiatric wards all over the world, about certain difficult patients, especially those who are being "manipulative", violent or who repeatedly indulge in self-harming behaviour, as to whether or not they are mentally ill as opposed to having a personality disorder. The practical consequences are that the difficult patient who keeps his illness label is allowed to stay on the ward, whereas if he acquires a personality disorder he may be discharged. The personality disorder label is usually favoured by the nurses who have to bear the brunt of the difficult behaviour. Doctors, on the other hand, who might have to bear the responsibility for what the person does when discharged (whatever the label) tend to favour the mental illness label. The way in which the diagnoses change is often somewhat arbitrary, resting more on some aberrant behaviour than any change in actual psychopathology.

Form and content
The confusion between form and content or the failure to distinguish between the two has been one of the most important sources of confusion and misunderstanding both within psychiatry and from without the discipline. It is pivotal to many of the charges with regard to the abuse of psychiatry. Diagnosis is based on the *form* of a symptom and not the *content*, so that what a delusional belief happens to be about is not relevant to descriptive psychopathology.

A 31 year-old woman periodically developed the delusional belief that she was under close police surveillance. She was Irish and active in the republican movement, and her brother was a member of the Irish Republican Army (IRA). Because she had developed a good relationship with a psychiatrist she usually presented at out-patients when she was becoming deluded. The psychiatrist would diagnose her as suffering from delusions of persecution and would prescribe trifluoperazine, which she would take with some reluctance.

The diagnosis of delusions of persecution was not based on the content ie the fact that she was under police surveillance (which one would presumably take for granted). It was based on the fact that there was a morbid basis for her belief, one of the criteria for delusional thinking. Thus she would see a traffic light change to red and know that was a signal to her, she would see a number plate with the letter

35

"R" in it and see that as a warning to her that she was being watched. If she was bumped into on the pavement she would interpret that as a further evidence. She became quite convinced that she was watched for every minute of the day on the basis of these different bits of evidence. They produced a state of constant fear, amounting to terror, and the belief that her life was in great danger. After taking trifluoperazine for a few weeks she would usually lose her delusional belief that she was being constantly followed by the police and revert to her normal belief that she was under routine police surveillance. The basis for her normal belief was that she was active in Sinn Fein, that her brother was in the IRA, and that she was visited from time to time by the police and that there were strange clicks and buzzes on her telephone. She resented the surveillance, but felt that it did not interfere too much in her life and, although she accepted there was some danger, she felt this was not excessive and it did not make her afraid.

Thus, it is possible to agree that a person is correct in their beliefs, indeed to share their beliefs, but still diagnose them as being deluded. There may, of course, may be some reluctance to consider someone deluded if what they say might be true or if one happens to believe the same thing. In practice, such cases are unusual, and they rarely present as real clinical problems. Moreover, it is not possible to make an absolute split between form and content, and Jaspers' notion of ununderstandability is not as clear-cut a criterion for delusional thinking as one might hope for.

Critics of descriptive psychopathology claim that content is often ignored and that this affects the relationship with the patient. Some of these criticisms reflect the observation of bad practice rather than faults inherent in the approach. The fact that a disorder is diagnosed on the basis of form does not mean that content has to be ignored. Indeed it is often necessary to concentrate on content to get at the form. It is also important that the social determinants of symptoms should not be ignored. Transcultural studies suggest that these can affect the form of symptoms, but the impact is most marked on content, especially on the content of delusional and obsessional thinking. Abnormal as well as normal thinking is influenced by what happens around you. This has been shown by a study carried out by Klaf and Hamilton (1961). Using case records they analysed the content of delusional thinking of two groups of psychotic patients, one from the 1850s and one from the 1950s. In the 1850s they found that religious ideas were prominent in the delusions of about half of the patients. In 1950 religion was no longer the major preoccupation of delusional thinking, having been replaced by sex and politics. The authors point out that in the 1850s Christianity played a much greater part in the life of the population as a whole (on Sunday the 30th of March 1851 40% of the people of England were at church!). Religion permeated family life, education and work and there was much emphasis on hell and punishment. It is still the case that certain communities, often in rural areas, are more involved with religion and anecdotal accounts suggest that this is reflected in the psychopathology of patients from those communities. The same seems to apply in fundamentalist Islamic communities. By the same token one would expect a much greater preoccupation with social and political issues in a mainly secular country such as the Soviet Union.

The issue of form and content is the key to understanding the controversy about the so-called "delusions of reform" which have been a focus of controversy in the allegations of political abuse. The point has already been made that these are diagnosed on the basis of the form of the delusion not the content. As such, to be present, the criteria for delusions must be met and Soviet psychiatrists maintain that their criteria are more stringent than those generally used in the West [15].

Classification

The most widely used classificatory systems used in the West are the World Health Organization (WHO) International Classification of Diseases, ninth edition (ICD-9) and the American classificatory system, DSM-III, the Diagnostic and Statistical Manual of Mental Disorders (third edition).

DSM-III is criticized in the Soviet Union on the grounds that it appears to have been devised for administrative rather than scientific purposes. It is considered to be arbitrary and unsystematic. There is some recognition of this in the USA where some psychiatrists see it as being a pragmatic tool, devised by committee, rather than having any empirical basis. Some critics suggest that it was devised to provide diagnoses for the purposes of billing patients and claiming from insurance companies. It is argued that by "naming" such a wide range of conditions DSM-III allows the psychiatrist to diagnose more or less anything and offer more or less anyone the possibility of having some form of treatment, especially psychotherapy. DSM-III is also criticized on the grounds that it is a heterogeneous system. There are "reductionist biological" concepts which are shown up in the large number of apparently clear disease-entities. There are also lingering psychodynamic concepts. DSM-III attempted to develop a classification based on descriptive psychopathology, the observation of form, rather than content, but a number of major anomalies slipped in. An example of the confusion of form and content is the classification of Depersonalization Disorder under the Dissociative Disorders (or "Hysterical Neuroses, Dissociative Type"). This includes Psychogenic Fugue, Psychogenic Amnesia and the somewhat dubious entity Multiple Personality Disorder. The inclusion of depersonalization here is theory-based rather than descriptive in that it assumes that there is a hysterical or dissociative mechanism for the symptom.

Social aspects of diagnosis and classification.

Although there is a social component to most aspects of diagnosis and classification there are instances when the social aspect is more immediate and obvious. This often relates to admission policies, especially when psychiatrists are encouraged to "play for safety". One of the criticisms of Soviet psychiatry, now being made by internal critics as well as the West, is that there has been excess caution with regard to admission and discharge policies [16]. However, few

---

15. There is greater emphasis in the Soviet literature on the disruptive nature of the delusion and the fact that it fully occupies the consciousness. Also, there is some tendency for English-speaking psychiatry to define a delusion on the basis of a false belief rather than adopting the German tradition which stresses the morbid origin of the belief (Fish, 1967). This applies particularly to the American literature. In the "Comprehensive Textbook of Psychiatry" delusions are described as "false ideas that cannot be corrected by reasoning and that are idiosyncratic for the patient; that is, not part of the cultural environment" (Lehman and Cancro, 1985). Linn (1985), also in the Comprehensive Textbook, has a similar definition, but perhaps approaches the idea of the morbid origin by describing a false belief which arises without the appropriate external stimulus.

Western psychiatrists are unfamiliar with social pressure, whether it be from family, neighbours, other doctors or the police, to admit or detain certain patients. Eisenberg (1988) gives an example of this happening at city level. On the 7th July 1986 Juan Gonzales, a homeless Cuban "refugee", killed two passengers and wounded nine others on the Staten Island ferry. What made the case a sensation was the fact that Gonzales had been seen at a psychiatric Emergency Room on the 3rd of July because of threatening behaviour and shouting "Jesus wants me to kill" but had not been admitted. As a result of the subsequent media outcry there was a massive increase in the number of referrals to Emergency Rooms and hospital admissions. Conditions in the city hospitals became so crowded that patients were being bussed out to old state hospitals many hundreds of miles out of New York. In addition the private sector was called in to house patients.

"What had happened?" asks Eisenberg (1988) ".. a municipal epidemic of homicidal psychoses? Hardly! What had changed were the administrative decisions made about the very same troubled and troublesome persons who had been on the city streets in the weeks and months before panic erupted."

It was nearly a year before hospital admissions settled down to their former level. It provides a clear example of the way in which social factors can influence psychiatrists to admit patients, for the most part against their will. It is all too easy to criticize psychiatry for this, despite the fact, perhaps because of the fact, that most psychiatrists were only too well aware that they were responding to social pressure and unnecessarily depriving people of their liberty.

Epidemiological aspects
The process of diagnosis and classification effectively determine the level of morbidity in the population. It also determines what proportion of patients fall into the different classes of mental illness. Endicott et al (1982) showed that the proportion of people earning a diagnosis of schizophrenia in a group of psychiatric patients varied between 7% and 26% depending upon which set of criteria were used. They later showed that none of the criteria were consistent in predicting outcome, in that none got to the notion of "core" schizophrenia in which there should be a deteriorating state (Endicott et al, 1985). Shmaunova (1985) quotes two studies in Moscow, one in 1972 and one in 1978, with the ratio of patients with schizophrenia to those with manic-depression changing from 24:1 to 13:1 over that period. She does not offer a view about which approach is correct but makes the point that epidemiology depends on diagnostic concepts and that these change [17]. Rotstein et al (1987) emphasize the problems of the different methodologies, for instance the fact that population studies show higher prevalence rates for psychiatric disorders than in-patient or dispensary studies. They comment on diagnostic differences, for instance with regards to schizophrenia.

It might be argued that criticisms of DSM-III are justified when the NIMH

16. This particularly applied at public holidays when there was a tendency to admit troublesome patients who could have been reasonably managed as out-patients. The issue is discussed in Chapter 13.

17. Shmaunova et al (1988) quote a number of studies to suggest an overall prevalence of about 1% for schizophrenia in the general population. They report that over the years 1967 to 1975 to 1981 the prevalence of schizophrenia dropped in the under 20 age group and somewhat less in the over 60 group. In the 40-60 age group the prevalence remained the same. There was also a drop in the prevalence of slow-flow schizophrenia. They argue that these results suggest that less severe forms of schizophrenia are not being admitted to dispensary lists, possibly because resources such as transport have been unavailable over this period.

study, using the Diagnostic Interview Schedule (DIS) based on DSM-III, appeared to show that one in six of the population had a significant mental illness at any one time (Regier et al, 1988). In the NIMH Epidemiologic Catchment Area Survey a total of 18,571 people were interviewed (in five areas: Los Angeles, Baltimore, St. Louis, New Haven in Connecticut and Durham in North Carolina) and reported that 15.4% of the population aged over 18 fulfilled the criteria for some form of mental disorder (which included alcohol or drug abuse) in the month before interview, with higher prevalence rates in people under the age of 45. The prevalence of schizophrenia was 0.7% with higher rates in men. The prevalence of affective disorders (including dysthymia) was 5.1% and higher in women. The finding of high levels of morbidity is not simply the result of using DSM-III as earlier studies have also revealed high morbidity rates [18]. Much of the reported morbidity is due to the inclusion of people with substance abuse and personality disorder. In a community sample in England, Casey and Tyrer (1990) reported a one-year prevalence of personality disorder of 28%.

Soviet epidemiological studies have reported widely varying results. One of the key studies is that reported by Rotstein (1977). This was a massive study undertaken by large number of psychiatrists in five areas, one rural and four towns, including Frunze (capital of Kirghizia) and Volgograd (formerly Stalingrad). Over 35,000 people were interviewed, and 1872 people were found to suffer from some form of psychiatric disorder, a prevalence of 5.3%. This included epilepsy, trauma, oligophrenia (mental handicap). The point prevalence of schizophrenia was 3.8 per 1000. Psychopathy and neurosis were the commonest disorders in the general population, but schizophrenia and epilepsy were the most commonly registered on the dispensary lists.

A result more analogous to some Western studies is that of Kornilov et al (1987) from the Kemerov Medical Institute. In a survey of 550 workers at a chemical plant they report that 73.2% of the workers had some form of neuropsychiatric morbidity! It is hard to make comparisons, however, because of lack of criteria. Certainly much of the morbidity is minor, for instance the presence of a single symptom such as asthenia or a somatic symptom like palpitations or abdominal pain. In a later report they elaborate on the findings (Kornilov et al, 1988), reporting that financial and domestic difficulties were commoner in those with depressive and neurotic reactions.

Epidemiology is only discussed briefly in this chapter because the differences in diagnosis and classification mean that is not possible to take comparisons much further. There has been much speculation about the influence of Capitalist or Communist systems on the prevalence of mental illness, drug abuse and alcoholism. The data which is currently available does not allow this to go beyond the realms of speculation.

---

18. Perhaps the most remarkable results were those of Srole et al (1962) which reported that 81.5% of New Yorkers had psychiatric symptoms and Leighton et al (1963) which claimed that 69% of the population of the town of Bristol, Stirling County, were "genuine psychiatric cases". Neither study used clinicians to make diagnoses.

Chapter Three

PSYCHIATRIC SERVICES

This chapter examines the structure of the psychiatric services within the Soviet Union. By way of background it begins with a brief description of the health service overall.

DEVELOPMENT OF HEALTH SERVICES

There was a strong tradition of social and preventive medicine in pre-revolutionary Russia. Nineteenth century physicians and surgeons such as Botkin, Pirogov, Mudrov and Zakharyn stressed the importance of the environment, in particular housing and work conditions. They laid emphasis on prevention and on treating the patient rather than the disease. In the nineteenth century, however, there was little opportunity to put these ideas into practice and the medical facilities in large cities like St Petersburg were rudimentary (Hyde, 1974). There were some instances of individual enterprise such as the out-patient department established by Botkin in St Petersburg. In the rural areas the Zemstvo system of local government, which began in 1864 after the liberation of the serfs, facilitated the introduction of limited health services. These varied widely, with much depending on the initiative of local officials or landowners. There were a total of 208,000 hospital beds, a ratio of 1.5 beds per 1000 population, and only 28,000 doctors, or 0.2 doctors per 1000 population. Central Asia was considerably worse off with many areas having virtually no medical facilities of any kind (Lisitsin and Batygin, 1978).

The Bolshevik government planned to introduce a nationalized health service after the October 1917 Revolution. Despite opposition from the Pirogov society (the main medical professional association), the People's Commissariat of Public Health was created and the decree of July 11 1918 proclaimed the first nationalized health service in the world. Semashko, a doctor who had been in exile with Lenin, became the first Soviet Commissar for health. The priorities of the service were to deal with the serious outbreaks of infectious diseases, in particular tuberculosis, cholera and typhus. Partly because of these priorities, but also because of the New Economic Policy (NEP) introduced at the Tenth Party Congress in 1921, the development of the health service, especially in terms of building and staffing levels, was restricted. Indeed, over the period of the NEP many doctors returned to private practice.

It was not until 1928, with the first of the five-year plans, that major changes took place. The number of doctors was increased and there were construction programmes for rest homes, sanatoria, hospitals and polyclinics (out-patient departments). The dispensary system, a series of specialized clinics, mainly run on an out-patient basis, to deal with specified disorders such as tuberculosis, venereal disease, cancer or mental illness, also started up at this time. Paediatric medicine was considered a high priority and resources were directed towards the training of paediatricians and the construction of childrens' hospitals and polyclinics. By 1940 there were 155,000 doctors and 790,900 hospital beds, with the greatest increases found in the Central Asian republics. Despite the impact of the Second World War the medical services continued to expand. By 1965 there were 554,000 doctors and 2,225,000 beds (Lisitsin and Batygin, 1978). In 1987 there were 1.2 million doctors, or 4.2 doctors for every 1000 people (Hyde, 1988) There are some differences across the republics with beds varying from 9 to 13 per 1000 and doctors from 2.3 to 4.6 per 1000 (Ryan and Prentice, 1983).

Despite the increases in services, for instance in terms of the numbers of beds, doctors and other health workers, there have been severe criticisms of the state of the health service. There have been numerous complaints in the Soviet Press about conditions in hospitals and polyclinics: buildings in poor repair, dirt, long periods of waiting, disorganization, poor standards of care. On a more objective level it appeared that various indices such as the infant mortality rate and the life expectancy, especially in men, started to flatten out and even dip [1]. In 1987 the new Health Minister, Chazov, criticized badly trained doctors, the shortages of drugs and equipment, the poor conditions in many hospitals. He argued for greater choice and for the introduction of the "family doctor" system, for more autonomy to the regions to determine their own planning and staffing levels. He attributed some of the problem to the fact that a smaller proportion of the national resources had been devoted to health in recent years, stating that this situation would be corrected.

Hyde (1988) summarizes some of the proposals for the development of health care in the twelfth five year plan, which aims to plan services up to the year 2000. Future measures are to be directed towards more preventive medicine, including controls on environmental pollution and safety measures at work. There are to be educational measures with regards to diet, alcohol, smoking and sex. It is hoped that by the turn of the century everyone will have regular health check-ups. Spending on hospitals and polyclinics is to be doubled and made more efficient by better evaluation and use of the principles of "cost accountancy". There is much greater emphasis on the quality of services. The recent changes in the Soviet Union will presumably result in the different republics developing their own priorities.

---

1. Average life expectancy for men over the past century:
   1897 = 31
   1913 = 32
   1927 = 42
   1939 = 44
   1956 = 63
   1972 = 64
   1986 = 64

41

Organization of the Health Service [2]

Planning and major administration was centred on the Ministry of Health in Moscow. The next administrative level for the health service was at the level of the health ministries of the fifteen republics (these are now largely independent). There may be separate ministries at the capitals of the autonomous republics which are administratively separate units within the biggest republic, Russia. There are health departments at the level of the province (*krai*), the region (*oblast*), which generally has a population of over one million, and the major cities. In turn the cities and rural areas are divided up into districts (*raion*). The raion is the key administrative area for providing health services and they have populations varying from 50,000 to 300,000, generally smaller in rural areas. In Leningrad, for instance, with a population of 5 million, there are 22 *raions*. The *raions* are then subdivided into *uchastki*, which I will translate as sector. Sectors are of various sizes, most commonly 3000-4000, although in some urban areas there are smaller zones of about 2000. This population is served by two *terapevts* (primary care physicians) and a paediatrician, with input from other specialties such as surgery and obstetrics. They are based in out-patient clinics (*ambulatoria*). In urban areas several of these might be sited in a polyclinic. In the rural areas some sectors are larger, possibly up to 12,000, served by a small rural hospital with resident staff. There are also be feldtsher-midwives, perhaps one per 1000 population.

Polyclinics serve populations of anything up to 50,000 people. Thus, there may be more than one polyclinic per *raion*. They offer a range of specialist services, but always include the *terapevt*, a surgeon, a paediatrician and a gynaecologist. Many polyclinics are attached to hospitals. Patients may go directly to the polyclinics or they may be referred there by the sector doctor. There is one childrens' polyclinic per population of 100,000, usually one per raion.

There are several levels of hospital. Small rural hospitals have a physician, surgeon, gynaecologist, paediatrician and dentist. Larger towns, those with populations of 100,000 or more, or those which serve as centres for rural populations, have the larger district hospitals of about 500 beds which provide a wider range of specialties. They will, when necessary, refer on to regional hospitals, usually situated in the regional capitals. There are specialist interregional centres for burns, cardiovascular surgery and other fields. The final level, the "fifth grade" establishments are attached to research institutes. Not all hospitals come under the aegis of the ministry of health as about 4% of them are run by organizations such as collective farms (Brod, 1984; Kaser, 1976).

Field (1967) and Davis (1989) also describes a number of separate, closed facilities such as the clinics for certain officials and hospitals and special facilities for the armed forces and bodies such as the Academy of Sciences. The largest group of people with separate facilities are workers in large industrial enterprises such as factories and mines. Apart from the different recreational facilities and sanatoria, there are hospitals and clinics attached to these enterprises. There is also full access to the state medical system.

Private practice has continued in various forms since the early days of the revolution. This was at its height during the period of the NEP and in the occupied

---

2. There are numerous sources for this section including Soviet textbooks, Medical Gazette, a number of Western books including Field (1967) and Hyde (1974).

zones during the war (Hyde, 1974). There has, however, been a gradual decline in private practice, although a number of "pay clinics" charge a fee for specialist appointments. More recently there has been a revival of private practice, mainly taking the form of a few health cooperatives which have been established in some of the larger cities. There has been some concern about these in letters to the press, both the lay press such as Pravda, Izvestia, Komsomolskaya Pravda and Trud and also in Meditsinskaya Gazeta or Medical Gazette (the "trade" journal for workers in health care). The main concern is about the ideological implications of having a private sector. Most authors, however, dismiss the private sector as being of little relevance, comprising less than 1% of the total health care system. According to Ryan (1989), there has been official resistance to the private medical cooperatives after some initial support.

THE PSYCHIATRIC SERVICES

Historical aspects

As in the rest of Europe and Asia, there were virtually no special facilities for the care of the mentally ill in medieval Russia. The Russian state was founded in the ninth century and, after Christianity was adopted as the official religion in 988 AD, a number of monasteries took on a role in the care of the mentally ill. Before this there were some regions such as Armenia which did have a tradition of caring for the indigent mentally ill, mainly through small religious institutions. The major developments took place at the end of the eighteenth century when several wards were opened in general hospitals and a number of asylums were built. The first asylums were established in St. Petersburg in 1771 and in Novgorod in 1776. In Moscow a ward in a general hospital was opened in 1779 and the first independent psychiatric hospital (the Preobrazhensky) in 1809.

In 1864 the Zemstvo (local government) movement took some responsibility for public health in some rural areas. Hospitals were built, some of which were in the form of farming colonies. As might be expected the distribution of care was patchy, with better facilities available in Western Russia and almost nothing in Siberia, Central Asia and the Caucasus. By 1892 the Zemstvos were responsible for 34 psychiatric hospitals with 9,055 beds and 90 psychiatrists (Wortis, 1950) [3].

There was a progressive tradition among nineteenth century Russian psychiatrists such as Kandinsky, Bekhterev, Balinsky and Sabler and they were able to introduce some policies of humane care and non-restraint. In 1887 Korsakoff, in his lecture to the First Congress of Russian Psychiatrists on "The question of the care of the mentally ill at home", raised the "patronage" system of care by which patients lived with their own family, or with some other family, and had daily care at a hospital. For a brief period this was attempted on a small scale in Moscow. At the First Congress of the Russian Union of psychiatrists and neuropathologists in 1911 the potential importance of the patronage system was recognized, but no steps were taken to implement it.

Although there were clearly pockets of excellence, the overall picture of psychiatric care in pre-revolutionary Russia is one of limited availability of

---

3. In "Ward 6", written in 1892, Anton Checkov describes the conditions in a charitable hospital in a small provincial town. The hospital has a psychiatric ward with five patients.

services. There was only one psychiatrist to every 332,000 population (just over 400 in all) with 0.3 psychiatric beds per 1000 population (Zharikov, 1983). Wortis (1950) quotes the figure of 36,240 psychiatric beds in 1913, which represented 0.26 beds per 1000 population.

Babayan (1985) writes that although Russian psychiatrists had recognized the importance of day care, both for early treatment and rehabilitation, it was not until the 1920s that out-patient care began to be properly developed. After the revolution a special psychiatric commission, which included the leading psychiatrists Kashenko, Gannushkin and Zakharov, was established in order to put some of the ideas of pre-Revolutionary times into practice, with the highest priority being to bring psychiatric care closer to the population. Psychiatric care was brought to many of the republics for the first time, especially to those in Central Asia. In 1928 the first psychiatric hospital in Turkmenistan was built, a 75-bedded hospital at first used mainly to treat opium addicts (Wortis, 1950).

It is claimed that the revolution led to the birth of Social Psychiatry, the aim of which was to allow patients to participate in society rather than to be isolated. In 1919 the First All-Union Conference on psychiatry and neurology emphasized the need for more decentralization. The first out-patient department was established in Moscow in 1919 (Babayan, 1985). At the Second All-Union Conference in 1923 the dispensary system was proposed as the basis of psychiatric treatment. Dispensaries were opened in many of the capitals, and the dispensary system grew from this time.

The civil war led to disruption of psychiatric care, and much of the effort of the Commissariat of Public Health was directed towards dealing with the epidemics of infectious diseases. Psychiatry had to wait its turn to a certain extent, especially for material resources, although major innovations took place in out-patient services and rehabilitation. There was patchy development of services throughout the 1920s. A number of small hospitals and general hospital consulting rooms were opened. The need for psychiatry to be based in the general hospitals was stressed, especially by another leading psychiatrist, Gannushkin. This happened to a limited extent from the 1930s onwards. Workshops were established and in 1927 a prophylactic workshop was set up in Kharkov which included a hostel for patients from out of the city. Production cooperatives of various sorts were also introduced. The first day hospital in Moscow began in 1932 (Babayan, 1985). Night "prophylactoria" were also developed under the initiative of Giliarovsky and Djagarov.

The main developments in the decade after the revolution were undoubtedly in the area of social and community psychiatry, partly because of the difficulties of the period and the limited resources available. Bed numbers actually dropped over the period from 1913 (36,240 psychiatric beds) to 1928 (30,016 psychiatric beds). Over the same period general hospital beds doubled (Wortis, 1950). The series of five-year plans which began in 1928 provided greater resources for psychiatry, both in terms of structures and personnel. Thus, in 1934 the 17th party congress declared that there should be an increase in the number of psychiatric beds by 55% as part of the 2nd five year plan which had begun in 1933. More hospitals were built and more psychiatrists trained.

The War dealt a severe blow to the development of services. Wortis (1950) reports that there were 81,996 beds in 1941, but that this number had gone down to 62,323 in 1948. Many psychiatric hospitals, including those at Smolensk, Minsk and Stavropol, had been destroyed and 20,000 psychiatric patients were killed by specialist units of the German army, assisted by local fascist militia. According to Sochneva (1985), in Latvia alone 2,000 inmates of psychiatric hospitals were executed by firing squad.

It was not until 1952 that bed numbers reverted to pre-war levels. In that year there were 81,200 beds, or 0.44 beds per 1000 population (Zharikov, 1983). Bed numbers continued to increase and in the 1970s they approached Western norms.

Table 2: *Numbers of psychiatric beds since 1913* [4]

YEAR	TOTAL BEDS	BEDS PER 1000 POPULATION
1913	36,240	0.26
1928	30,016	0.2
1932	42,600	0.27
1941	81,996	0.42
1948	62,323	0.35
1952	81,200	0.44
1961	175,000	0.78
1965	205,200	0.9
1968	222,000	0.9
1975	312,600	1.25
1980	314,300	1.17
1985	334,300	1.2
1989	347,000	1.2

There are rural/urban differences. Zharikov (1983) writes that the number of beds may be about two per 1000 in the larger cities but less than one per 1000 in many rural areas. In addition to the general psychiatry beds there are also specialist drugs/alcohol beds which have increased from 69,600 in 1980 (0.26 per 1000 population) to 127,200 in 1989 (0.44 per 1000 population).

Psychiatric beds as a proportion of all hospital beds
In 1913 17.4% of all hospital beds were for psychiatric patients. This reflected the relatively low number of beds overall, and, with developments in the service, the proportion fell to 10.5% just before the Second World War. After the war, the proportion fell again because of the specific destruction of psychiatric hospitals. The percentage has gradually climbed back to around 10% and has remained at this figure. Table 3 shows the proportion of psychiatric beds to general hospital beds since 1940 (Field, 1967 and "National Economy", 1987). If "narcological" beds are included the proportions are about 30% higher, eg 12.6% for 1987.

4. This has been drawn up from the following sources: National Economy (1987), National Economy (1989), Zharikov (1983), Gorman (1969), Field (1967), Hein (1968), Hosking (1985), Hyde (1973), Lisitsin and Batygin (1978), Ryan (1982), Sigerist (1937), Wortis (1950).

Table 3: *Psychiatric beds as percentage of all hospital beds*

1913	1940	1950	1960	1980	1987
17.4%	10.5%	7%	9.3%	9.4%	9.1%

Current policies

The size of the Soviet Union inevitably means that the provision of psychiatric care is patchy, although central planning aims to ensure some uniformity in the level of services. All parts of the country have access to psychiatric care, including in-patient facilities, but in some rural areas the nearest psychiatric hospital may be many hundreds of miles away. In some of these areas there are local general hospitals which usually have psychiatric wards.

The system of care is diverse and is made up of a network of different kinds of service. Zharikov (1983) writes that the hub of the service is the dispensary, and that this facilitates continuity of care, allowing ready movement of patients between the different services, especially the transition from in-patient to out-patient. The level of treatment should be determined by the nature and severity of the disorder, and the general trend is towards treatment out of hospital whenever possible. This requires good out-patient facilities and social treatment.

The system of care can be described as a chain with a series of interconnected links. Figure 1 depicts the full chain of services in the better served parts of the country (Holland, 1975; Zharikov, 1983; Zenevich, 1986).

The telephone "hot-line" services are patchily available. They are a relatively new feature in the Soviet Union, modelled to a certain extent on the Samaritans service in Britain. They are not organized by the voluntary sector, but by psychiatrists, psychologists and psychotherapists. The "hot line" in Moscow went into operation in 1982. There is a centre which is staffed by a team of 21 psychiatrists, all working as psychotherapists, and psychologists. The centre has 24-hour cover and has 13 offices. Some of the team work by telephone, but there may also be direct referrals to the psychotherapy unit where patients can receive immediate treatment. This is generally brief, problem-oriented psychotherapy. Most of the calls are related to problems within families, generally communication problems between husbands and wives (Ogonyok, 1984).

I visited one of these centres in Leningrad in 1985. This offered a "social-psychological consultation service". The staff comprised one psychiatrist and five psychologists. There were at least two staff present at any one time. There was a phone-in service, where callers could remain anonymous if they chose to. Some problems were dealt with on the telephone, but callers were usually invited to attend the centre. Most would be offered group and individual psychotherapy. Most of the patients had family problems. About one in six patients were referred on to the psychoneurological dispensary with more difficult problems, usually more severe neurotic disorders. Another example of this kind of service is the crisis centre at the Bekhterev Institute where people can phone in with family and personal problems.

There are various types of counselling service. They may be attached to institutes, industrial enterprises or be part of a service such as the telephone service described above. Psychohygienic counselling centres are generally situated in polyclinics and are for people with "emotional problems" or those finding themselves in difficult situations (Zenevich, 1986). Psychologists rather than psychiatrists are mainly involved. The services described are relatively new in the Soviet Union and at present they are concentrated in the major conurbations. As part of the drive for preventive medicine and psychoprophylaxis, there are plans to extend similar facilities to other parts of the country.

Figure 1: *Psychiatric services in the major cities*

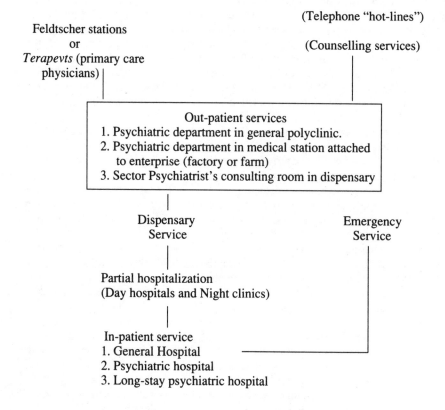

Out-patient services

Most patients with minor psychiatric disorders, especially the neurotic disorders, are seen and treated in polyclinics by primary care physicians and neuropathologists (essentially neurologists). In rural areas they will be seen by feldtshers [5]. The first point of contact with the psychiatric services is either the

5. The Feldtsher is a health worker with an extra year of training on top of the basic nursing course. They act as general auxiliaries and, in some rural areas, are essentially primary care physicians.

out-patient department in the polyclinic or the consulting room of the sector psychiatrist, usually in the dispensary. All the out-patient services are linked to the dispensary, which is responsible for a defined area, usually covering a population of 300,000-400,000 people. Thus, depending upon the size of the district (*raion*), one or more will be served by one dispensary. There are 19 psychoneurological dispensaries for the 17 districts of Moscow, and 12 dispensaries for the 22 districts of Leningrad.

The district is divided into a number of sectors which is covered by a sector psychiatrist and a group of two or three other psychiatric workers, usually two nurses, or a nurse and a nurse/social worker. There may be a feldtsher. These make up the sector team, which might be based in the dispensary, especially in urban settings where the dispensary is close to the population that it serves. In rural areas it may be attached to a hospital where there may also be a psychiatric ward.

Consulting rooms are also sited in the psychiatric departments of the polyclinics and the medical stations of enterprises such as factories, mines and farms. In addition, factories may have their own psychiatric units. Gorman (1969) described the Likhatov Motor Plant in Moscow which employed 70,000 workers. There was a psychiatric unit which carried out about 30 visits per day on workers and their families.

There is a separate system of out-patients in the general polyclinics where there are psychiatrists, psychologists, psychotherapists and neuropathologists. It is hoped that this move will improve accessibility and availability, especially to patients who are reluctant to visit a dispensary. Patients suffer from the same range of disorders as those seen in the dispensaries, but, on the whole, are less ill. In the prophylaxis department of the polyclinic there may be a psychiatrist, nurse and psychotherapist (generally a psychologist). In particular, patients with neuroses, personality disorders, various types of psychosomatic disorder are seen, as well as the organic conditions such as epilepsy. Psychotherapists do not necessarily have psychiatric training, although they are usually medically trained. Some Soviet psychiatrists are worried by this trend, arguing that poorly trained psychotherapists might miss the more serious psychiatric disorders. However, there is direct liaison between these departments and the dispensary, generally through the sector psychiatrist.

Sector psychiatrists treat the whole range of psychiatric disorders, but tend to concentrate on the severe end of the spectrum, essentially those with chronic psychotic disorders. The psychiatrist or some other member of the sector team visits patients in their own homes after discharge from hospital. One of the main aims is to try and prevent patients developing defect states. Attention is paid to living conditions and providing the basic necessities to allow someone to continue living in the community.

The psychoneurological dispensary is the main facility for the treatment of patients with psychoses and the more severe borderline disorders. Most new patients are referred there from the polyclinics or general hospitals. It is thought that the close links with the general hospitals and psychiatric hospitals enable the overall service to manage with fewer beds (Zharikov, 1983). Dispensaries must have at least five doctors. Thus, many small towns have them, but they are not found in rural areas with low density of population. In such areas the main regional hospital takes on a more important role. Most regional hospitals will have a dispensary and a department for borderline (neurotic) disorders. Psychiatrists from the hospital go out to the rural areas to see patients.

The dispensary system

Zakharyn introduced the concept of the "dispensary method" in the nineteenth century [6] The system is based on the principle that illness is the result of the interaction between the individual and the environment, thus the social context and the progression of an illness over time are critical. This accounts for the different components of the dispensary system: the provision of care for a defined population, allowing for close observation of people within a social context, the keeping of detailed medical records and long-term follow-up. Ryan (1985) argues that the practical aspects of the approach were linked to the dispensary concept in Britain and France in the nineteenth century.

The dispensary system has been used in different specialties. Kaser (1976) reported that there were 1,373 dispensaries for the treatment of tuberculosis, 722 for venereal diseases and 242 neuropsychiatric dispensaries. There were also dispensaries for the treatment of malignant disorders and several other categories, and it was planned to widen the system to cover all specialties. The throughput of patients having regular observation at the dispensaries rose to 50 million in 1982 and to 115 million for those having periodic examinations (Ryan, 1982). With the expansion of the dispensary system more community services were planned, for instance having groups of specialists (eg cardiologists, rheumatologists, gynaecologists) visiting workplaces. The practical benefits of the dispensary system are the opportunities it gives for early diagnosis, supervision of treatment and social treatment, especially the emphasis on working and living conditions. This is seen as particularly valuable in psychiatry, where it is thought possible to prevent relapse by early intervention, either in the form of drug treatment, or psychosocial measures such as practical counselling. The system also facilitates welfare services and home nursing. Prophylactic work outside the dispensary, for instance in industrial enterprises, hostels, schools, collective and state farms, tractor stations, is considered important. Dispensary records are helpful in planning services, and also for research, particularly for long-term follow-up studies. The wide availability of this kind of information goes some way to explaining the strong emphasis on long-term development and outcome in Soviet research.

The dispensary is the central point for the coordination of the psychiatric services necessary. The consulting rooms of the sector psychiatrists may be located there. There are workshop facilities which are available for inpatients at the dispensary and for day patients. In rural areas there may be a link with a farm. Patients discharged from hospital are encouraged to return to their former work, but those who are unable to do so have training for alternative employment. There are different types of social and psychological treatment, including various activities and group psychotherapy. Lauterbach (1984) reports that the facilities at the dispensaries may include the services of psychotherapists specializing in sleep disorders. There are cultural activities, including music, drama, reading. There may be "clubs" for ex-patients. The welfare work includes arranging for various

6. The actual term was probably coined by Semashko, the first "People's Commissar of Health Protection".

49

types of social assistance, help with job transfers and improvement in housing conditions. Social intervention includes trying to help settle conflicts at work or within the family. There are a number of specialist functions such as the treatment of patients with speech disorders. The services for children and adolescents are separated off from the main activities of the dispensary.

The emergency psychiatric team, which is available in many parts of the Soviet Union, might also be based at the dispensary. Larger dispensaries have an emergency service with 24-hour ambulances (Holland, 1975). The larger cities may also have a separate facility for dealing with emergencies. In Leningrad, for instance, one of the ambulance sub-stations, sub-station 13, has a team of psychiatrists and feldtshers to deal with patients who are psychotic or suicidal.

Some dispensaries have night clinics or "prophylactoria" for up to 50 patients. These represent a modified form of hospital admission. There is always a day hospital [7]. Day hospitals and night clinics treat the same type of patients as those who are admitted, including those with acute psychoses (they do not, however, handle aggressive patients). The night "prophylactoria" may be used for patients who are in full-time employment during the day but need more extensive support; they are also suitable for patients with family problems. These are more common in the specialist narcological dispensaries for alcoholics.

It is argued that the role of environmental factors in precipitating episodes illness is better understood because patients are seen at home and work. It is also possible to predict early relapses. This improves the prospects for overall rehabilitation in that family and employers are confident of observation and early treatment, thus reducing anxieties about the consequences of having someone with an acute relapse of a psychotic illness at home or in the workplace. The contact with relatives and the trade union is considered to be critical.

The proportion of patients with psychiatric disorders who are registered with dispensaries varies. Rotstein (1977) examined the populations of one rural area and four towns. Only 18.6% of those with some form of mental illness were on the dispensary lists [8]. As dispensary services have developed a higher proportion of patients, especially those with more severe forms of illness, have been registered. Recently there is a policy to remove the less severely ill from dispensary lists.

I have visited several dispensaries in Moscow and Leningrad. The dispensary in the Moscow district of Leningrad has seven LTMs (workshops), six of which are independent, with one being sited in a nearby factory. There is a separate department for children and adolescents and also a speech therapy department. It is a large dispensary with ten sector psychiatrists, each of whom has a consulting room in the dispensary. Each works with two other staff, either a nurse (*medsistior*) or a nurse/social worker (*sotsistior*). There were two psychologists,

---

7. Hein (1968) reports on the usage of places at a psychoneurological dispensary from the Ryazan oblast. On average, there were 300 places occupied every day. The breakdown was as follows:
   30 in the day hospital
   15 in the night clinics
   190 in the workshops
   50 in both day hospital and workshops
   15 in both night clinic and workshops

8. Patients with epilepsy and schizophrenia were most likely to be registered with 57.6% of epileptics and 55.% of schizophrenics registered. Of those with slow-flow (sluggish) schizophrenia only 27.8% were on the list. 6% of neurotics and psychopaths, 28% of manic-depressives, 37.5% of those with oligophrenia and 21.1% of those with organic disorders due to trauma were on the list.

two psychotherapists (also psychologists) and a physiotherapist.

A smaller Leningrad dispensary, the Oktiabraskaya, has only three sector psychiatrists. This serves a population of 127,000. The dispensary has 10 doctors overall, also 17 nurses and 14 junior "sanetari" (health workers). There is also a speech therapist, a nurse-social worker and a nurse dealing with guardianship issues. There is a 100-place day hospital with two psychiatrists, four nurses and two work instructors. In the next building, attached, is a 150-place LTM (work-therapy workshop) consisting of three workshops, staffed by two psychiatrists, three nurses and one instructor. There is a physiotherapy department and there are rooms for hypnotherapy and autogenic training. This dispensary had no psychologist, but was planning to get one. There were two in the two polyclinics with which they were associated. There are three sector psychiatrists, each with a nurse, one child psychiatrist and nurse and one adolescent psychiatrist and nurse for this population.

I sat in for several days with one of the sector psychiatrists who had a sector population of 40,000 [9]. The basic working week was Monday to Friday. The working day of seven hours was broken into five hours in the out-patient room in the dispensary followed by one or two one-hour home visits [10]. On average there are about twenty home visits per month. Every fourth Saturday she was on duty for the whole district. Occasionally on Sundays she was on the ambulance service. There was no problem with patients getting appointments and it seemed that anyone who turned up from the sector was seen more or less straight away.

The system of registration allocates patients to one of five groups on the dispensary list:

1. In-patients.
2. Acute patients and those recently discharged from hospital are supposed to be seen within three days.
3. New patients and those with frequent relapses or on maintenance treatment, also patients who had recently attempted suicide, are seen monthly, either in the dispensary or at home.
4. Patients with chronic disorders who do not relapse frequently but do not function normally are seen every three months.
5. Patients who do not need any treatment or active rehabilitation, also patients with head injury who are functioning well, are seen every six months.

The system is flexible and patients move between the categories. After a psychotic illness they normally remain in group two for one to five years and then move into group four. Patients should come off the registry when they achieve normal work capacity. Thus, patients with a reactive psychosis may come off after a year. On the whole patients with borderline disorders (neurotic and personality disorders) are not registered unless these suffer from long-standing disorders which result in an invalidity category.

Out-patients appointments in specialist Institutes are more difficult to get, and seems to be somewhat arbitrary. Patients come from other out-patient departments,

---

9. About half the patients had an organic diagnosis of dementia, trauma or epilepsy or disorders such as diencephalitis or arachnoiditis (discussed on page 191). The other half were patients with schizophrenia or depression.

10. This is rather heavy on resources in that there is a driver allocated to the job. He waits outside whilst the psychiatrist may spend an hour in the patient's flat.

even other cities and regions. One patient that I interviewed at the Bekhterev Clinic had come from Estonia because she was dissatisfied with the local treatment and had persuaded the local Professor to refer her. I tried to find out why she had been referred, wondering if she had any special connections. There were none that the responsible psychiatrist knew of. He thought that it was just because she had insisted on coming and had a high level of motivation, rather than having any connections. The psychiatrist did say these might play a part in some cases. Patients from some of the Southern republics who had influence might arrange to have treatment at specialist units in Moscow or Leningrad. The out-patient department at the Bekhterev also gives second opinions for Leningrad dispensary psychiatrists. The psychiatrist would usually come along with the patient and there would generally be a commisia of two to three academic psychiatrists with particular expertise in the field.

Futiryan (1990) describes the pattern of services in Novomoskovsk, a town of 147,000 a few hundred miles south of Moscow. He writes that it began 26 years earlier with an out-patient department that he ran in the town's polyclinic. This has developed into a dispensary, a home service (community care), a day hospital, workshops (run on profit-making lines), a preventive department (essentially a club for young people with recreational facilities but also planned discussion on drugs and alcohol) and an emergency medical team. The day hospital treats up to 400 patients a year and the average stay is 31 days. He stresses how important it was to have the cooperation of town officials and industry and stresses that the service is now part of the infrastructure of the town. He writes that it was particularly helpful that the dispensary opened in one of the "liveliest streets of the town".

Inpatient facilities

There are different inpatient facilities, but the majority of beds are in specialist psychiatric hospitals which are based at regional or district level. The optimum size for these specialist hospitals is considered to be 500-600 beds according to the Ministry of Health, and it is hoped that the large hospitals, some with more than 1000 beds, will soon be a thing of the past (Babayan, 1985). At present the average number of beds in the psychiatric hospitals is 630 (Ryan, 1983).

Other psychiatric in-patient facilities include the psychiatric wards in dispensaries and general hospitals, also the "dom-internats" (roughly the equivalent of nursing homes). Psychiatric wards are more common in general hospitals in rural areas, where the specialist psychiatric hospital may be a considerable distance from the population served. All told it seems that about 10% of psychiatric patients are in the wards attached to dispensaries or in the psychiatric wards in general hospitals.

The psychiatric hospitals are seen as being distinct from the old asylums. Babayan (1985) writes that after the revolution most of the asylums or "colonies", many of which were geared around agricultural production, were reorganized into mental hospitals for active treatment and rehabilitation. They were also reorganized along geographic lines, so that they were as near as possible to the populations that they served rather than standing as self-contained units, isolated from the rest of the community.

Despite this, to some extent because of the size of the Soviet Union but also because of a failure to implement agreed policies, there are still hospitals which are a considerable distance away from their catchment areas. In addition, some patients, especially those with chronic disorders which appear unlikely to respond to treatment and rehabilitation, are transferred from the main psychiatric hospitals to these more traditional asylums. Wing (1974) reports that there are two of these for the city of Leningrad. About 5% of psychiatric beds are in these old "long-stay" hospitals (Kaser, 1976).

There are separate in-patient facilities for adolescents, and sometimes for the elderly. In some regions there may be hospitals with specialist functions, for instance for patients with epilepsy or chronic alcoholism. There tends to be specialization within the hospitals, and most psychiatric hospitals have a department for the treatment of borderline disorders (neuroses and personality disorders). At the Bekhterev Institute in Leningrad there is a separate ward with 16 beds for this purpose. They tend to admit more difficult patients, often coming in from the region.

Psychiatric hospitals vary with regard to the facilities associated with them. Some have a day hospital and dispensary attached. There are rehabilitation services in the form of occupational therapy and workshops. There may be special workshops in local factories or other enterprises. In addition, some enterprises have outlying workshops at dispensaries and hospitals. They all have recreation areas with film projectors and libraries.

There are some hostels attached both to dispensaries and to the hospitals for patients who could otherwise be discharged but who have no family ties or no definite place of residence. The old "patronage" system is also used on rare occasions. This might be by the patients own family, another family or an agricultural establishment. This used to have a prominent place in the psychiatric services, but more recently has had only a small role in the overall pattern of care. An additional facility is the sanatorium which is a kind of nursing home. Thus the Kashenko hospital in Leningrad has a 100-bedded sanatorium outside the city. Patients only stay there for a month at a time, and each dispensary has the right to send a certain number of patients there each month (Wing, 1974).

There is strict legislation about the facilities and conditions within the hospitals. For instance, a Ministry of Health decree (Korsakoff Journal, 1988) states that there must be a range of facilities (open-door, partially open and closed). It states that all hospitals should have a workshop, library and sports hall. Patients should sleep for more than 8 hours and there must be less than 13 hours between supper and breakfast. There should be a daily bath. Diagnosis should be made within 10 days. It goes on to give procedures for complaints and the appeal and review procedures.

Holland (1977) reports on the Kashenko hospital in Moscow, a massive complex of 3,000 beds in various buildings in one set of grounds. She worked in a 100-bedded acute admission unit for women, most of whom were acutely psychotic. There were two wards with fifty patients each, one for disturbed patients and one for convalescent patients. The dormitories housed ten to twenty patients and there was one 10-bedded dorm for suicidal patients, with a nurse continuously on duty. Four psychiatrists covered the routine care of the two wards, and there were also four psychiatrists from the Institute who worked there and carried out clinical research. There was a ward round at 9am every day at which new patients were interviewed and there was discussion of admissions and transfers [11]. Other patients were seen for treatment plans and discharges. There was a twice-weekly round with the Director of the Institute (at that time Snezhnevsky) or Associate Director at which difficult cases were reviewed. In teaching settings it is typical to have a ward round or case conference once a week on the wards. One or two patients will be discussed over 2-3 hours. Once a month there will be a bigger case conference with just one patient. Ponomareff (1986) writes that the resident (ordinatura) does the full examination and this is reviewed by the chief of the service. Difficult problems go to a "grand round" with residents, the chief of service and a visiting consultant, generally a professor.

   I visited psychiatric hospitals in Moscow, Leningrad and Smolensk and spent most of my time at the largest hospital in Leningrad [12]. This served a population of two million people and was also the site of the admission wards for all adolescents from Leningrad, and all army invalids. Patients aged 15-18 are admitted to adolescent wards. Altogether there were 32 wards in the hospital with up to ninety patients in a ward [13]. I spent some time on an acute female ward which served a sector of half a million as well as covering all the cases of puerperal psychosis from the catchment area. The ward had been intended for 40 patients, but had up to 85 beds. Like all acute wards this was locked. The staff consisted of one senior doctor and two other doctors. There were 3-4 nurses on duty per shift. Patients were admitted for about two months on average, and went out on leave for progressively longer periods towards the end of the admission. The ward was divided into sections for acute patients, patients soon to be discharged and chronic patients. Apart from the necessary living functions there was a small area for working and also a room for the procedures, various drug treatments and private interviews with patients and relatives. The nurses were all female, as they were on the equivalent male ward across the corridor. The only wards with male nurses were the hospital's two wards for disturbed patients.

General hospital Psychiatry
The treatment of patients in general hospitals rather than specialist psychiatric hospitals has been considered as the next stage in the development of psychiatric services (Snezhnevsky, 1983). Zharikov (1983) writes that there is still a role for the specialist hospitals, but also argues that there is a strong case for having beds in

11. The history and mental state required were similar to the West. Relatives were always interviewed and there was emphasis on the level achieved at school and work. She reports that there was a cautious attitude to discharge, with the aim being to have patients free of symptoms. There was little on the psychodynamic aspects of the patient and almost nothing on the psychosexual. She writes: "there is reluctance and embarrassment to present and discuss psychosexual difficulties in a case history." My own experience does not bear this out in that I found psychiatrists in Moscow and Leningrad ready to discuss the sexual experiences of a patient, although, as with most Western psychiatrists, they rarely attributed aetiological significance to these.

12. Hospital Number Three in the North of the city. It had been founded in 1870. There had been 2,695 patients in the hospital at one time, but when I visited, with the effects of the new legislation, the numbers had reduced to 2,400 places. There were 100 doctors, most of whom were psychiatrists, 12 psychologists, 856 nurses and 155 sanetars. The working day for psychiatrists is 9am to 3pm, with a duty day twice a month. There are five other hospitals in Leningrad. These have smaller catchment area populations of about half a million.

13. The wards are not exactly comparable to wards in Britain in that they are often divided into different sections, for instance for acute and chronic. They are, however, covered by the same team. Adolescent wards are smaller, but still occasionally go up to 60 beds. Most specialist institutes have smaller wards. At the Bekhterev Institute the acute admission ward had 60 beds, 45 female and 15 male, all of whom are psychotic, although there are no aggressive or suicidal patients. The medical input was greater and there were 4-5 nurses on per shift.

general hospitals, mainly on the grounds that this brings services nearer to patients and also tends to reduce the stigma associated with mental illness. This is especially important in the rural areas where the psychiatric hospital is some distance away from the population. Progress, however, has been slow. Gorman (1969) reported that the Ministry of Health had planned to have more general hospital units, but that there was resistance from local health ministries. Babayan (1985) reports that the Ministry of Health requires that all general hospitals with 300 or more beds should have a psychiatric ward. There is a standard design for general hospital psychiatric departments incorporating a 60 bedded psychiatric ward. These units should concentrate on diagnosis and on the treatment of patients with organic disorders, those with neuroses, psychogenic reactions and borderline disorders. However, especially where a district has no other psychiatric facilities or the psychiatric hospital is some distance away, the department should be able to deal with fresh mental cases of "nearly all categories".

There has been more tangible progress in establishing out-patient facilities in the general hospitals and polyclinics, and there is an increasing role for psychiatry, psychology and psychotherapy. In 1975 the Ministry of Health decided that psychotherapy services in the polyclinics should be developed. It was recognized that more psychotherapists were needed and that there should be additional centres for training (Karvasarsky, 1980). As in the West, several studies have shown that a high proportion of patients attending general medical departments have psychiatric symptoms. Smulevitch et al (1985), reporting on a study carried out at Moscow Polyclinic Number 171, found that 38.4% of patients with somatic disorders had some psychiatric symptoms. They found that brief courses of treatment, pharmacological, social and psychotherapeutic, were helpful. They argued that the network of psychiatric departments in polyclinics should be expanded further.

I visited Polyclinic Number 51 in Leningrad. This served a population of 70,000 as a general polyclinic, but, in its specialist role as a rehabilitation unit for patients with brain injury (strokes and trauma), served a population of one million. There were extensive facilities for physical treatment of this group of treatment and a wide range of staff. In addition there was a psychotherapist (medically trained) and two psychologists. They had recently carried out a study on a large group of patients with brain damage. One group of patients were given the full range of physical treatments eg pool, massage, exercise, specialist activities such as the workshop or "driving bay" (simulated driving of cars or lorries). The other group has the same programme, but also psychotherapy. As might be expected, this group fared better. They also arranged a "Phoenix group" of patients from the community, both older patients and those with recent brain damage, who met every two weeks on the premises for tea and general conversation.

The narcological service
Many patients with alcohol-related problems are dealt with by the ordinary psychiatric services, but there is also a narcological service which has its own range of facilities, both in-patient and out-patient.

Special hospitals
There are nine special psychiatric hospitals for the criminally insane which were

under the administration of the Ministry of Internal Affairs but which have recently moved over to the Ministry of Health.

Services for the elderly

The pensionable age for women in the Soviet Union is 55 and for men 60. There is no distinct specialty of psychogeriatrics, although there are specialist departments in most of the main institutes [14]. Patients admitted to psychiatric hospitals may go to general wards or special wards for the elderly. Patients diagnosed as demented may return home or be admitted to dom internats which are nursing homes with full medical and nursing cover if relatives are unwilling to have them at home [15]. There are different attitudes to the elderly across the republics and regions of the Soviet Union. There is a greater role for the extended family in Central Asia and areas such as the Caucasus, and, as might be expected, relatives in rural areas are considered to be more tolerant of the elderly.

According to Medical Gazette (27.7.1988), there is a shortage of nursing-homes, with queues for places in some cities, for instance Sverdlovsk and Archangelsk. Many old people have to wait for suitable places in places with inadequate facilities. The same article, however, describes some excellent small units, for instance a 60-bedded home on Sakhalin Island. It discusses various plans such as temporary relief units and day units.

Preventive psychiatry

There is a distinction between "psychohygiene" and "psychoprophylaxis". Zharikov (1983) defines psychohygiene as the branch of general hygiene which deals with mental health and the development of personality. It aims to determine the optimum conditions which enable individuals to manifest their full potential and function in all spheres of activity. The absence of mental illness does not necessarily mean that mental health of the population is optimum, just as actual absence of disease does not mean that people are healthy. The social conditions for individuals and the collective are important. These are essentially the concepts of the World Health Organization definition of health.

Psychoprophylaxis refers to the prevention or amelioration of psychiatric illness. It is divided up in the usual way into primary, secondary and tertiary. Primary prophylaxis refers to the prevention of psychiatric illness. The aim is to lower the actual number of new cases (ie reduce the incidence). Secondary psychoprophylaxis aims to prevent acute illnesses developing into chronic forms. Tertiary psychoprophylaxis refers to the rehabilitation of patients with established chronic disorders. Secondary and tertiary prophylaxis are mainly centred in the dispensaries and workshops.

Primary prophylaxis aims to improve the general physical health of the population, and this includes measures to combat infections that might have an aetiological role in psychiatric disorder. It is also about social conditions and the

14. The Bekhterev Institute in Leningrad has a chair of psychogeriatrics and a large, well-established department. There is emphasis on rehabilitation with orientation and memory training and an attempt to keep elderly patients, even those with dementia, in work. There are various clubs for patients and relatives.

15. There are social pressures to keep relatives at home in the major cities as they bring square metres of accommodation with them. Even in Moscow and Leningrad there is a relatively small proportion of the elderly (less than 1%) in the dom-internats. There are only nine of these in Leningrad. By contrast, Gurland et al (1979) showed that 4% of old people were in residential accommodation in New York and London.

provision of facilities to promote general interests and activities. This is particularly critical during pre-school and school age.

Microsocial factors, which refers to family life and conflicts in personal relationships, are considered as important aetiological factors in borderline conditions and thus within the scope of primary prophylaxis. There has been considerable work on the psychological aspects of family life. The Western approach is criticized on the grounds that relationships are studied purely within a psychoanalytic framework and without consideration of the social context. Old age is another area which is considered in need of more psychohygienic work. Zharikov (1983) writes that this has been a neglected area, but is a pressing problem. Work needs to be done on helping people to cope with the changes brought about by retirement, the loss of a partner and children leaving home. Physical health is especially important in this age group.

Primary psychoprophylaxis involves lectures to general organisations such as *Knowledge* (something like a popular science club which takes an interest in a wide variety of topics, often related to health, psychology and sociology). There are also smaller-scale lectures to specialist groups such as teachers. Ponomareff (1986) describes an evening group for young adults with a psychiatrist and a psychologist leading the group. The group meets once a week for an hour and a half and mainly discusses relationships. There are also workers' clubs with lectures on how to improve relationships, work better and achieve personal goals.

At the dispensary in the Moscow district of Leningrad which I visited there seemed to be a strong emphasis on prophylactic work. People were referred in from nearby factories if they were considered to be under stress because of the work. Members of the dispensary team would visit the person at home and at work and try and evaluate the causes of the problem. In addition there was more general work in the form of lectures to local societies and enterprises. They also made educational material available.

The "prophylactoria" attached to mines, factories and other establishments are seen as having a beneficial effect on mental health. There are 24 day programmes during which people might work, but also have various types of treatment including exercise, heat treatment, different sorts of baths. Conditions are designed to be "stress-free" eg no slamming of doors. They are said to make almost everyone feel better and reduce absenteeism from work by 40%. There are 20 such places for every 1000 workers in mining and 15 for those working in the steel and oil industries.

Future directions

In recent years there has been an increase in the range of services to those with less severe disorders. There are, however, some concerns about this policy. An article in the Journal of Psychiatry written jointly by psychiatrists at the Ministry of Health and the Serbsky Institute argues that too many patients with less severe conditions, especially the borderline disorders are registered at the dispensaries (Churkin et al, 1987). The authors say that these "on the whole normal" people should not be registered if their links with society are intact. Moreover, patients with head injuries who have adapted well and those with schizophrenia who have had a good outcome should also be removed from the lists. They write that it is not possible to claim that the patients have been fully rehabilitated until they are off the register altogether. Registration has to be justified on social and clinical grounds, and in general only those with psychotic illnesses need to be registered. The reasons that they give are that unnecessary registration places social restrictions on some patients. A more pragmatic reason is that it also means that resources in psychiatry go into the treatment of neurotic and other borderline disorders rather than those with more serious disorders. The authors show that the number of patients with non-psychotic disorders registered with dispensaries has increased by 400% since 1968 whereas there has been relatively little change in the number of psychotic patients being registered. They claim that there is a danger that psychiatry will change from the psychiatry of psychosis to the psychiatry of borderline conditions [16].

The policies of the Central Committee for the development of the health services leading up to the year 2000 include an improvement in quality of services as much as quantity (MG 15.8.1987). There is also a strong emphasis on the drugs and alcohol services and there are plans for more services in the rural areas, with emphasis on dispensaries and community care. There is also awareness of the changing patterns of family life and the need for more nursing homes, although this is not yet a priority. Recent planning has shifted emphasis from quantity to quality. The concern is to improve standards, both in terms of the actual fabric of the buildings and also in terms of the quality of care. It is hoped to bring this about by improvements in the training of staff and in general motivation, and to this end the salaries of medical and nursing staff are being raised.

Recent changes in the Soviet Union have led to attempts at private enterprise. These have generally been in the area of counselling and psychotherapy (MG 24.2.1988). A collective in Kharkov called *Marriage and the Family*, related to a teaching institute, offers a diagnosis, psychotherapy and sex therapy service (MG 26.2.1988).

Comparative aspects

There have been two main approaches, the quantitative and the qualitative. The quantitative approach, the traditional Soviet approach, has been to quote numbers of beds, day hospitals, doctors and so on in the Soviet Union, and to contrast these to the numbers of people who do not receive adequate care in the West. The Western approach has traditionally been more qualitative, pointing out the problems and deficiencies in the Soviet health service, individual cases of hardship or injustice [17]. This section and the next chapter will attempt to steer some kind of middle course between the two approaches. The main emphasis here will be on comparing the services in the Soviet Union and the USA, essentially a comparison of a socialized versus a pluralistic service (Field, 1989).

In the USA the pattern of psychiatric care in the public sector is more easily

16. According to Medical Gazette (2.3.88), the removal of patients from the dispensary lists will be done on an experimental basis to avoid blunders. A number of regions, including Moscow, Leningrad and Latvia, have been chosen for the experiment. The plan is to reduce the list by 30%. If there are positive results after two years the measures will be applied more widely.

17. Of recent years there has perhaps been something of a reversal in these trends. Far more emphasis is being placed upon quality of services in the Soviet Union. By contrast, both in Britain and the USA, there is a shift towards a more quantitative approach, at least in evaluating the services. The so-called "performance indicators" and "diagnosis-related groups" refer mainly to numbers of admissions and out-patient appointments, lengths of stay etc.

understood in the context of the different types of funding. The three main sources of revenue are federal (central government), state and local (county or city). Each State has traditionally been responsible for providing the basic safety-net facility, the State psychiatric hospital. These are intended to provide for intermediate and long-stay patients. In addition there is variable provision of care at a more local level in the form of county hospitals which are intended to handle more acute admissions, theoretically on a short-term basis. The widest divergence is in the provision of out-patient facilities. Despite legislation and the availability of federal funding, many parts of the USA have virtually no facilities for out-patient treatment and rehabilitation. In many areas the only public provision is the state hospital, and critics claim that this is no more than a measure to ensure that the clearly insane, especially those who are a public nuisance, are dealt with.

The state hospitals have undergone major changes over the past few decades. Since the 1950s there has been a massive decrease in the number of state hospital places, largely because of deinstitutionalization. There are, however, contrasts between different states, mainly due to demographic factors. The State of New York has a total of 60,000 beds in 38 state hospitals. Five of these hospitals are in the city of New York which is made up of five boroughs, each one of which has one state hospital. Thus, one borough, the Bronx, with a population of 1,200.000 people, has a 630 bedded state hospital. In contrast, the State of Vermont is planning to manage without a state hospital by discharging patients to the care of community mental health centres and admitting to county hospitals or contracted private hospitals when necessary.

The county hospitals usually serve large catchment areas. A few of the major cities in the USA, in particular New York, have city hospitals which are roughly equivalent to the county hospitals. Many have psychiatric wards intended for the assessment and treatment of patients with acute psychiatric disorders. There are varying numbers of beds, but the average city hospital might have three wards of about 30 beds. Patients requiring long-term admission are generally transferred to the state hospitals.

There are two main types of psychiatric hospital in the private sector. The non profit-making hospitals are run as charitable institutions, although they are generally self-financing and charge for their services. Many operate restrictive admission policies, often taking only those patients with adequate private insurance. Other hospitals may be contracted to the public sector and therefore admit patients from certain geographical sectors, essentially acting as a back-up service to the county or city systems.

The profit-making hospitals are run as commercial concerns and may be subsidiaries of large enterprises. One particular chain is part of a cosmetics group. They actively compete for business and make use of various commercial techniques, including television advertising. Profit-making hospitals have been increasing in numbers steadily since 1975. According to Dorway and Schlesinger (1988), the proportion of beds in the private sector has increased from 10% in 1970 to 35% in 1986 and in the corporate profit-making sector from 1% in 1970 to 15% in 1986. These profit-making units rarely treat patients on the government back-up insurance scheme, Medicaid. In the past these units have concentrated on voluntary patients, generally those with less severe disorders, relying mainly on patients with private insurance schemes. Because clear diagnoses are required to justify payment critics have argued that the American diagnostic system, DSM-III, have been tailored to cover almost any kind of human distress. A newer trend has been to deal with troublesome adolescents and this is discussed on page 249. Psychiatrists working in the private sector admit patients directly to these hospitals which then charge the patient for board and additional services. The psychiatrist may continue to treat the patient and then will charge for each visit that he makes to the patient whilst in the hospital.

Although the concept of community care was advocated as early as 1913 by Adolf Meyer, there was no significant progress until the 1963 Community Mental Health Act legislation. This provided central funding to establish centres for treatment, rehabilitation and prevention. The aim was to serve a catchment area, offering a wide range of services near to the population and to encourage multidisciplinary work, continuity of care, consumer participation and prevention. Each centre had a catchment area population of 75,000 to 200,000 people. The 1965 Act provided federal funds to try and achieve these aims. To qualify for federal funding the centres had to provide in-patient, out-patient and "community" services and also have a 24-hour emergency service. They were also supposed to provide partial hospitalization in the form of either day or night care and were encouraged to provide aftercare and rehabilitation.

The aim of creating over 2000 Community Mental Health Centres was never achieved and at present there are about 600 centres unequally distributed across the country, many of them with no input from psychiatrists. The 1975 Public Law 94-63 meant that any qualified mental health professional could be in charge of one of the programmes. The majority have only part-time psychiatrists and are headed by psychologists or social workers. There are problems with funding so that many of the centres are too overstretched to provide adequate community services. The result is an understandable shift away from the more seriously disturbed patients and the chronically sick to a greater provision for the "worried well". Langsley (1985) writes that community psychiatry, the child of the 1960s and the "third psychiatric revolution", has suffered over recent years. Fiscal support for the community mental health centres has decreased and there is poor morale amongst the staff, with many psychiatrists leaving. The number of psychiatrists working in them since has halved since 1970.

There have been a number of attempts to compare the Soviet and American systems of care. Several accounts of the 1960s and 1970s, mainly from American psychiatrists, praised the Soviet psychiatric services (Auster, 1967; Hein, 1968; Sirotkin, 1968; Visotsky, 1968; Fuller Torrey, 1971). They comment favourably on the organization of the service, especially community care, day care, workshops, staffing levels. There was generally a rider that the conditions were fairly basic. Fuller Torrey (1971) was impressed by the ambulance service and the fact that the police are rarely involved in hospitalization. Allen (1973) compares various aspects of Soviet and American psychiatry and concludes that the advantages of Soviet psychiatry are the greater availability of care, irrespective of economic status, good staffing levels, the rehabilitation service, work treatment and day hospitals, also the emergency and preventive services. On the negative side he points out the lack of psychodynamic concepts, little psychotherapy, inflexibility and the civil liberty issues, the fact that there was no legal redress in court with regard to commitment. Holland (1975) draws up a table of comparison and concludes that the Soviet system comes out favourably in terms of the pattern of the service. Thus, there is better distribution and availability of the service and the facilities for follow-up and emergency service are also superior. The negative aspects, as she sees them, are the lack of confidentiality and the quality of the doctor-patient relationship, the relative lack of psychotherapy and the fact that there are fewer non medical or nursing professionals working in the field.

Davis (1989) maintains that there are inherent problems in a centrally planned, socialized health service. Health care may become a lower priority, compared, say, to defence. He argues that this is borne out by the relatively small proportion of the GNP spent on health in the Soviet Union in comparison to the USA [18]. Central planning may result in difficulties in predicting local needs, poor distribution, shortages and deficits. The results are crowding due to insufficient space, a lack of modern equipment and even drugs and a slow pace of development. The deficits in turn promote corruption. In recent years there has been much criticism along similar lines within the Soviet Union.

However, it can also be argued that the American system, which spends a high proportion of the GNP on health, does not meet the needs of a large section of the population, especially seriously ill, long-term psychiatric patients. It might also be argued that many of the apparent innovations in the West are either unproven psychotherapeutic methods or new "me-too" drugs rather than technical developments of real benefit to patients.

In-patient facilities
The Soviet Union has always had fewer psychiatric beds per head of population than the developed Western countries. Hein (1968) reported that in 1965 the USA had three times as many beds as the USSR. Thus, there were 0.9 beds per 1000 population in the USSR and 2.9 beds per 1000 in the USA. The differences were even more dramatic during the early to mid 1950s: at that time there were three-quarters of a million psychiatric in-patients in the USA (Katz, 1985) whereas there were about 100,000 for the larger population of the Soviet Union.

Over recent decades in-patient numbers have decreased dramatically in the USA, with the most obvious decrease being in the number state hospital places. In 1955 there were 560,000 patients in state hospitals but by 1977 this number was down to 184,000. There had, however, been an increase in beds in other sectors and in 1978 there were 301,000 psychiatric beds in all mental health facilities. What constitutes a psychiatric bed is not always clear, particularly with regard to the elderly. Thus, in 1978 there were also 425,000 beds for people with psychiatric disorders in places which would not be classed as mental health facilities. These included nursing homes with a wide range of patients, including chronic schizophrenics (Katz, 1985). Beers et al (1988) report that of the many elderly patients in nursing homes over half receive psychotropic drugs, and 26% are on neuroleptics.

The following table gives some indication of the shifts in the pattern of

18. The Soviet Union with 4.6% and Britain with 5.2% spend a lower proportion of their GNP on health than most European countries and notably than the USA at 10.8%.

institutionalization in the USA over the past four decades.

Table 4: *Patients per 1000 population within different facilities in the USA (Kramer, 1989)*

	Patients in mental institutions	Patients in homes for the aged or dependent
1950	4.06	1.96
1960	3.51	2.62
1970	2.14	4.56
1980	1.13	6.3

In the Soviet Union, the proportion of people in specialist homes for the elderly and invalids is much lower by comparison to the USA and Western Europe, although there are plans to increase this [19]. The trend in Britain has been very similar to that in the USA. According to Jones (1972) there were 3.77 in-patients per 1000 population in Britain in 1914. This dropped to 3.09 per 1000 in 1919 and the figure remained around this mark until deinstitutionalization began in the late 1950s. The proportion dropped to 2.1 in 1970 and is currently about 1.2. Thus, up until the mid 1950s there eight times as many psychiatric beds per head of population in Britain as there were in the Soviet Union, whereas the figures are now roughly comparable.

These differences are not accounted for by overall numbers of hospital beds. Over recent decades the Soviet Union has had a higher proportion of hospital beds for its population than either the UK or the USA. The latest estimate is 3.5 million beds, or 12.8 beds per 1000 population. The proportion of psychiatric beds to general beds, however, has been consistently lower in the Soviet Union than in the West. In the Soviet Union psychiatric beds have accounted for about 10% of the total number of hospital beds (Field, 1967; Hyde 1973; Ryan, 1982; National Economy, 1987), and there has been no real change in this proportion since the 1950s. By contrast, in the late 1960s, the proportion of psychiatric beds to all hospital beds was 33.1% in the USA and 49% in Britain (Hein, 1968; Hyde, 1973). Even in 1985 25% of all hospital beds in Britain were psychiatric (Abrahamson, 1988)

The graph in figure 2 shows the number of psychiatric beds over the past century in England/Wales, the USA and the USSR.

Up until the 1960s there were significant differences in the pattern of services in the West and the Soviet Union. In the West psychiatric care relied heavily upon in-patient facilities, whereas the Soviet Union had far fewer psychiatric beds and employed an extensive network of out-patient and community facilities.

With the shift to community care in the West there has been a tendency to move beds into general hospitals and to have smaller specialist hospitals. Britain, in particular, now has a high proportion of psychiatric beds located in general hospitals. There is a similar trend in the rest of Europe and in the USA, although

19. The minister responsible for the *dom-internats* or nursing-homes for the elderly and the invalids in the Russian Republic,19stated that there was a serious shortage of such places in the Russian Republic 1(MG 27.7.1988). He said that the aim of the twelfth five-year plan was to increase available places to about 50,000. This would mean a nursing home to psychiatric hospital bed ratio of 1:3 as compared to 5:1 in the USA.

progress is slower. Moreover, hospitals still tend to be larger in the USA and mainland Europe than in Britain. About one in six psychiatric hospitals has more than 1000 beds. The USA still maintains the large State hospitals, many of which also have more than a 1000 beds. Current policy in the Soviet Union is to reduce the size of the psychiatric hospitals. Over the period 1970 to 1978 the average number of beds increased from 581 to 630 (Ryan, 1982), but more recently this trend has been reversed.

Figure 2: *Psychiatric beds in England/Wales, the USA and the USSR*

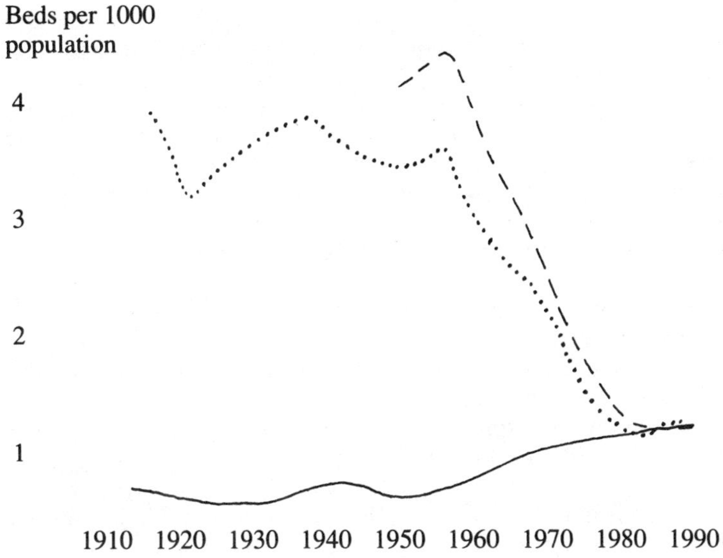

Beds per 1000
population

beds per 1000 in England and Wales
beds per 1000 in the USA (excluding nursing homes)
beds per 1000 in the USSR (excluding drugs/alcohol)

Asylums: in or out?
There are two opposing views about the asylum era, just as there are two views about the new policy of community care. Institutionalization has been described as a measure to deal with people that society wanted out of way, the "great confinement" of Foucault. However, it can also be seen as a humane attempt to provide for a group who up till that time had been neglected or ill-treated. Similarly, the move into the community can be seen as a libertarian initiative to defend patients' rights and welfare. On the other hand, it can also be seen as an economic expediency which results in a cut-price service with a callous disregard for the needs of some of the weakest members of society. Each side has had its horror stories: brutality and intimidation in the institutions; neglect in the community with patients either homeless or exploited by unscrupulous landlords, patients having to be heavily

sedated to be maintained in the community. There has also been the carers' lobby who have highlighted the burden placed upon the families of patients.

In the USA some of the patients discharged from psychiatric hospitals went to the private sector, generally to the nursing homes. Thus, Fagin (1985) reports that 19% of the 1.3 million people in nursing homes in the USA had a psychiatric disorder as their primary diagnosis. Many more had some psychiatric symptoms. Conditions in nursing homes are sometimes considerably worse than they were in the original asylums, and there is little evidence to suggest that they offer a more therapeutic environment. Linn (1985) studied a large group of patients with schizophrenia or organic brain syndromes who were randomly assigned to community nursing homes or other psychiatric wards; they found that outcome in terms of mental state and behaviour was worse in those patients who went to the nursing homes.

Another result of the policy of deinstitutionalization has been that many ex-patients have found their way into the prison system, and this issue is discussed further in chapters 12 and 13. Critics of deinstitutionalization argue that society has moved back to the pre-asylum era, where patients were essentially left to their own devices, and thus became vagrants or were dealt with by the prison system. On the other hand, it is clear that community care with adequate resources provides a good standard of care. Unfortunately, for most of the USA and Britain adequate resources are not available.

As is apparent from the above graph there have been more gradual changes in the in-patient population in the Soviet Union. Unlike the West, Russia never really had its era of "confinement", and there was no spate of asylum building over the nineteenth century and early twentieth century. After the Revolution, psychiatric care was developed outside the hospitals, although it was also thought desirable to "catch up" with the West, and a series of five- year plans aimed to increase the number of beds and build more psychiatric hospitals. Despite this, in the mid-1950s there were about eight times more beds per head of population in Britain and America than in the Soviet Union. After the drastic, rapid policies of deinstitutionalization in the West and the increase in beds in the Soviet Union the proportions became roughly comparable. At present the number of psychiatric beds per head of population in the Soviet Union is similar to Britain. It is not possible to make a direct comparison with the USA, where there are as many psychiatric patients in nursing homes as there are in psychiatric hospitals.

Table 5 shows the current position with regard to psychiatric beds.

Table 5: *Psychiatric beds per 100,000 population* [20]

USA (designated):	120
USA (all):	280
England and Wales:	120
Scotland:	319
USSR:	121
USSR (including alcohol):	165

20. From Katz (1985), Kendell (1989), Kramer (1989), National Economy (1989)

A recent development in the West is the increasing pressure from various bodies, including relatives and carers' organizations, for the retention of in-patient facilities. In many American cities the demand for beds is increasing and in some parts of New York patients are admitted directly to the state hospitals, some of which are hundreds of miles outside the city. There are plans to open more beds at these hospitals. It is possible, therefore, that after three decades of deinstitutionalization, there may be some trend towards a reversal of the policy [21]. Paradoxically, at the same time in the Soviet Union, there is a swing in the other direction. Having caught up with the West with regard to numbers of beds per population, there has been a reevaluation of policies, with renewed emphasis on community care. There are plans to reduce beds and to have more general hospital psychiatry in smaller units nearer to the populations served. Thus, just as the curves that describe the numbers of beds per population were about to meet they may start to diverge again.

Day and Community Care
It is generally agreed that Soviet psychiatry has led the way in various aspects of community care and rehabilitation. Day care has had a role in rehabilitation, but has also been considered as a real alternative to admission. In many ways this happened for pragmatic rather than theoretical reasons in that the basic infrastructure in terms of buildings was simply not there to provide what, at the time, was considered to be the proper system of care. Thus, the first day hospital for psychiatric patients was set up by Djagarov in Moscow in 1932.

In the West there were some early experiments with day clinics, for instance in Montreal and London in 1946 (Farndale, 1961). In the USA the first day clinic was opened at Yale in 1948. However, despite these early endeavours, day care played only a limited role in psychiatry until recent years. The policy of deinstitutionalization has changed this and in Britain there are now extensive day care facilities, although many fulfil a more general rehabilitation role rather than providing an alternative to admission. In the USA, the Community Mental Health Centres provide day care in certain parts of the country.

One criticism of the dispensary system is that it represents a threat to civil liberties [22]. The criticism is essentially related to the fact that records are kept and patients can be traced and followed-up. As such it represents a more general challenge to the concept of keeping medical records. The risk of abuse can be laid at the door of any system of medical records. In the West, as with the Soviet dispensary system, patients' records are kept whether or not the patient attends. In Britain, the white paper on community care, "Caring for people", suggests that tracing defaulting patients and closer follow-up of all patients will be an expected feature of good practice. There are already districts with mental health case registers, sometimes computerised (eg Fagin and Purser, 1986). Most psychiatrists would regard these as desirable, providing valuable clinical and research information. The potential for abuse lies in what is done with the data rather than

---

21. An article in the American Journal of Psychiatry might be seen as an indicator of this turning point. Bennett (1988) describes how coming into hospital helps patients with severe mental illnesses!

22. This criticism has been applied to the neuropsychiatric dispensaries rather than those dealing with oncology, tuberculosis and venereal diseases.

with the data itself. Denmark holds records on a nationwide cohort of psychiatric patients. Every patient admitted over the course of one year, 1970-1971, was kept on a register (the equivalent of the dispensary list) and information collated. A recent study (Kastrup, 1988) reported on the ten-year follow-up of this cohort [23].

Babayan (1985) writes that the dispensary system provides a chain of services, with social treatment and work therapy available at each link in the chain. The advantage of a centrally planned socialized system is that, theoretically at least, it provides a comprehensive and extensive system of care. The American system may have other advantages, but it fails to provide a basic network of care for many psychiatric patients, certainly most of those in the public sector. Essentially there is little in the way of continuous care except in those few areas with adequately funded community mental health centres. In Britain, on the other hand, patients who are within the system are often well provided for. Community psychiatric nurses now work in a similar way to the Soviet dispensary staff in doing home visits after discharge and working to prevent admissions.

Emergency services

The Soviet system for emergency admissions seems to be relatively effective. Police are rarely involved and there are fewer involuntary admissions than in the West (see chapter 12). Part of the reason for this is long-term follow-up and the relationship that develops between sector psychiatrist and patient. However, the emergency duty system and ambulance service are also important.

In the USA emergency provision for patients presenting with acute disorders is limited. Ambulance services, which are privately operated, are only used by those with insurance and may avoid patients with psychiatric problems. The police have a major role in dealing with acutely disturbed psychiatric patients. In rural America most involuntary patients are admitted directly to locked wards in the county or state hospitals. In the larger cities patients are brought to the emergency room (ER) of the city or county hospitals. Patients are brought to the ER, often by the police, and may then be admitted to the locked ward of the same hospital. Unfortunately, there are often no beds available and ERs become clogged up. There are instances of patients waiting around ERs for days, even weeks, and in New York there is a complex, bureaucratic system for trying to arrange suitable placement. Doctors have to telephone the State Office of Mental Hygiene and inform them which patients need to be admitted. Beds are then allocated in various scattered city and state hospitals. This might mean that patients are admitted to state hospitals several hundred miles away from where they live.

---

23. The nationwide cohort of 12,737 patients admitted over the year 1970-1971 was followed-up for 10 years. An interesting finding was that 7.4% of the patients became long-stay and 11% became "revolving door" (Kastrup, 1988).

Chapter Four

CONDITIONS AND STAFFING

In recent years there have been widespread criticisms within the Soviet Union of nearly all aspects of health care, psychiatry included. Criticisms range from charges of incompetence, inefficiency and corruption through to condemnation of the crowded conditions, decaying fabric and poor availability of modern equipment and drugs. Some critics maintain that the service is uniformly bad apart from the special clinics for certain groups of officials and military personnel. Ironically, however, there is also criticism of these establishments. The material conditions are generally good but the personnel, having obtained the posts through dubious means, are considered inferior.

Psychiatric facilities
Conditions in the psychiatric hospitals vary. Most are large, having about 600 beds on average. Zharikov (1983) writes that there are plans to improve the conditions in the activity areas of hospitals and also the dormitories, in particular to reduce the number of beds per ward. He hesitantly refers to the "open door" policy, which, he writes, is progressive and valuable in trying to break down the barriers and the isolation of patients from rest of society. He writes that while many hospitals have adopted such policies they cannot be extended to all.

There have been several descriptions from a comparative angle from Western visitors. Gorman (1969) writes that conditions in psychiatric hospitals vary and describes a rural hospital in Vinnitsa, 150 miles from Kiev. This was a large institution with 1,900 patients and he found that conditions were shabby and cramped, with 80-90 patients to each ward. The new director was planning to introduce smaller wards with 4 to 8 beds. Bloch and Reddaway (1977), reporting the views of ex-patients, report poor conditions in psychiatric hospitals, emphasizing the cramped accommodation and poor temperature regulation. Holland (1977), who spent eight months attached to an admission unit at the Kashenko Hospital in Moscow, describes old buildings and large, crowded wards. She condemns the lack of seclusion rooms and the limited occupational therapy and recreational space. Patients tended to sit around, taking occasional walks in an enclosed area. Visiting was restricted to a few hours a week. She says that the facilities were just adequate, basically clean and simple, but with no privacy. A recent visit by a British camera crew [1] reported that conditions in the hospital were reasonable and found that there were Orthodox and Baptist voluntary groups working on the wards which had improved morale and activity levels (Dispatches, 1989). They also reported from Kaluga hospital outside Moscow where they found pleasant conditions in the hospital work-shops with reasonable wages for the work done. The same programme was less complementary about the Leningrad Special Hospital where they found the conditions to be sparse and crowded. One patient said that there had been no difference since the hospital was transferred to the Ministry of Health in 1988. However, another patient interviewed was satisfied with the conditions. Patients interviewed in the Serbsky Institute were pleased with conditions, remarking that the staff were warm and treated you well. However, this was a comparison with the crowded Krasnodor Special Hospital where, according to the patient, the male staff treated patients "like animals".

I have spoken to a number of Soviet psychiatrists about their experiences in different hospitals. The general view is that the basic structure and furnishings are poor and conditions cramped, with too many patients per room. There is wide variation. Hospitals in the remote rural areas have the worst reputation. There tends to be much bureaucracy and too few staff to spend time with patients. Doctors may be poor quality, often not psychiatrically trained. Other staff are often ignorant and there are reports of drunkenness and brutality. Hospitals might be hundreds of miles away from the populations served. Although most Soviet psychiatrists admit that conditions in the rural areas are often worse than in the cities, they also point out that there are some newer, smaller hospitals in the rural areas which are less crowded and much pleasanter than anything found in the big cities. In a major article in "Medical Gazette" there is criticism of many of the traditional psychiatric establishments, especially with regards to their over-cautious approach and the fact that many are distant from the populations served (*MG* 2.3.88). The article maintains that the basic fabric of the buildings is often neglected, that wards are too crowded and there is a shortage of drugs. It singles out Dnieperpetrovsky psychiatric hospital [2] for praise as being well-equipped with good staff and excellent conditions. There are permanent "open-door days" for relatives and there is a positive attitude from the local population.

My own impression, based upon attachments to several hospitals and dispensaries, along with visits to specialist institutes, general hospitals, polyclinics and other facilities, is mixed. Several of the visits were arranged privately and I often found that the conditions and atmosphere in these places was better than those in the establishments that I visited more officially. This perhaps belies the view often expressed by visitors to the Soviet Union that if what they've seen is the best there is then the rest must be terrible. The reasons why some establishments and not others are shown are complex, often as much to do with the personal contacts of the person organizing the visit. Moreover, Soviet and Western doctors tend to be looking at different things. The reason why there is pride in a particular place is often not appreciated by the Western visitor, because of a different set of expectations. The lack of space is striking, with beds too close together and little room for personal possessions. There tends to be insufficient room in the rest of

1. Cohen (1989) gives a fuller description of this visit.
2. Dnieperpetrovsk is a city in the Ukraine, about two hundred miles north of the Black Sea.

the ward for adequate day activities. The situation is always worse in Winter when patients are more likely to be indoors. Leningrad's largest hospital clearly suffers from the shortage of space, and this was widely recognized by the staff there. The acute wards, which were intended for 40 patients, often had up to 90 beds. There was little going on in the ward. Some patients sat in a small work area, doing occupational therapy. In the male ward patients were sitting in the corridor and there were at least four games of chess in progress. The Bekhterev Institute has a pleasanter ambience, although conditions are still cramped. The wards are light and nicely furnished and dormitories have 6-8 beds. There is more room for general activities. There are pictures on the walls, as well as various lists, such as which patients are in particular psychotherapy groups. Again, the ward is locked. There are limited visiting hours, a couple of hours three times a week, and doctors meet relatives once a week. The door to the ward has a list of the foods and quantities which it is permitted for relatives to bring in to the patients.

In contrast to the hospitals, out-patient departments and day hospitals in the dispensaries are relatively spacious. In many cases the buildings were purpose built, so that there is enough floor space for the various activities including the work-shops. The rooms for the sector psychiatrist are generally of a good size. The ones that I saw were comfortable and personalized with pictures, books, rugs and flowers.

Soviet psychiatrists generally consider it more important to concentrate on the facilities for patients out of hospital in that it is hoped that patients are only going to be admitted for relatively short periods of time.

Comparative aspects

Although it could be argued that the basic framework of the Soviet psychiatric system is superior to that of the USA, many American psychiatrists would claim that in terms of quality American psychiatry is superior to anything found within the Soviet system. Many, especially those with psychoanalytic leanings, would make similar claims with regard to the British "socialized" system. It is certainly the case that conditions within the Soviet Union are markedly inferior to what is available in private psychiatric hospitals and clinics in the USA. In particular, the conditions in the profit-making hospitals often border on the luxurious. Ironically, these may be found in hospitals with extremely restrictive regimes, particularly the newer ones which treat troublesome adolescents. The non profit-making hospitals vary according to their location. In the inner city areas they often acquire a rather run-down feel, unlike the profit-making hospitals. The wards are generally locked.

By contrast, Soviet hospital conditions are comparable to those within the public system in the USA, although how this is evaluated is problematic. Judgements about quality and standards of care are influenced by a number of different factors. It probably depends more on what has happened there than on the colour of the walls or the number of feet between each bed. As a parent whose mentally handicapped son was treated both within the American and Soviet psychiatric systems, Davidow (1976) gives an account of his son's four years of treatment in the Kashenko Hospital in Moscow. He reports a high staff ratio and good facilities and is particularly complimentary about the caring attitude of the staff and the respect and opportunities given to patients. He compares this favourably with American system. He is particularly bitter about the abuse and neglect of the American institutions, condemning what he calls the "hellholes" of state institutions and the cheaper private establishments. He writes about the guilt felt by relatives because the only good care in the USA is very expensive.

This might be considered a highly subjective account, but it is one of the few descriptions from personal experience of the two systems. There is no doubt that conditions in many of the hospitals in the American state system are still poor, although they have improved dramatically since the early scandals which raised public awareness. Perhaps the most celebrated early account was given in "The Shame of the States" by Deutsch (1948). This was a graphic account of conditions in state hospitals. A passage reads: "In some of the wards there were scenes that rivalled the horrors of the Nazi concentration camps - hundreds of naked mental patients herded into huge, barn-like, filth-infested wards, in all degrees of deterioration, untended and untreated, stripped of every vestige of human decency, many in stages of semi-starvation." Not even the most extreme critics would suggest that such conditions are found today. Cohen (1988), however, commenting that there were 4,000 American psychiatrists in 1948 and 35,000 in 1987, writes that conditions in the psychiatric hospitals are still appalling. He reports that there is overcrowding, that hospitals are often like prisons with netting and barbed wire. Mail and telephone calls may be stopped. He also reports violence within hospitals with frequent complaints from patients of physical and sexual abuse by staff.

The state system essentially provides for most patients with severe, chronic psychiatric disorders, either from the beginning of the illness or once the insurance cover runs out. What is available depends upon the location. Some states have no public facilities apart from the state or county hospitals and psychiatric care may amount to no more than periodic or long-term admissions to state hospitals, sometimes disparagingly referred to as "warehousing". New York is one of the few cities in the USA that has something approaching a system of public health care.

I visited a number of state and city hospitals, mainly in New York. Most are large buildings with many floors. Most wards are locked and there tends to be emphasis on safety and security, for instance the double windows being covered with wire mesh. The wards are generally bare, with little in the way of furniture or personal possessions. Floors are covered with linoleum, not always clean. In some wards staff liven up the walls by putting up prints or patients' art-work. In several wards the strip fluorescent lights are on during the day because the wards are dark. There may be fifty patients per ward, although the numbers sometimes run over. Conditions are more spacious than in Soviet hospitals, with more smaller rooms, for instance with two to five beds. Most patients were milling around in their blue pyjamas and there were few activities. There were young adolescents on adult admission wards. Most of these were "conduct disorders" and it was not uncommon for children of twelve or thirteen years of age to be in such wards for up to three months, either waiting for a place in another hospital or to go home. One of the most serious gaps in the USA is the lack of separate facilities for adolescents. The problem is compounded by the fact that fear of litigation means that many young patients who have made minor parasuicidal gestures are admitted. Indeed in some American hospitals all such patients are admitted automatically, whereas in Britain the vast majority would not become in-patients.

I spent time in two city Emergency Rooms (ERs). The first was small and had a friendly but slightly chaotic atmosphere, with the staff complaining about the lack of cleaning wax for the floors and the fact that the telephone, vital for phoning around to arrange admissions, was not working properly. Many patients remained in cramped conditions for several days, sleeping on stretchers or trolleys in side cubicles. One morning there were eight patients waiting and one, who was psychotic, had been there for ten days. The larger ER that I visited was located in a seedier part of town. It often dealt with violent patients and there are always at least two security guards on duty. For much of the time there are also numbers of police waiting around, usually because they had just brought someone in. Violent patients were handcuffed to chairs bolted to the floor and were transferred to the wards or other hospitals in strait-jackets. The atmosphere was not conducive to good relationships between patients and staff and was generally combative rather than therapeutic.

My impression of conditions in British hospitals is relatively favourable by comparison, although perhaps it is not fair to compare a system in which one works with systems visited for short periods. The basic fabric of some of the older buildings is far from satisfactory and many patients still sleep in large dormitories. However, the fact that wards are generally not locked and patients are often involved in activities off the ward during the day means that one is less likely to create the atmosphere of aimless milling around which seems to be a feature of American and Soviet hospitals. There have been many criticisms of British hospitals, for instance by Cohen (1988). More extreme criticisms of conditions in psychiatric hospitals are made by various pressure groups, especially those with anti-psychiatry leanings. There are allegations of abuse and neglect and poor conditions [3].

Staffing

Psychiatrists

The number of psychiatrists in the Soviet Union has gradually increased over the course of the twentieth century. Before the revolution there were just over 400 psychiatrists, comprising 1.5% of the total number of doctors. The numbers dropped slightly over the period of the Second World War. By 1963 there were 8,600 psychiatrists out of a total of 443,300 doctors, that is about 2% of all doctors (Field, 1967). At present there are 37,300 psychiatrists in the Soviet Union [4], comprising 2.8% of all doctors, and giving a ratio of 1.3 psychiatrists per 10,000 population.

There are similar numbers of neuropathologists, who treat neurological disorders, but also some neuropsychiatric conditions such as epilepsy. They might also treat various disorders such as diencephalitis which might be considered a neurotic disorder in the West. Some general physicians do psychotherapeutic work in general hospitals and polyclinics, although this is generally only with patients

3. For example Beardshaw (1981), Healy (1983), Dalton (1983), Hospital Doctor (8.11.1984). These are discussed in more detail on page 238.
4. National Economy (1989) quotes 37,300 psychiatrists and narcologists for 1989 compared to 23,800 in 1980.

with psychosomatic disorders and minor neurotic disorders.

Gorman (1969) and Hyde (1973) review the results of the literature and various visits and commissions. In general there appear to be good staffing levels in most hospitals [5]. Although the ratio of psychiatrists to hospital patients should ensure adequate staffing levels there is evidence that there are problems in rural hospitals, mainly because of reluctance on the part of psychiatrists to work in the more remote areas of the country.

What might be considered a disadvantage of the Soviet system, by comparison to that in Britain, is that different psychiatrists are involved with in-patient and out-patient care (the same applies in the public sector in the USA). There does, however, tend to be close communication and cooperation. There is provision for good staffing levels for out-patients and day hospitals. At the sector level one doctor serves a population of about 30,000 adults.

Psychiatry is a relatively popular speciality in the Soviet Union in comparison to its status in the West. This is partly related to the fact that pay and holidays are better. There are 42 days of leave per year and every 5 years there is a period of 2-3 months of study leave.

The training of psychiatrists
There is less undergraduate teaching in psychiatry than in the West. Two weeks in a mental hospital and about a hundred hours of lectures seems to be a typical programme. Future psychiatrists first qualify as doctors at a medical school [6]. This lasts for six years including the intern year during which half the time is spent working as doctors and the rest at lectures and seminars. This is followed by two or three years in training, either at a specialist institute or at a hospital, in order to become a practising psychiatrist or *ordinatura* [7]. The next step for a psychiatrist would be to head a department, for instance to become the chief psychiatrist on a ward. Psychiatrists are eligible for a period of ongoing training once every five years. Holland (1976) criticizes the training for being heavy on organic psychiatry and psychopathology and light on psychotherapy.

The academic stream involves three years of research as an *aspirant* which leads to the defence of a dissertation for the title of *Candidate of Medical Sciences*. This may lead to a post at a university or institute, either as a *Junior Scientific Worker* or as a *dotsent*, roughly equivalent to a lecturer. A period of more intense, independent research may lead to the title of *Doctor of Medical Sciences*, usually in the late thirties. This makes one eligible for the rank of *Senior Scientific Worker*. Becoming a full Professor involves supervising a number of *aspirants* for their Candidate degrees and is usually achieved in the mid to late forties.

There has been much internal criticism of the standard of Soviet doctors, some directed at the basic quality of students and training. In an article in Pravda in July

5. The Kashenko hospital had 160 psychiatrists and 800 nurses for its 2,600 patients. Most hospitals should have a similar proportion of nurses for this number of patients. There would be fewer doctors as many of the psychiatrists at the Kashenko are from the Institute of Psychiatry.

6. Paediatrics and public health are very prominent in the Soviet health system. Of the 1,231,700 doctors in 1987 there were 151,300 paediatricians and 62,900 public health doctors (National Economy, 1987). At medical school level one may enter into a general medical school or a specialist medical school for paediatrics or public health. It is possible to become a psychiatrist after qualifying from any of these.

7. Training has improved recently. In the past it was possible to start working as an *ordinatura* in a hospital immediately after qualifying and be eligible to promotion to head of department without any specialist training.

1986, two professors of medicine called for a greater readiness to throw out incompetent students, as well as better funding, equipment and books for teaching institutions. Psychiatrists have been criticized for incompetence and unimaginative approaches to treatment, for instance the excessive use of drugs at the expense of psychotherapy (MG 12.2.1988 and 23.11.1988).

Nursing

The general training for nurses lasts for three years which includes only two or three weeks of psychiatry. There is no special psychiatric training, but this starts in a hospital post. In order to work in a dispensary nurses must first spend six months in a psychiatric hospital. My impression is that in general nurses are seen as having a relatively non-specific role, essentially subservient to doctors and involved in carrying out instructions and ensuring that the administration of a unit is in order. An article in the Soviet nursing journal (*Med Sestra*, July 1984) lays out in great detail the duties of senior nurses on psychiatric wards, to the extent of providing a sample timetable. Duties include leading the inter-shift discussion, supervision of treatment regimes and checking meals, bedding and paperwork. It also stresses that nurses should be aware of the various stages of the patients' treatment regimes in order to ensure that these are progressing satisfactorily. There are shortages of nurses in the Soviet Union, especially in the rural areas, and it is rare for there to be a full complement of nurses on a ward. Even in the major cities there may be 3-4 nurses on an admission ward with up to 90 patients.

The training of feldtshers involves the basic nursing training followed by an extra year. In rural areas, working in primary care, they treat patients with psychiatric problems.

Other disciplines

Compared to the West there are fewer non-medical or non-nursing staff involved in the care of psychiatric patients. A nurse may receive additional training and become a *sotsistior*, working in roughly the same way as a social workers but with emphasis on social rehabilitation. The main additional group of mental health workers are the industrial/ occupational supervisors who work in the special workshops in hospitals, dispensaries and special industrial sites [8]. There are also *sanitars*, who carry out general domestic duties in hospitals and dispensaries.

Until recently psychologists have not been widely employed in psychiatry [9], although specialist institutes such as the Institute of Psychiatry in Moscow and the Bekhterev Institute in Leningrad have always had a good complement.

Comparative aspects

Psychiatrists

In the Soviet Union there are 37,300 psychiatrists for a population of 282,000,000, compared to 35,000 for a population of 240 million in the USA. The proportion of psychiatrists per capita population is somewhat lower in Britain [10].

8. Wing (1974) details the staff at a dispensary in Leningrad: 27 doctors, 56 nurses and 50 "occupational supervisors".

9. Psychology is an important and popular discipline in the Soviet Union. There are probably more psychologists per head of population than in any other country in the world. Traditionally they have had only a limited role in psychiatry. They work in various fields, however, including industry, education, sports.

A number of issues make it difficult to compare the figures directly. In the USA more psychiatrists go for options such as liaison psychiatry or private out-patient work. The shift to "office" based, private psychiatry began in the 1930s and presently about half of all American psychiatrists are involved primarily in this type of work. The number of psychiatrists working with the bulk of the psychiatric patient population is considerably less proportionately than in the Soviet Union. The input in the USA is further reduced by the fact that most American psychiatrists in the public sector also do private practice. There is a marked contrast in the level of care in private hospitals and the state hospitals. Private hospitals have a high staff-patient ratio and patients are seen on a regular basis, perhaps daily, by psychiatrists. In the state hospitals there may be one psychiatrist for two large wards and patients may be seen less that once a week [11].

Private medicine has had less of an impact upon the psychiatric service in Britain (with the exception of psychotherapy). This is partly because the National Health Service was established more or less at the same time as major changes were taking in the practice of psychiatry. Developments in social psychiatry and community care were happening in the context of the newly-formed health service and tended to be incorporated into the public sector. The resources available for the public sector have been adequate, and staffing levels reasonable. Although there is a lower ratio of psychiatrists to population than in the USA, the majority of these psychiatrists work within the public sector.

Training
Mombaur (1984) compares the training of psychiatrists in several countries and is impressed with the comprehensiveness of the American training [12]. However, the divorce from medicine and, especially, neurology has meant that little neurology is taught, and, in the past, little medicine. According to Rudy (1985), it was only in 1977 that the American Board of Psychiatry and Neurology (ABPN) decided that it was necessary to have a one year internship in medicine before going into a psychiatry programme. There are still several generations of "non-medical" psychiatrists. On the other hand, the American psychiatric training is strong on psychology, especially psychodynamic psychology. During training there may be more than ten hours of psychotherapy and psychoanalysis per week along with individual psychotherapy with patients. The Soviet training is perhaps stronger on basic medicine and neurology, but there are deficiencies in the amount of general theory and psychology taught. The training schemes are far less structured, with much of the experience gained in post.

Nursing
Staffing levels for nurses in the Soviet Union do not compare favourably with most of Western Europe where one would expect 3-4 nurses per shift on a 30-bedded

---

10. In Britain there were 3,869 psychiatrists in 1985, an increase of 34% since 1976 (Abrahamson, 1988). This represents about 6% of all doctors.

11. In hospitals with medical school links there are usually a number of wards designated as teaching wards. These are much better staffed. Thus there may be 4-5 residents on one ward of 24 patients, each having about five patients each. The other wards in the hospital will have one attending psychiatrist for two wards.

12. The programmes can be so comprehensive that future psychiatrists may end up with as little as six months of general psychiatry in their training.

acute admission ward. However, the problems in the public sector in the USA are considerably worse. A ward of up to 50 patients often has only one nurse per shift and the staff complement is made up with 4-5 mental health workers. One reason why it has been possible to maintain an open-door policy on admission wards in Britain is that there have been sufficient numbers of nurses with high professional standards and abilities [13].

Other disciplines and case management
Some of the developments in the West in terms of the multi-disciplinary approach and the practice of case management have meant that assessment and even treatment may be carried out by staff without adequate psychiatric training [14]. This is particularly a feature of the community mental health centres in the USA, some of which have no psychiatric input at all. There is evidence that non-medical personnel are prescribing in the USA (Sturt and Waters, 1985) and in Britain Community Psychiatric Nurses (CPNs) are increasingly involved in making decisions about drug treatment. Although they are not legally entitled to prescribe, many of those working in primary care are called upon to give advice on drugs and dosages by general practitioners. The pharmaceutical industry has recognized this and its representatives now visit CPNs regularly with product information. Powerful psychotropic drugs are effectively being prescribed for patients, often for many years, by nurses [15].

One criticism of the Soviet system has been that it is mainly doctors and nurses who are involved in the care of psychiatric patients. The Soviet response is generally that this is appropriate and that it is necessary to have proper medical or nursing training to treat mental illness. Soviet psychiatrists argue that patients should be seen by doctors and criticize the lack of proper medical care for some patients in the West, giving this as another example of the mentally ill getting a poor deal in comparison to other groups of patients.

---

13. Both Soviet and American psychiatrists tend to express surprise that it is possible to manage acute admission wards without locked doors. They tend to attribute it to the nature of society and issues of litigation.

14. In the ER I saw a trainee social worker do an assessment on a depressed patient. He then presented his findings to the attending psychiatrist, along with his view that this was a "biological depression" and that the patient should be admitted. A compulsory admission was then arranged.

15. This also happens in some new patients. I have seen a young patient with manic-depression who was admitted to hospital with severe extra-pyramidal side-effects after having been given 100mgm of Modecate one day and 400mgm of haloperidol, much of it intravenously, on the next by a general practitioner on the advice of a CPN.

Chapter Five

AETIOLOGICAL THEORIES

As might be expected from the Soviet concept of disease, it is assumed that psychiatric disorders have a multifactorial aetiology and that there is an interaction of biological and psychosocial aetiological factors. The fact that there is a neural substrate for the psychiatric disorders, including the neuroses, does not imply that there is always a "biological" cause. Psychosocial factors such as distressing life events or interpersonal conflicts influence the course of a disorder, but do so by affecting the brain. They act upon the neural substrate, directly influencing the function of the higher nervous system, also affecting endocrine function, the autonomic nervous system and the immune system.

There has been more emphasis on the biological basis for psychiatric disorders for a number of reasons, including a reaction to what was described as Western trends in "psychogenesis" during the middle decades of the twentieth century. However, biological theories have tended to play down the role of genetic factors until recent years. The resistance to genetic theories was not simply due to Marxist ideology but has to be understood in the context of historical events. The relationship between psychiatry and genetics has been uneasy, partly because of the eugenics movement. Babayan (1985) criticizes what he calls "eugenic illusions" and writes that in the Soviet Union there was a short-lived eugenics movement in the immediate post-revolutionary years but that this soon proved erroneous and disbanded. He claims that in the past in other parts of the world the movement went astray. He writes that in the USA laws were passed for the compulsory sterilization of "hereditarily ill persons and criminals" and that in Nazi Germany it led to the notorious "racial hygiene" system [1].

In place of heredity theories there has been considerable interest in physical environmental factors, especially during the intra-uterine and peri-natal periods. There is a large body of literature about the role of birth trauma and of various infectious, inflammatory and auto-immune processes of the nervous system. Manifestations of this include the fact that mild, compensated forms of hydrocephalus are diagnosed much more than in the West, especially in child psychiatry. At the other end of the life-span the effects of the early stages of arteriosclerosis and of hypertension on the brain are more widely recognized than

1. The Nazi law of July 14 1933 called for the compulsory sterilization of schizophrenics as part of the campaign to wipe out hereditary diseases.

in the West.

Snezhnevsky (1983 and 1985) writes that in psychiatry it is particularly difficult to establish links between cause and effect, stressing the importance of multifactorial aetiology. He writes: "The origin of illness, including mental illness, as well as the development, course and outcome depend on the interaction between the causes (aetiological agents), various harmful influences in the environment and the condition of the organism. It is a combination of outer (exogenous) and inner (endogenous) factors." He makes the point that endogenous factors should not be taken to refer only to the genetic predisposition but should include various properties such as immune status and brain damage resulting from past events. Clearly there is a balance between the relative influence of endogenous and exogenous factors and this varies with the individual and the disorder. He argues that a particular aetiological factor only results in illness if there is a confluence of a particular set of circumstances. Thus, an infectious agent must be considered in the context of the host organism and related factors, which might be psychosocial. Similarly, a life event provokes a reactive disorder in the context of the biological vulnerability of the host. He argues that even in the infectious psychoses there are often significant endogenous features. This is in contrast to the views of the traditional "Leningrad" school which held that there were specific noxious agents causing particular psychoses. Snezhnevsky's criticism of this concept is sometimes misinterpreted as him saying that "everything is schizophrenia."

The role of heredity

As discussed above, the genetic aspects of mental illness have been relatively neglected in the Soviet Union and there has been little research in the area. The relationship between heredity and environmental factors is considered unclear. Despite this, the role of genetic factors is recognized, and Vartanian (1983) writes that the clear role of genetic factors is one of the arguments for the biological nature of the endogenous psychoses. The Western twin studies and adoption studies are quoted widely, partly because few such studies have been carried out in the Soviet Union. He suggests the following figures as a summary of the concordance rates in monozygotic (MZ) and dizygotic (DZ) twins for schizophrenia, manic-depression and epilepsy.

	schizophrenia	manic-depression	epilepsy
MZ	44	56	48
DZ	13	16	10

There is an attempt to quantify the actual variance that is accounted for by genetic factors by a process referred to as "genetic-correlation analysis". This appears to suggest that the index for heritability for endogenous psychoses varies between 50 and 74 percent. Figure 3 shows the coefficients of heritability and of "genetic correlation".

Figure 3: *Coefficients of heritability (N) and "genetic correlation" (g) in the endogenous psychoses.*

Diagnosis	C S	E-P S	R S	MDP
C S	N = 50%	g = 0.40	g = 0.13	g = 0.0
E-P S		N = 74%	g = 0.31	g = 0.27
R S			N = 56%	g = 0.78
MDP				N = 61%

(CS= continuous schizophrenia, E-PS= episodic-progressive schizophrenia, RS= recurrent schizophrenia, MDP= manic-depressive psychosis)

The coefficient of heritability indicates the contribution of environmental factors. Thus, if the coefficient of heritability is 50% for continuous schizophrenia that leaves 50% of the variance to be accounted for by environmental effects. The figure also indicates that recurrent schizophrenia is nearer to manic-depressive psychosis (with a coefficient of genetic correlation of 0.78) than it is to continuous schizophrenia (with a coefficient of genetic correlation of 0.13). This is said to pose a nosological problem in that recurrent schizophrenia and manic-depression have a similar genotype but differ clinically. It is therefore argued that it is better to think of this group as a "nosological class" of illness. It is argued that this view is supported by various psychopharmacological studies, for instance the finding that lithium is effective in the prophylaxis of recurrent schizophrenia, but not of the episodic-progressive form (Minsker et al 1977). Similarly, it is noteworthy that there is often some immediate environmental provoking factor in recurrent schizophrenia and manic-depression, but not in the continuous form. That said, however, the interaction of hereditary and environmental factors is stressed in all these disorders. The microsocial environment - family and interpersonal relationships in early childhood, upbringing and individual experiences - are important (Vartanian, 1983). This is especially so because intervention may help in preventing onset of illness.

Although molecular biology is now one of the major areas of psychiatric research in the West there appears to be little work in this field in the Soviet Union. This is partly related to the limited level of technology, but also reflects the fact that genetics still has a relatively low priority. There seems to be something of a wait and see attitude. Although some Soviet psychiatrists are hopeful that this approach will establish clear-cut disease entities, most appear to hold the view that the studies will eventually confirm their position: that there are no clear-cut genetic causes. It is thought that advances in molecular biology will establish the role of environmental factors, and demonstrate that what is inherited is a vulnerability to develop a wide range of different disorders.

Environmental factors
Environmental factors include those in the physical environment as well as psychosocial factors and one of the major differences in approach between Soviet and Western psychiatry has been the relative emphasis on physical factors. A body of research has accumulated on the aetiological significance of trauma and various toxic and infectious agents. The findings will be discussed in more detail below in the sections on the aetiology of schizophrenia and the neuroses. According to Sternberg (1983), over 20% of the dispensary population who are over the age of 60 have psychiatric disorders due to arteriosclerosis, hypertension or other vascular causes. These may present as psychotic disorders, but also with neurosis-like, psychopathic-like and affective symptoms. The clinical picture is often polymorphic and shifting, generally showing mild features, notably sleep disturbance, and moving on to one of two main syndromes: vascular dementia or the vascular psychoses.

One result of the emphasis on external agents and organic pathology is that there are fewer diagnoses of neurosis and affective disorder, especially in patients with a late onset of symptoms. Some younger patients who would be considered neurotic or depressed in the West might also receive a diagnosis of encephalitis, diencephalitis, arachnoiditis or vegetative disorder. These disorders, generally thought to have an infectious aetiology, are discussed in chapter 10. It is recognized that psychosocial factors may be important in these "organic" disorders, presumably by affecting the immune response.

Psychosocial factors are discussed in greater detail in the section on the aetiology of the neuroses in chapter 10. Personality is generally included and this can be understood in terms of the broader concept of personality which comprises a person's system of relationships with the outside world. The social component of personality, the "ensemble of social relationships", means that personality changes over time and responds to changes in the environment. The interaction between personality and life events is illustrated in the study of Dragunskaya (1987) who investigated personality structure in patients with MDP using a semi-standardized psychological interview. She reports problems in several areas, but the striking ones were motivation and rigidity. She writes that this particular personality constellation would mean that any demanding life changes could be pathogenetic in that they require effort and adapting to the change. Psychotherapy should therefore be geared towards helping the patient cope with life's difficulties and will involve improving motivation and the patient's attitude to changes in his life.

The influence of early environment
Traditionally Soviet psychiatry has placed less emphasis on the importance of the early psychosocial environment as compared to early physical environment. There are a number of theoretical reasons for this: the dialectical materialist concept of mind, the concept of personality, resistance to the ideas of psychoanalysis, the influential ideas of Makarenko on the effects of the social environment on deprived orphans.

This has also applied to Soviet psychotherapy. Pathogenetic psychotherapy, based on Miasishchev's psychology of *otnoshenia* (a word which implies both attitudes and relationships) is not particularly concerned with the impact of early upbringing and childhood separations [2]. On the other hand, Lichko (1977) argues that early childhood is critical for the formation of important attitudes towards family and towards other people. The early school period will determine attitudes to work and also the sense of duty and responsibility towards society. The pubertal period will determine sexual attitudes. Soviet psychology and psychiatry now put more emphasis on the significance of early psychosocial environment and is integrating this into the concepts of development and personality.

Social factors and "life events"
Social factors are considered important in the aetiology of psychiatric disorders, especially the borderline conditions. Indeed it used to be said that these social factors were responsible for the high rates of psychiatric disorder in the West. There has been little work on the influence of social factors within the Soviet Union, although education-related problems and job satisfaction have been examined. On the other hand there is a fair amount of work on life events and these are recognized as often being due to social pressures. The term psychotraumatic factor is generally used in the Soviet literature. Smulevitch (1983) writes that psychotraumatic factors which are of aetiological significance are rarely sudden, severe mental traumas such the death of someone important or a situation of extreme danger. They tend to consist of prolonged periods of emotional tension which produce inner conflicts. They are often situations which create uncertainty about the future or require decisions to be made. Frustration is also important. He quotes situations such as dislike of job and not being able to get divorced because of the children.

Psychotraumatic factors are thought to be of importance in the borderline conditions (neuroses and personality disorders) and to have less importance for the endogenous psychoses, despite the general emphasis on multifactorial aetiology. Vishnevsky (1984 and 1988) investigated the aetiological significance of life events in a prospective study of 48 women who had children with infantile cerebral palsy. This is regarded as an "objectively unsolvable psychogenetically traumatizing situation". In an 8 year follow-up he demonstrated the shift from depressive reactions (acute, labile affect) to depressive neurosis to a depressive personality development (a monotonous affect, reduced mental activity and hope). Anxious-dysthymic traits, vegetative dysfunction and psychosomatic diseases developed. There were two variants, depending on the premorbid personality traits of introversion or extroversion.

Aetiological mechanisms
Infectious agents and immune function
There has been much interest in the role of infectious agents (especially viruses), immune function and auto-immunity in psychiatric illness. This is discussed in more detail in Chapter 8. Auto-immune processes are postulated as aetiological mechanisms in a number of disorders. It is suggested that altered cell antigens, possibly proteins from brain tissues, provoke the production of autoantibodies which have a destructive influence on normal neurones. There are many reports of changes

---

2. This is not to say that the theory of *otnoshenia* ignores the importance of early experiences. Miasishchev is quoted as saying: "In human beings as distinct from animals the role of traces of past experience is so great that reactions depend much less on the immediate stimulation that on the relevant experiences in the past; indeed, the effect of stimulation depends mainly on one's attitude as determined by the past . . ." (Winn, 1962).

80

in immune function in patients with schizophrenia and, to a lesser extent, epilepsy and other disorders. It is argued that a more general process such as auto-immunity can better explain the global nature of the deficits in a disorder like schizophrenia than isolated biochemical or receptor abnormalities.

Biochemical theories

The Soviet literature contains studies on neurotransmitter and receptor function. The dopamine hypothesis of schizophrenia and the amine hypotheses of depression are widely quoted. There is some Soviet work on enzymes, for instance creatine phosphokinase. This is linked to the study of membrane permeability which is considered significant in the endogenous psychoses. Increased levels of enzymes reflect increased membrane permeability due to cell damage. This is thought of as a non-specific process and fits in with the viral and immune hypotheses.

Neurophysiology

The main aetiological theories in the 1950s and 1960s were based on Pavlovian neuropsychology, and there is still considerable emphasis on neurophysiological research. From this perspective, psychiatric disorders, either psychoses or neuroses, are the result of faulty sets of conditioned reflexes. These are due to environmental influences on the organism. These might be physical agents or psychosocial factors, but the basic typology of the nervous system is also important. It was thought that if one could eliminate the noxious environmental factors, whether these were physical or psychosocial, the conditioned reflexes could be modified. This is complicated by the fact that there are also thought to be secondary processes which are due to the organism's adaptive responses.

Comparative aspects

It might be argued that the differences between Soviet and Western aetiological theories are more a matter of emphasis than any fundamental difference in approach. It is certainly the case that there might be bigger disagreements about aetiology between psychiatrists within the Soviet Union or within the USA than there would be between some Soviet and Western psychiatrists. That said, however, a number of trends do emerge, as one would expect from the different concepts of mental illness. For a number of reasons, early upbringing is seen as less important by Soviet psychiatrists. The role of social factors is given similar weight in Britain and the USSR. By contrast, these are virtually ignored in the USA where there tends to be a split between the biological theories and the psychological, often psychoanalytic, theories of aetiology. An important difference between the Soviet Union and the West is the greater emphasis on physical environmental factors such as trauma and viral infection and the body's response to these.

The issue of multifactorial aetiology provides another contrast between the Western and Soviet approaches to aetiology. There is a tendency in the West to consider that something is either organic or psychological. Thus, the psychoses are seen as organic, which generally implies a genetically determined biochemical disorder, whereas the neuroses are seen as "psychological" or to do with "problems of living". The Soviet position is theoretically more holistic in that it assumes a biological process which is influenced by psychosocial factors.

Chapter Six

ASPECTS OF TREATMENT

This chapter will outline some of the principles of treatment in the Soviet Union and then describe a number of specific forms of treatment [1]. There is further discussion in the chapters on the various disorders.

Most Soviet authors stress the importance of combining biological, social and psychological aspects in any one patient. In theory few patients would receive only drugs or only psychotherapy. It is recognized, however, that one might sometimes use drug treatment alone for pragmatic reasons, for instance because of the difficulty in getting the right psychotherapeutic help. Smulevitch (1983) writes that social treatment is important in all patients, irrespective of diagnosis, and helps to reduce the amount of time spent in hospital. Avrutsky and Neduva (1981) write that the progress in psychopharmacology over the previous decades has been the real turning-point for psychiatry, changing it from a descriptive to a therapeutic discipline, but that social-rehabilitation measures are of equal importance in the treatment of all psychiatric disorders.

General principles of drug treatment

Avrutsky and Neduva (1981) write that safety is of prime importance in any regime of drug treatment and that the first consideration should be to do no additional harm. It is considered important that doctors should be familiar with all the effects of any drug that they prescribe, both the beneficial and the harmful effects and there is a relatively large section on side-effects in the Handbook (Smulevitch, 1983).

Emphasis is laid on knowing the wide range of actions of each drug along with its spectrum of psychotropic activity. It is argued that drugs from the same group have common effects, but that each one has its own selective actions, for instance with regard to their being stimulatory or inhibitory. The drug profile is critical in targeting particular syndromes. Vovin (1986) makes the point that psychotropics have short-term and long-term effects. Short-term effects, those appearing over hours up to several days, tend to be thymoleptic, stimulating, sedative, stabilizing. Long-term effects tend to be those which have direct influence on the course of the

1. The main sources are: Karvasarsky (1980), Avrutsky and Neduva (1981), Smulevitch (1983), Bacherikov et al (1989) and Voronkov et al (1990). The texts vary in their orientation. The "Manual for psychiatrists" (Voronkov et al, 1990) is closest to the Western approach with regard to drug use. A more comprehensive list of drugs is given in the Soviet pharmacopoeia, "Medical Preparations" (1985).

disorder. The indirect effects of a drug are that they facilitate the restructuring of the personality by reducing the severity of symptoms.

It is helpful to be clear about the distinction between form and syndromal presentation to appreciate the Soviet view on the efficacy of psychotropics. According to Smulevitch and Panteleeva (1983) psychotropics not only affect the syndromal presentation, but influence the course of the disorder by "enhancing favourable trends in the development of the pathological process." They do not, however, think that they change the basic stereotype of the course, that is the way in which the pathological process progresses. The view, essentially, is that the psychotropics influence symptoms rather than the basic pathological process. They treat acute episodes and facilitate rehabilitation.

The dynamic principles of treatment are emphasized in that drugs and dosages should be modified as the disorder progresses. The treatment should change with the changing clinical picture, both those related to the disorder and the drug-induced changes. Changes in psychosocial factors may also require changes in prescribing. They also stress the interrelationship between the biological and psychosocial, making the point that a drug also has an important psychotherapeutic effect ie the placebo effect.

Avrutsky and Neduva (1981) make the point that it is important to be aware of drug-induced mental states (in that psychotropic drugs affect mental function). The drug itself produces a clinical picture, with its own course and syndromal presentation, and this interacts with the endogenous clinical picture. The drug creates new "symptoms", hopefully a favourable modification of the existing ones.

Early treatment

Soviet psychiatrists believe that early intervention and treatment are effective. This applies particularly in schizophrenia where there is progressive personality disintegration. It is thought that early treatment facilitates adaptive processes by developing healthy "lacunae" in the personality at the expense of pathological processes. The result is that there tends to be a more intense approach to treatment, especially in the early stages of an illness, often with longer admissions than considered necessary in the West. The same applies to out-patient treatment. A day hospital, for instance, might have a daily period in which some patients receive intravenous neuroleptics and then have a quiet period of two or three hours in a side ward where they rest or sleep before resuming their activities. This generally continues for several weeks, after which they would move on to oral preparations. Vovin (1986) writes that a recent trend for the early stages of treatment is "rapid neuroleptizaton", often with intravenous drugs, and that this approach removes symptoms faster than traditional approach.

It is claimed that this early intervention disrupts the pathological process and leads to quicker resolution of symptoms, longer periods of remission with less severe defect states. There is only anecdotal evidence for this. My impression from a spell at a day hospital was that patients with severe psychotic symptoms did make a relatively rapid symptomatic response, and that they were able to move on to the rehabilitation stage quickly. In general this would involve the workshop attached to the day hospital. Defect states in general also seem to be less severe, although this might be a function of the more contained environment that the patients were in. Unfortunately there is as yet no convincing evidence, in the West or the Soviet Union, that early intervention and treatment changes the eventual outcome of the serious psychiatric disorders.

Theoretical aspects
Soviet and Western approaches to drug treatment appear to be similar because psychotropic drugs are often used in the same sort of way. There is, however, a different theoretical underpinning, and the use of neuroleptics does not mean that the dopamine hypothesis of schizophrenia is accepted. Infectious, inflammatory and immune processes are considered more significant than changes in neurotransmitters and the literature contains many references to the immunomodulatory properties of the neuroleptics. For instance, Mikolaisky (1988) reports on correlations between clinical state, immune status and the efficacy of treatment in a group of schizophrenic patients. The measures included various non-specific parameters such as antibody levels, complement activity and the Mantoux. There were also measures of "neuroallergy" and neuroauto-immunity, including brain auto-antibodies. Inflammatory processes are thought to damage the cell membrane permeability, one manifestation of which is increased lipid peroxidation. One approach to treatment, therefore, is to limit this damage and lithium is said to normalize cell permeability and reduce lipid peroxidation. Other preparations, for instance vitamin E, are also thought to have the same effect. Other theory-bound treatments arise from the greater emphasis on vascular disorders, leading to the idea of treatment with hyperbaric oxygen and the organic, "toxic" theories leading to the detoxification treatments.

Drugs in use

Neuroleptics
The range of neuroleptics is similar to that used in the West. Chlorpromazine is described as being more sedative, and trifluoperazine and haloperidol as having greater anti-psychotic properties, being useful in resistant paranoid states. Majeptil (thioproperazine), a phenothiazine with a similar profile to chlorpromazine, but less sedating, is also widely used. Neuleptil (pericyazine), a phenothiazine in the same group as thioridazine, is thought to be useful in psychopathic and psychopathic-like states when there is no defect state. It has mild anti-psychotic properties, but is most useful in aggressive, disturbed behaviour and is acceptable as it is not too sedating. Teralen (trimeprazine), a phenothiazine related to promethazine with anti-histaminic and mild anti-psychotic properties, is considered useful in a range of neurotic disorders, particularly when there are obsessional or phobic features, also in psychosomatic disorders and syndromes such as hypochondriacal-senesthopathic disorders. Depot neuroleptics, most commonly fluphenazine, are used, but less widely than in the West.

Clozapine (leponex) is considered to be a useful neuroleptic, particularly in cases where other drugs are ineffective, and was used in the Soviet Union over the years in which it was unavailable in many Western countries. Doses of 400-600mgm per day would be used. It is considered useful in schizophrenia, but also severe depression-depersonalization syndromes (Nuller and Mikhalenko, 1988). In severe forms, for instance febrile schizophrenia, it is considered invaluable.

Tranquillizers
Smulevitch (1983) gives a table showing the efficacy of a range of tranquillisers in different syndromes. They appear to be most effective in the following syndromes: asthenic-vegetative (similar to neurotic depression) , obsessional-phobic (similar to phobic disorder) and hysterical syndromes. They are least effective in anxiety and obsessional states. Lorazepam seems to be the most effective across the range of disorders with diazepam slightly less so, but better than lorazepam in the asthenic-vegetative and hysterical syndromes. Fenazepam is a benzodiazepine with a more pronounced and longer-lasting effect than diazepam. It is said to have a powerful therapeutic effect in a wide range of neurotic, neurotic-like and psychopathic-like disorders. It may be used in severe obsessional disorders which do not respond to other measures.

Mebicar is a Soviet preparation, a bicyclic biocarbamide, a group of drugs with a wide range of psychotropic properties. Mebicar itself is a tranquilliser, mainly affecting subjective anxiety and without peripheral effects or sedation (Yenikeyev et al, 1989). It can be used in a range of neurotic and neurosis-like disorders, also in some psychoses and organic disorders as an adjunct to neuroleptic treatment. It is said to improve concentration and memory.

Raevsky (1985) reports on the use of sodium valproate, in anxiety. He argues that its GABA-ergic properties give it useful tranquillising properties in various neurotic and neurotic-like disorders. There is not the sedation or ataxia found with the benzodiazepines. Older tranquillisers are still in occasional use, for instance valerian and the bromides in the neurotic-like disorders (Zaviliankskaya, 1987)

Antidepressants
There is a similar range of drugs to those used in the West with amitriptyline and imipramine being commonly used. These drugs are also used for persistent anxiety, when the anxiety/fear is not a brief stress reaction. The Soviet tricyclic antidepressant, azafen (pipofezine), is reported in Medical Preparations (1985) to be thymoleptic and sedative, and to have few anticholinergic effects. It is considered to be a useful stimulant antidepressant, and may be used when there is an asthenic picture. It is more suitable for mild to moderate depression and in more severe cases should be used in combination with other tricyclics. The tetracyclic inkasan (metralindole) is also thymoleptic and stimulating, thought to be most useful in depression with mainly adynamic (anergic) syndromal presentation. There is also an atypical Soviet tetracyclic, piradizol (pirlindole). Nuredal (nialamide) is the only monoamine oxidase inhibitor (MAOI) listed in "Medical Preparations".

Lithium is widely used and carbemazepine has been in use in manic-depression for some time, indeed before this role was widely recognized in the West. It is also recognized as a treatment for schizophrenia. Vovin (1987) records five years experience in using carbemazepine on 73 patients with endogenous psychoses. He reports a beneficial effect in 83% with complete loss of all phasic course in 28%. The results were markedly better in schizophrenia than affective disorders. A range of drugs, including the neuroleptics and benzodiazepines, are used in addition to antidepressant drugs.

Nootropes

These drugs stimulate the metabolism of the nerve cells and have a direct, positive effect on mental function, improving memory and perception. The main indication for their use is when there is evidence of "mental insufficiency". They are thought to be useful in asthenic, adynamic, depression and the vegetative syndromes. Thus they may be part of the treatment of endogenous psychoses or the borderline conditions, often in combination with psychotropics. They may, for instance, improve intellectual function in schizophrenics with defect states. They are also thought to help with the general exhaustion, lack of drive and motivation of late stages of chronic alcoholism. An interesting, potentially important use for the nootropes is in the condition febrile catatonia, when it is given intravenously.

Their main use is in organic disorders, where there are reversible changes in consciousness: infection, toxic states and cardiovascular disorders, but they are not helpful in dementia. They may be used to stimulate mental activity in children with degrees of mental retardation. The main drugs are pirasetam (nootropil) and atsefen (meclofenoxate hydrochloride). Other drugs with metabolic activity, classed with the nootropes, include aminalon (GABA) and sodium oxybate. Aminolon has been tried in patients with dementia, but there is no clear evidence of its efficacy. Piriditol, a nootrope with some antidepressant and sedative properties, is thought particularly useful in the elderly.

They are considered to be useful in patients with asthenic and adynamic syndromes. However, because of limited availability, they are often used only in patients with organic disorders such as trauma and diencephalitis.

Psychostimulants

These include the amphetamine-like substances and are said to increase the level of vigilance and stimulate intellectual activity. They are thought to be useful in a number of syndromes: asthenia, astheno-depression, apathic and adynamic states. They are less used than the nootropes and there are doubts about the duration of effect and the long-term consequences. Sidnocarb (mesocarb) is the only one in general usage, because, unlike the amphetamine-like substances, there is a gradual therapeutic effect and it does not produce motor excitement or euphoria. It has a different chemical structure and different pharmacological properties to the amphetamines and is thought to have a specific stimulant effect in the neurosis-like disorders. Hypochondriacal syndromes and alcoholism are other possible indications. Because of the stimulant effect, possibly some antidepressant effect and, theoretically, lack of dependence, it is a popular drug.

Vitamins

Vitamins are widely used in Soviet psychiatry, not just in alcohol-related disorders. Many patients with borderline conditions and neurosis-like disorders, as well as those with the organic disorders, are put on vitamin preparations. Korkina (1989), from the Patrice Lumumba Medical School, reports on the treatment of patients with anorexia nervosa with carnitine and cobamamide (a form of B12). Compared to control patients who had no vitamins they report weight gain, improvement in fatigue and increase in the cerebral mass, with increase in the thickness of the neocortical layer.

Hormones
Vovin and Aksenova (1982) report on the use of various hormone preparations in the endogenous psychoses, especially affective disorders. A paper from Kiev by Sinitsky et al (1988) attempts to show a relationship between changes in mood and changes in the neurohumoural system. There is an attempt to treat different depressive profiles with antidepressants combined with various biologically active substances, for instance T4, T3, insulin, vasopressin, somatotrophin and sodium succinate. The actual treatment depends upon the clinical picture, which is analyzed in detail, but also on the EEG findings and various indices such as catecholamines and serotonin metabolites, thyroid function, electrolytes. The exact rationale for using the different combinations was not clear from the paper. Other papers in the literature also report on different indications for various preparations, including the use of intranasal oxytocin in acute reactive depression.

Immunomodulation
The immunomodulator levamizole has been used to stimulate immune function in patients with schizophrenia. It has been shown that in vitro it improved the phagocytic properties of lymphocytes of schizophrenic patients (Vetlugina et al, 1989). It is reported as being useful in some patients with schizophrenia, but not improving the symptoms in the most severe form, juvenile malignant progressive schizophrenia (Mikheeva et al, 1987). Sekirina et al (1988) report that as an adjunct to neuroleptics levamisole normalized immune parameters and improved clinical state in young patients with slow-flow schizophrenia, especially those with depressive-asthenic features. They used doses of 150mgm of levamisole twice a week over a period of six weeks. Semenov et al (1988) from the Ministry of Health Research Institute in Moscow report on the use of levamisole in treatment-resistant schizophrenics. They report an improvement in symptoms, both productive (positive) symptoms and those of the defect state and also improvement in extrapyramidal side-effects. Various immunological parameters improved, and they consider the changes in humoral immunity to be significant. In about a quarter of the patients who had serum antibrain antibodies [2] these disappeared after treatment. There was an increase in the number of T-cells, which were low in absolute numbers and also as a percentage of total white cells. In about a third of patients there was some worsening of symptoms after 2-3 weeks, but this reversed spontaneously after 3-5 days.

Two substances are mentioned by Zavilianskaya (1987) for their immunostimulant properties as being useful in the treatment of neurosis-like disorders are splenin, an extract of cattle spleens, and proper-mil, a yeast preparation. They are listed in Medical Preparations (1985) under "general biogenic preparations" and proper-mil is mentioned as having been used in the treatment of multiple sclerosis. A substance which is thought to be promising is timalin, a bioregulator which is obtained from the thymus gland of calves and has now been isolated and manufactured (Druzhinina, 1989). The active component, a

2. These antibodies were present in 74% patients with schizophrenia and 4-12% normals.

polypeptide, activates the thymus and stimulates immune function. It is thought that it might slow down the ageing process, having been shown to increase the life expectancy of some laboratory animals by one third. It also reduces mortality rates in birds with infections. Other "bioregulators" have been isolated from various organs and are currently being studied in clinical trials.

Use of drugs

Some of the principles of drug use have already been discussed. Compared to the West lower doses tend to be used and there is greater readiness to use drug combinations. Indeed, it is argued that there is a link between these two. Thus, Mosketi et al (1984) from Odessa, comment on the combined use of fenazepam, lithium and haloperidol in patients with schizophrenia. They write that treatment is more effective when combinations of various preparations are that this allows lower dosages to be used. Thus, haloperidol, normally used in doses of 15-30mgm per day according to the authors, was used in an average daily dose of 3mgm. They report that the treatment was highly effective in treating symptoms (the syndromal presentation), but that on a four year follow-up it did not appear to alter the course of the various forms described. Thus, the "pathological process" continued despite the fact that the symptoms were arrested. It was, however, successful in treating subsequent relapses. An important point was the lack of extrapyramidal side-effects. The same group also report good results from a combination of benzodiazepines, small dose haloperidol (up to 3mgm per day) and lithium (up to 450mgm per day) in adolescents with tics and obsessional movements (Aksentiev et al, 1987).

Drugs are more often given parenterally, most typically by intravenous drip, especially at the beginning of treatment. This often means that drugs are given once a day, in day hospitals, for instance, in the afternoon. Intravenous barbiturates with caffeine are reported as being useful in catatonic and certain stuporous states. According to Tsaritsinsky (1984) it is important to take into account circadian rhythms. In a trial of several different regimes he reported that haloperidol was more effective in paranoid schizophrenia when taken at night. The remission was more stable and there were fewer side-effects.

Treatment resistance

Zharikov (1983) advises caution with high doses of drugs, mainly because of the side-effects and suggests that if a drug appears to be ineffective it is probably wiser to change to a different drug or attempt combined treatment rather than increasing the dosage. Another approach is a sudden cessation of all drug treatment, with a gap before starting the drug again.

Vovin (1986), writing on treatment-resistant depression, suggests that after changing drugs one should move on to intravenous drug preparations. The next stage should be to stop all treatment for one week and then start a new treatment regime. At this stage, if this had failed, one might move on to sleep deprivation or the administration of an injection of intramuscular reserpine in addition to the tricyclic anti-depressants. Other possibilities are ECT, and (not now in use) pyrogenic therapy or atropine coma therapy. Nuller and Mikhalenko (1988) suggest ECT as a treatment in resistant depression but do not mention either atropine coma therapy or pyrogenic therapy. One possible reason for changing antidepressants might be if patients develop antibodies to a particular drug (Oskolkova, 1985).

Sleep deprivation
Vovin and Aksenova (1982) report on the use of sleep deprivation. The methods include total deprivation for 36 hours or partial deprivation, with patients either being woken at 1am or during REM sleep. The important factor is the prevention of REM sleep. They suggest various activities during the night of sleep deprivation, including talking, music, playing games. There should be an improvement in mood and motor function after the first session, but this usually only lasts for the day after the deprivation. Further reduction in symptoms usually follows repeated deprivations. A course of sleep deprivation is generally 3-8 nights, usually with an interval of 2-3 days at first and then once a week. The benefits of the treatment are its simplicity and the lack side-effects. In general, however, it is necessary to combine the treatment with anti-depressants to maintain its effect. It is thought useful in the prevention of chronic states of depression.

"Physical" treatments
Physical treatments such as ECT are used more sparingly in the Soviet Union than in the West. In the treatment section of the Handbook, Smulevitch (1983) writes that the introduction of psychotropics has meant that there is significantly less need to use ECT or insulin coma therapy. Psychosurgery has not been used since 1954 when it was banned by the Ministry of Health.

ECT
Avrutsky and Neduva (1981) write that the use of shock therapy is regulated by resolutions from the Institute of Psychiatry and the Ministry of Health. It can only be given in hospitals. They write that because of the "apparent brutality" of the treatment and the consequences for the brain it is used rarely, and, in some places, not at all. Although they note the opposition to the treatment, they state that in their view the treatments do have a place, especially in the treatment of patients with resistant depression or obsessional states. They say that tranquillisers (especially fenazepam) have changed the outlook in persistent obsessional states, but that shock therapy is still valuable in certain cases. ECT is generally given two or three times a week for a course of 3-5 or 9-10 treatments.

Vovin and Aksenova (1982), in a monograph on the treatment of resistant depression, advocate caution in using "powerful treatments" such as ECT or insulin because of their major effect upon the patient. They are especially opposed to their use as a therapeutic trial in that the treatments will distort the clinical picture and thus hinder adequate treatment. They quote foreign authors on efficacy, but stress that studies indicate that if patients have not responded to drugs such as imipramine they are less likely to respond to ECT. They also oppose giving repeated courses. The Handbook (Voronkov et al, 1990) does not mention usage in mania or but says that 3-5 sessions of ECT might be indicated rarely in severe depression which is treatment-resistant. A rare indication is "hypertoxic" or febrile schizophrenia.

Smulevitch (1983) writes that mechanism of action of ECT is unknown, and stresses the contraindications and side-effects. Caution is necessary in old age and if there are any physical illnesses. Snezhnevsky (1985) writes that ECT should never be used in children who are under 15 years old. The main indications are severe, treatment-resistant depression and, less commonly, other psychotic disorders. Caution about ECT is not just related to its side-effects, but also the fact that it is thought to produce less enduring results. Smulevitch and Panteleeva (1983) write that psychotropics produce complete rehabilitation in 74% of patients, which is 10-22% more than with ECT.

By contrast, Nuller and Mikhalenko (1988) consider ECT to be an effective and relatively safe form of treatment in severe depressive illness. They comment that it provokes fear in many patients and unjustified caution in some psychiatrists. They argue that it should be more widely used, but advise caution in patients with depression with features of depersonalization in whom the treatment is less effective and more likely to produce intellectual and memory disturbances.

Attitudes to the treatment vary within the Soviet Union, with many psychiatrists still opposed to the treatment. In one hospital in Leningrad the treatment was used widely on one ward but not at all on the next ward where there was a different doctor. Babayan (1985) writes about ECT as "...another harsh method used in clinical practice... repeatedly subjected to critical analysis." He reports on experimental studies on animals at the Institute of Psychiatry under Giliarovsky which showed that ECT produced "grave" morphological changes to nerve cells and glial tissue. He says the result was a reduction in the use of the treatment in practice and his view that there should be the "strictest limitations on the use of ECT." This attitude is perhaps more characteristic of an older school of Soviet psychiatry, and the literature shows that there are exceptions. Thus, Mosolov and Moshchevitin (1990) describe use of ECT several times a day in patients who had been in continuous psychosis for more than five months. There is a tendency for psychiatrists with greater "Western" orientation to use the treatment more widely. Thus there appears to be wider usage of the treatment in Leningrad and the Baltic republics than in Moscow and most other parts of the Soviet Union. This does, in part, reflect diagnostic practice, in that the same psychiatrists are perhaps more ready to diagnose depression than schizophrenia.

Insulin coma therapy
Sakel described the use of mild coma in the treatment of drug addiction in 1930, and in 1933 reported a dramatic improvement in the psychotic symptoms of a schizophrenic patient treated with deep coma. During the 1930s the treatment was gradually introduced into different European countries, including the Soviet Union. After Sakel was brought over to the USA in 1936 to demonstrate his technique the treatment gained acceptance in the USA. It became widely used and its popularity continued up until the mid-1950s. In Britain it continued to be used on a wide scale up to the early 1960s. The treatment is now virtually never used in the West, although small doses of insulin, insufficient to produce coma, are sometimes, used to stimulate appetite in patients with Anorexia Nervosa.

In the Soviet Union the treatment is still used. Many psychiatrists consider it to be valuable in the treatment of schizophrenia, and argue that it has fewer harmful effects than ECT. It is considered particularly effective in apathetic forms of the disorder. Avrutsky and Neduva (1981) write that the treatment is less used now that now the psychotropics are available, arguing it is no better than properly used psychotropics, especially as the treatment requires much input of medical and nursing time. They write that there is a greater risk of side-effects, for instance cardiovascular complications, fits and psychomotor excitement. There are a number of contraindications, mainly related to physical health. They write, however, that one cannot ignore the beneficial effects in many patients and that there are instances where it has produced prolonged remissions where drugs have had no effect. It is used in severe schizophrenia, especially paranoid schizophrenia, which is resistant to treatment. In the Handbook (Voronkov et al, 1990) its usage is suggested in treatment-resistant depression. Holland (1977) describes the treatment in use at the Kashenko Hospital in Moscow where it was considered to be useful in the treatment of both continuous and episodic-progressive schizophrenia, although drugs were usually the first line of treatment. It is now used less frequently and many centres do not give the treatment at all. It seems to be more widely used in the Baltic Republics, possibly because staffing levels are higher than in many parts of the Soviet Union. Kontsevoi and Kolesnikov (1987) describe a modified form of insulin coma therapy. They report positive results in patients with severe forms of schizophrenia, claiming that ll out of 15 of the patients were not psychotic and were free of relapse on follow-up at eighteen months. Modifications of the treatment include the induction of sub-comatose states.

Atropine coma therapy
This treatment was introduced by Forrer in 1950 and, according to Avrutsky and Neduva (1981), a number of different authors in the past reported that it was helpful in some resistant hallucinatory-paranoid states and also severe, treatment-resistant obsessional disorders. Its use is now banned.

Pyrogenic or "fever" therapy
Pyrogenic or fever therapy is based on the apparent success of malaria treatment in cerebral syphilis [3]. Malaria is no longer used, but a fever is induced with the drug sulphazin, which was first introduced in 1924. Avrutsky and Neduva (1981) write that the benefits of this treatment are not due to the fever but are mainly related to the immunological changes that it brings about. The treatment is used occasionally in patients with chronic alcoholism, in syphilis and resistant psychosis. Sulphazin is given by intramuscular injection which produces a rise in temperature after a few hours. Two to three injections are given over two or three days. They comment that in some clinics the treatment has been used to correct forms of disturbed behaviour and against some types of excitement. It is recognized that the treatment has been abused as a "punishment" to control difficult or violent patients and this is considered to be highly unacceptable.

Smulevitch and Panteleeva (1983) remark that the treatment has been used "without any particular success". Bacherikov et al (1989) in "Clinical Psychiatry"

---

3. The idea of treating mental illness by means of fever or infection is one that dates back for many centuries. In 1917 Wagner Jauregg introduced malaria therapy as a treatment for cerebral syphilis. He was awarded the Nobel prize in 1927.

(a Ukrainian textbook) continue to advocate its usage, but this has been overtaken by a general ban on its use within the Soviet Union [4].

Other methods of treatment

There are a number of treatment approaches which are either unknown or virtually never used in the West. Soviet medicine in general tends to rely upon a wider range of treatment methods than those found within mainstream medicine in the West. More conventional drug treatment is often used alongside these approaches. The treatments include exercise, massage, the use of baths, oxygen therapy, the drinking of koumiss (fermented mare's milk), acupuncture. Many of these approaches are used in the West, but tend to be available from non-medical practitioners and considered to be fringe medicine.

A wide range of preparations which stimulate various metabolic processes are in use in the Soviet Union, both within psychiatry and in other branches of medicine. Many of the herbal remedies seem to be similar to the preparations used by herbalists and homeopaths in the West. Soviet preparations include various tonics or "general strengtheners" such as fitin, calcium glycerophosphate, glucose and vitamins. There are stimulants such as ginseng, pantokrin, lemon, aloe. In psychiatry many of the preparations are aimed at the treatment of asthenia. In the stage of hypersthenia mild sedatives such as valerian or the bromides may be indicated. In the hyposthenic stage stimulants such as jinseng, lemon extracts, sidnokarb are used as well as vitamins and "general strengtheners" such as extracts of aloa. In addition nootropes or minimal doses of insulin are sometimes used.

Hyperbaric oxygen

This treatment has been used in various psychiatric disorders, mainly those where it is thought that there is vascular insufficiency [5]. Isakoff et al (1987) report on its use in cases of treatment-resistant schizophrenia. They report that patients have 10-12 sessions of the treatment and that negative symptoms, especially apathy, are helped. It is also reported as being an effective adjunct to treatment in alcohol withdrawal (Epifanova et al, 1988).

Detoxification

Various methods for "detoxification" have been used in patients with psychotic disorders, especially when there is thought to be an organic component. Haemabsorption has been used in patients with schizophrenia, alcoholic and toxic psychoses and vascular disorders of the brain. Markovsky and Fel (1986) report on the use of haemabsorption, combined, in some patients, with hyperbaric oxygenation, in a group of 50 elderly patients with vascular psychotic disorders. The patients had a range of psychotic symptoms with different degrees of cognitive impairment. They would be classified under various groups in the West: early dementia, schizophrenia, paraphrenia, psychotic depression. They show that this combination is more effective than the traditional approach to treatment with

4. With the devolution of health services to the republics this might not necessarily apply. The 1991 visit by the WPA team reported its use in the Ukraine, commenting that it was only used with the patient's consent.

5. The Action for Research into multiple sclerosis, based in Glasgow, claims that hyperbaric oxygen is effective in general functioning, especially bladder control, in multiple sclerosis (Lancet 1989a).

psychotropic preparations (this would include neuroleptics, antidepressants, and nootropes). They claim that there is striking improvement in the areas of attention, thinking, praxis and memory. They consider that improvement is due to normalization of metabolic processes, reduction of hypoxia and reduction in levels of triglycerides and toxins in general.

Reducing-diet treatment

Avrutsky and Neduva (1981) describe reducing-diet therapy (RDT) which was introduced by Nikolaev in 1948. The treatment consists of a period of starvation, possibly for up to three weeks, aiming to achieve 10% weight loss, followed by a purging with water and magnesium sulphate followed by the gradual introduction of a special diet consisting of fruit and milk products along with vitamins and restricted salt intake. They stress that patients' motivation and, above all, consent is important. The main indication is certain forms of schizophrenia, slow-flow and episodic-progressive schizophrenia, especially when there is the depressive-asthenic syndrome. It is said to improve drive and motivation. This treatment is now very rarely used. A patient I met on a home visit in Leningrad described having had this treatment many years previously, claiming that it helped her considerably, making her more animated. She asked if it was still being used. The sector psychiatrist said that she didn't know if anyone was using it now.

Dehydrating agents

Rollin (1972) reports on the use of magnesium sulphate and other dehydrating agents in hydrocephalus, even in its mild, compensated forms.

Electrosleep [6]

Electrosleep is a method by which relaxation and eventually sleep is induced by the rhythmical application of small electrical current to the brain. It is occasionally used in psychosomatic disorders such as duodenal ulceration, hypertension and asthma, also for insomnia and chronic anxiety.

Acupuncture

Acupuncture, or reflexotherapy, is widely used in Soviet medicine, and there is a Ministry of Health Research Institute of reflexotherapy in Moscow. In psychiatry there are a number of indications, depression being perhaps the commonest. The rationale for its action is thought to be the links between the nervous system and humoral system [7]. Acupuncture is considered useful in disorders where immunological factors are important. According to Hundanov, a leading exponent (MG 24.2.1988) the theories have moved away from the simplistic notions that there were particular points for particular diseases. He states that the mechanism is still unclear, but that it is known that external stimuli, such as electromagnetic forces, influence behaviour and that acupuncture is thought to modify these.

   Poliakov (1987) writes that reflexotherapy has been used in endogenous depression in the past. He reports on its use in 167 depressed patients with either

6. Although little known in the West it is used by some psychiatrists, and there is a review by Haslam (1987).

7. Acupuncture is used in the West, although relatively little in psychiatry. However, one placebo-controlled study (testing the effects of acupuncture on specific and non-specific points) found that the treatment was effective in the treatment of severe recidivist alcoholism (Bullock et al 1989).

manic-depression or schizophrenia, claiming that it has a range of effects like the antidepressant piradizol, with greater stimulatory than sedative effects. He claims that it is effective in some resistant cases and that it normalizes the EEG [8]. Markelova et al (1986) report on changes in blood and urine levels of various neurotransmitters and their metabolites after reflexotherapy in patients with depressive syndromes. In anxiety-depression there are high serotonin levels which returned to normal on recovery. In astheno-depression there were low levels which did not return to normal on recovery. Dudaeva et al (1990) recorded changes in the EEG and evoked potentials in patients with endogenous depression treated with reflexotherapy. They demonstrated activating and stimulating effects, and found a correlation between clinical improvement and the neurophysiological state.

Physiotherapy
This covers a much wider range of activities than would be considered as physiotherapy in the West. It includes exercise, massage and various types of baths. One of the most widely used of the physiotherapy treatments is "electro-phoresis". A pad is applied to parts of the body, for instance the arm, shoulder or neck, and a small ionizing current passed through this. Various substances, for instance calcium chloride, are placed between the pad and the skin and the idea is to introduce beneficial ions. The effect is a pleasant, tingling sensation. This may be used in neurotic disorders, especially obsessional and phobic disorders, and is thought to help with general weakness and tone. The placebo effect is recognized as being of positive value. It is also possible to introduce drugs, for instance local anaesthetics, by this method and this is thought to be less invasive than injections and also produce a more localized effect.

Mugutdinov (1985) comments that non-drug methods are becoming increasingly important in treatment, especially for the neurotic disorders. He describes successful results with thermal pulsation, a treatment which involves the application of pulses of heat of varying intensities and frequencies to circumscribed areas of the body. Most improvement was found in insomnia, depression and in vegetative symptoms. Andriushkiavechene and Visotskas (1986) from Vilnius report that a vigorous physiotherapeutic regime, including exercise and weight-reduction, led to improvement in mental state in a mixed group of psychiatric patients all of whom had atherosclerosis.

The recent upheaval in Soviet society has resulted in a spate of publicity for all kinds of treatments. These include various mystical/psychotherapeutic approaches, often promoted by cult figures such as faith healers and television healers. Some of these methods are being studied in scientific establishments such as the All-Union Centre of Psychoendocrinology in Moscow.

Hospital admission
Snezhnevsky (1983) writes that admission to observation wards should be as brief as possible, covering the acute stage when large doses of neuroleptics are being used. It is desirable to move patients as quickly as possible to open wards, periods

---

8. Perhaps surprisingly the best results seemed to be in melancholic patients, although not those who were anxious or apathetic. It was not effective in psychotic depression in which intravenous antidepressants were most effective. The study was not double-blind.

of leave and out to day hospitals. He advises caution about transferring depressed and suicidal patients to open wards. In practice there is greater caution about discharging patients than there is in most European countries, although American psychiatrists, influenced by the threat of litigation, tend to exercise a similar degree of caution. Psychiatric admissions in the Soviet Union tend to be longer, and this is not necessarily regarded in a negative light. The Western view that admissions should be as short as possible is not shared. This perhaps reflects a different attitude overall with regards to in-patient treatment. Many Western psychiatrists appear to regard admission as a kind of defeat and strive to keep patients out of hospital at all costs, these generally borne by patients and relatives.

"Milieu therapy" and the ward regime
Considerable importance is attached to the fact of being admitted to hospital. The interaction with staff and other patients is thought to be critical in treatment and outcome. As might be expected there is a tendency to prescribe or regiment the ward programme and the various stages of treatment. An article the Soviet nursing journal (Med Sestior, July 1984) carries details of treatment regimes. In patients with depression, for example, it states that only after the retardation phase is over should patients begin to move around and take part in ward activities. With return of mood and interests a more active treatment regime is instituted.

Rehabilitation
Rehabilitation has a special place in Soviet psychiatry, particularly in Leningrad, and the reasons for this are perhaps as much to do with the history of Soviet society as with psychiatry. Zharikov (1983) quotes the WHO definition of rehabilitation as the use of medical, social, educational and work measures with the aim of adapting a patient to the maximal possible level of activity compatible with his level of disability. He writes that rehabilitation cannot be separated from medical treatment or psychotherapy and that it begins with the first contact with the patient, essentially as soon as a tentative diagnosis is made. It continues until there is no further improvement in the patient's social or professional status. It aims to provide alternative abilities to compensate for the defects produced by the illness.

As already discussed there is much emphasis on the individual in working out the programme of treatment. Volovik (1986) writes that this depends on the level of social functioning and adaptation. These in turn are determined by psychological factors, especially personality [9], social factors (the pattern of relationships) as well as the course of the disease. The important implication of this approach for rehabilitation is that one does not have a programme of treatment for a certain form of schizophrenia, but for an individual. One individual with a particular form of schizophrenia might be unable to do even a mundane job, but someone else with the same condition might be able to hold down a responsible job. According to Kabanov (1986) systems theory is more helpful in making this kind of evaluation than employing simple psychoanalytic or behavioural models. These allow one to avoid the dichotomy of social versus biological. He writes that rehabilitation "presents an arena for systemic activity where the interacting

9. Abramov et al (1987) examine the nature of the personality change in schizophrenia and attempt to break this down into components. As might be expected the marked deficits are in the areas of emotion and motivation.

participants are a patient as an organism that is an open system and his social and biological environment."

According to the Bekhterev model there are three stages of treatment, with the details of the programme being worked out in a partnership between the psychiatrist and patient. The acute stage of treatment is mainly biological and includes drug treatment and a wide range of other measures which are aimed at improvement in physical and mental health. These include physiotherapy techniques such as massage and electrical stimulation of the muscles. The biological measures are combined with psychosocial measures: psychotherapy [10], occupational therapy, social skills training. The second stage involves the return to social activities and more collective treatment is applicable: work therapy, group therapy and education. Drug treatment has less of a role. On the wards there is an "activating regime" in which patients take part in social, cultural and sporting activities. There may be groups for discussion, support or more structured such as those discussing particular books, television programmes or newspaper articles. In the third stage, full rehabilitation, the patient takes his place in society again and the critical factors are work and accommodation.

The approach is tailored to the individual and leads to a flexible, graded approach which aims to produce a gradual, but stable, change in the patient's system of relationships and his level of social functioning. A treatment such as group therapy should suit the patient rather than remaining a fixed modality which a patient should slot into. Kabanov and Zachepitsky (1982) describe group discussion therapy which illustrates this. A patient with severe problems in social skills and communication might start group discussion therapy by being given a few sentences of dialogue to complete. The next stage would be structured discussion on a particular topic, preferably one relevant to their circumstances. The final stage would be an open discussion about any topic. They describe this approach as having behavioural elements, but say that it is much more than this in that it requires active participation and a change in basic attitudes/relationships.

Rehabilitation deals with the consequences of serious mental illness, in particular the changes in personality and the level of social functioning. It is also concerned with the social consequences of chronic illness, including the effects of institutionalization. Krasick and Logvinovitch (1977) from Tomsk examine the factors involved in "hospitalism" or institutionalization in a large group of chronic patients. They consider that it is due to the interaction between the individual, the course of the illness and various iatrogenic factors - including inadequate medical treatment and excess caution about discharge or "hyperguardianship". Gladishev (1977), from the Bekhterev Institute, describes the results of active rehabilitation in 100 chronic patients who had been in a long-stay rural hospital for years. He demonstrates that a combination of drugs, work therapy, psychotherapy, exercise and occupational therapy resulted in improvement in 82%, leading to discharge in 30%.

---

10. Poliakov et al (1987) stress the importance of the psychological correction of the defects in schizophrenia. They argue that it is necessary to find the intact areas in the emotional-motivational sphere and to create new social behaviour and enable the patient to find a new social niche. They quotes different approaches to this. Their approach is to use individual discussion to start with and move on to "psychocorrection" groups run by a psychologist. The group meets regularly, say two to three times a week during the in-patient stay and then once a week as out-patients. The early stages of the work concentrate on relationships within the group.

Work therapy
Babayan (1985) writes that the experience of both pre-revolutionary and Soviet psychiatrists has proved the value of prescribing work on an individual basis in the treatment of psychiatric patients, especially those with chronic psychoses. Work therapy has been a part of Soviet psychiatry from the early days [11]. Many Western commentators have remarked upon the major emphasis upon work in the system of Soviet psychiatry, especially rehabilitation. An American psychiatrist, Sirotkin (1968) wrote: "I would like to underscore a distinctive aspect of the Russian system which varies from our traditional concepts concerning psychiatric services and therapy. This distinction can be summed up in one word, 'work'."

There are theoretical as well as empirical reasons why work has such a key position in Soviet psychiatry. Mental processes are determined by external activity and relationships according to Soviet psychology. Man is defined by his activity and thus by the work he does. Work therapy, therefore, is not just something to do after the disorder has been treated and the mind sorted out, but is a fundamental part of the sorting out process. Work therapy is used for in-patients and out-patients. The idea is to prescribe the work according to the stage of the disorder. Initially it has a therapeutic purpose. It is then used as a preparation for discharge, possibly teaching new vocational skills. The final step in the rehabilitation process is a rational job placement. Workshops are present in all hospitals and also most dispensaries have attached treatment workshops. These are often organized as independent units which try to create the atmosphere of an ordinary factory by resembling production workshops.

Work is supervised by the workshop team, and this involves psychiatrists, nurses and the job supervisors. Work should never be purposeless as patients recognize this, often responding negatively or refusing to do it. The nature of the work may be simple or complex. Skilled work includes the carrying out of repairs, electronics, bookbinding, the use of drills and lathes, and clerical work. Patients' skills are sometimes used in a pragmatic way. A patient who approached me in a Leningrad hospital turned out to be a teacher of English from Sakhalin Island. He was working in the radio workshop, but also used to translate psychiatric material from English into Russian, although he was rather slow at this.

My impression of hospitals in Leningrad and Moscow was that the work therapy was at a more basic level than at the dispensaries. As patients spend much more of their time at the dispensary than they do in hospital this would seem to make sense. The treatment-workshops in the dispensaries have 50 to 200 places. They generally occupy large buildings, often a large floor space, something which is at a premium in the major cities. A surprising feature is that the workshops are staffed by doctors and nurses as well as job supervisors. In 1985 the workshop at the Bekhterev Institute had 350 patients, with a staff of 4 psychiatrists, 8 nurses, one psychologist and a varying number of instructors who guided the work procedures. Many of the patients lived in Leningrad and came in on a daily basis and there were twenty patients from the Institute itself. The work regime was

11. Many pre-Revolutionary psychiatrists, including Korsakoff, had written about the importance of work therapy and in the mid-nineteenth century Sabler introduced a form of this in Moscow. It was incorporated into Soviet psychiatry from an early stage. Work therapy was organized by Giliarovsky in Moscow in 1920, by Ilion and Chegodayev in Gorky in 1927 (Babayan, 1985). As already mentioned a workshop was established in Kharkov in 1927 with a hostel for those living out of the city.

decided by the doctors and depended upon the patient. Patients might work all day or just in the morning. I was told that there were also about fifty work-therapy departments in different factories in Leningrad. Some out-patients work at home, generally under the supervision of the home nursing team. Work assignments such as knitting might be left for them.

Rehabilitation is not just the responsibility of the health services and social services, but also of industry, which is obliged by law to provide sheltered working conditions and employ patients who have completed treatment. There may be special workshops in factories or a work unit may be based at a hospital. Psychiatric care may be given by a psychiatrist from the medical department of the enterprise, if this is a sufficiently large one, alternatively by the local polyclinic or dispensary psychiatrist. The VTEK, a board concerned with the medical aspects of work, determines the work capacity in liaison with psychiatrists. It can lay down the conditions under which someone with a disability works: possibly shortening the working day to four hours, specifying the type of placement.

Rural areas pose special difficulties because of the lack of a wide range of rehabilitation measures. However, many state farms have experience of rehabilitation and patients may live and work there, some of them from urban areas.

Disability levels
There are three categories of disability for pension purposes (Lisitsin and Batygin, 1978)

1st level: The patient is unable to work and requires constant care.
2nd level: The patient is unable to work, but does not require constant care.
3rd level: The patient is able to work to a limited extent.

Patients on 3rd level disability will be recommended to work and may be given new jobs in ordinary enterprises. Patients with 1st and 2nd levels might not work or it might be suggested that there is a change of work or adapted working conditions. Thus, there are special workshops for invalids with shorter working days and individual production rates. Alternatively, there may be no obligation with regard to norms or production rates. Working conditions will be adapted to the stage of the disorder. It is clear that changes in the nature of Soviet society will affect such measures, particularly if there is a shift to the market economy away from the norms and production rates which are a feature of a planned economy.

Prophylaxis
The acute or first stage of treatment is concerned with the removal of symptoms. The second stage requires stabilization of the condition, reduction in sedation and the prevention of chronicity. The third stage is about rehabilitation, getting people back into society, and the prevention of relapses (Zharikov, 1983; Vovin, 1986).

There are a number of different approaches to drug treatment in prophylaxis. Lithium is used widely. A number of different regimes are used, sometimes involving cycles of treatment, with drug-free intervals, also brief periods of treatment such as "weekend therapy". The depot neuroleptics are also used, but less so than in the West. It is unusual for patients to be on these for many years without interruption, an increasing tendency in the West.

Babayan (1985) writes that the social work of the home nursing team (which is part of the sector service) is important in preventing relapses and even defect states. Thus, in addition to regular review of mental state, there is a regular check, at least twice yearly, on the patients' material welfare and housing conditions. When necessary they may be given material assistance in cash or kind, for instance bedding or clothing. The amount and duration of assistance depends upon the patient's need and, perhaps surprisingly, the budget of the dispensary. There is a regular review of the necessity for home nursing by a permanent commission, chaired by the chief doctor at the dispensary.

Treatment in practice

There are 37,000 psychiatrists in the Soviet Union and it would be impossible to guess at how many of them treat patients according to the principles outlined. Certainly the psychiatrists that I met held a wide range of different views about treatment. Some psychiatrists, especially those with more interest in Western psychiatry and genetics, appear to think more along the lines of the disease-entity model, that there are specific treatments for particular disorders. Many acknowledge the theoretical aspects of the approaches discussed above but thought that in practice treatment was often limited to drug treatment and the most basic rehabilitation measures eg work therapy. This clearly varies from centre to centre. Treatment also varies considerably from one psychiatrist to the next. Some of the treatments mentioned above might be available because of the interest of a particular ward or dispensary doctor. However, even with conventional treatments there is greater heterogeneity than in the West.

At different hospitals and dispensaries that I visited in Moscow and Leningrad I saw a range of different treatments. Common to all were drug treatment, work and occupational therapy along with various forms of physiotherapy and exercise. Many also carry out one or more types of psychotherapy, most commonly group therapy. Additional treatments such as acupuncture or hypnosis generally depend upon the interests of the staff working there. Psychotherapy is less used within hospitals than in dispensaries, although there are notable exceptions such as the Bekhterev Institute.

One unfortunate factor which influences treatment is availability of drugs, especially outside the major centres. Many of the drug treatments described will not be available to provincial psychiatrists and even sector psychiatrists in major cities.

Comparative aspects

As discussed in Chapter One there are two main concepts of disease: the realist or "Platonic" and the nominalist or "Hippocratic" concept. The nominalist approach, the theoretical approach in the Soviet Union, attaches less importance to the diagnosis given to a patient and is more concerned with matching treatment to the individual profile of the patient (made up of the syndromal presentation, personality and psychosocial factors). Thus, Smulevitch (1983) writes that treatment depends upon the stage that the disorder has reached, the balance between the biological and psychosocial aspects and between the clinical presentation and individual features of the patient. Thus, a patient might be described as suffering from a particular form of schizophrenia but also as having features of an anxiety state with certain abnormalities of personality development. Treatment is influenced by each of these aspects. Perhaps the main difference between this approach and that of the English-speaking world is that treatment is targeted at symptoms and syndromes, irrespective of the main diagnosis. Thus, a patient with depression may receive anti-depressants, but also stimulants if there is an asthenic component and neuroleptics for psychotic symptoms.

By contrast, there is a tendency in Western psychiatry, probably because of the influence of the realist disease concept, to prescribe specific treatments for specific "diseases". Thus, a diagnosis of depression carries with it the implication that any drug treatment should be with the anti-depressants. The hierarchical approach implicit in the realist concept means that disorders at the top of the hierarchy prevail over other syndromes for the purposes of treatment. A patient with schizophrenia who also has anxiety symptoms is treated for the schizophrenia, not for the anxiety symptoms. Critics of this approach argue that it leads to an over-simplification of treatment. Once a diagnosis has been established it is simply a question of turning to the specific treatment for that disease, even if the disorder happens to presents with atypical features. The problems arise when the treatment does not work and one consequence of this approach has been the tendency to use increasing dosages of drugs, rather than matching drugs to symptoms. The argument goes that if the diagnosis is right then the drug must be right and more needs to be given.

One danger of the Soviet approach to drug therapy is that it can lead to idiosyncratic and unsystematic treatment. There are, however, attempts to correlate particular syndrome patterns and other factors with drug regimes. Mosolov et al (1989) give a table with the different syndromes, mainly those in the psychotic spectrum, on one axis and a list of drugs and drug-combinations along the vertical axis. The results appear to suggest that a combination of lithium and an anti-psychotic is the most useful treatment across a range of syndromes, irrespective of diagnostic grouping. Another danger is that it might encourage unnecessary polypharmacy with the risks of drug interactions. However, most Soviet authors argue that combinations of drugs are more effective than single drugs and also allow smaller dosages to be used, thus reducing the likelihood of side effects (Smulevitch and Panteleeva, 1983; Mosketi et al, 1984). Another consequence of treating symptoms rather than diseases is that a wider range of treatments is used in the Soviet Union, some of which would be considered to be "fringe" by Western psychiatrists.

Soviet psychiatrists have traditionally been more conservative in their use of physical treatments, especially those which are considered to have potentially damaging effects. It is claimed that the materialist approach, which sees the brain as the substrate for all psychological processes, normal and abnormal, naturally leads to greater respect for the brain and caution about treatment. Soviet psychiatrists have specific criticisms of Western practice in this respect. They consider that the overuse of physical treatments is, paradoxically, the result of the disregard given to biological treatment. This is said to have arisen because of the emphasis on the social or psychological approach (even the influence of the anti-psychiatry movement of the 1960s) resulting in lingering dualist notions that drugs actually make very little difference to the mind. In this context biological treatments are seen as an admission of failure rather than a complementary part of treatment. Ignorance of the principles of biological treatment means that psychologically or socially oriented Western psychiatrists use these treatments badly, relying on excessively high doses of drugs or inappropriate use of ECT.

It does seem that some Western psychiatrists have a sceptical view about the role of drug treatment. This can result in a rather haphazard approach to prescribing, with patients taking the same drugs in similar doses whether they are in-patients or out-patients, possibly for long periods of time. Decisions are often left to relatively junior doctors, the role of senior doctors being to confirm diagnoses. Observers of American psychiatry have criticized the approach to drug treatment used by analytically-oriented psychiatrists, perhaps a reflection of the training of an earlier generation [12]. In Britain the move towards the "multi-disciplinary" team has meant that in some units there appears to be little difference between the role of the psychiatrist and that of other members of the team, for instance social workers or psychologists. Much of the work is concerned with social and family processes and "medical" decisions are reduced to whether someone needs an antidepressant or a neuroleptic.

Psychosurgery
Various attempts at treating psychiatric disorders by brain surgery were carried out in the late nineteenth and early twentieth century (Clare, 1980). In 1935 Moniz performed the first prefrontal leucotomy in Portugal [13]. Largely through the efforts of an American psychiatrist, Walter Freeman, the treatment became widely used in the 1940s and 1950s in the USA [14]. At that time about 5000 operations a year were being carried out. In Britain over 10,000 operations had been performed by 1954 and soon afterwards Japan, India and many other countries began to use the procedures. According to Valenstein (1986), there was little opposition to the procedure at first and many psychoanalysts managed to integrate the procedure into their conceptual framework. A leading American psychiatrist, Smith Ely Jeliffe, argued that the frontal lobes were the site of the Freudian fixations. He argued that a more selective procedure would be beneficial, essentially an operation that could severe the connections from the anus to the frontal lobe (to deal with anal fixation). There was opposition from many quarters, including psychiatrists like Grinker and the psychoanalyst Harry Stack Sullivan. Subsequently the voices of protest became more strident, with media involvement and some restrictive legislation. Concern was particularly great about the its use children and also as a means of social control [15].

In 1977 the National Commission for the Protection of Human Subjects of

12. The American literature does supply examples of this from time to time. Wylie and Wylie (1987) discuss a thirty-nine year-old divorced woman who was being treated in psychoanalysis. The treatment was not going well because she could not develop a transference. The analysis was therefore "modified" with phenelzine which led to dramatic changes in her private life. She started up a new sexual relationship and also developed a transference relationship with the psychiatrist. The authors suggest that the changes were brought about by the psychoanalysis which had been modified by the phenelzine. One might, of course, speculate that the patient's depression had been treated by the phenelzine with the result that she regained her sexual drive and her interest in men, including the analyst.

13. Moniz was shot in the spine by a patient, although not, as is often stated, by one that he had operated upon. He received a Nobel prize for his work in 1949.

14. The late psychiatrist and medical historian Richard Hunter argued, facetiously perhaps, that the upsurge in psychosurgery in the late 1940s and 1950s was due to the fact that neurosurgeons were short of work after the war.

Biomedical and Behavioural Research carried out an investigation of psychosurgery and concluded that some forms were useful in certain disorders. Despite the reservations, the treatment has remained in use, although has decreased in popularity, and the annual number of operations carried out in the USA has been in the hundreds rather than the thousands. More recently there appears to be an increase in interest in the procedure (Valenstein, 1986). In Britain psychosurgery continues to be used in a number of centres, with the main indication being refractory depression and obsessional disorders. Lovett and Shaw (1987) also suggest that the procedure might have a place in the treatment of hypomania [16].

Bridges (1987), reviewing 1,200 operations over 20 years at the Geoffrey Knight Surgical Unit in London, claims a 50% rate of improvement. He claims that the newer stereotactic techniques cause few problems although they find that progressively increasing the size of the lesion (destroying more brain tissue) results in a higher proportion of patients having a good outcome. The indications, according to him, are patients with severe depression, anxiety, tension and obsessional disorders. He attacks crisis intervention, psychotherapy and community care, saying that they are of limited value, whilst claiming that "...contemporary psychosurgery is simply an indispensable therapy." A supporting letter from Snaith (1987) argues that psychosurgery remains an effective treatment for depression and that it should be used more often. He writes that "they have surely the thanks of many hundreds of people who would otherwise have had to endure their lives in a pit darker than hell itself" (perhaps not the scientifically objective language one might expect from the champion of so radical a treatment). He argues that consent should not necessarily pose a problem in that such patients cannot give informed consent and that desperate cases require desperate measures.

One of the central problems about psychosurgery, over and above the unease about ethical issues, has been the lack of proper evaluation. Reports of its efficacy are purely anecdotal and there are no double-blind trials. The subjective evaluation used in the "studies" would be unacceptable in any trial of a new drug treatment. In 1972 Levy asked "Is it too much to ask that the same stringent criteria (as used for new drugs) should be adopted in dealing with potentially more dangerous, and certainly more expensive, surgical procedures?" This question remains unanswered.

Psychosurgery was banned by the Ministry of Health in the Soviet Union in 1954, at the very peak of its usage in the West. Soviet psychiatrists generally maintain that this was because it proved to be an ineffective treatment with intolerable side-effects. However, the reasons are probably more complex than this. It was very much the time of the cold-war and also the height of the Lysenko

15. Some psychiatrists and neurosurgeons advocated the use of psychosurgery in criminal behaviour. Valenstein (1986) quotes a Californian neurosurgeon as saying: "The person convicted of a violent crime should have the chance for a corrective operation....Each violent young criminal incarcerated from 20 years to life costs taxpayers perhaps $100,000. For roughly $6000, society can provide medical treatment which will transform him into a responsible well-adjusted citizen." In "Violence and the Brain". Mark and Ervin (1970) argued that brain pathology was the cause of much of the violence in society and that neurosurgery could help to provide the answer. There was considerable controversy as these views were put at a time of urban rioting, predominantly in black areas. Clare (1980) summarizes some of the other controversial aspects. He quotes Breggin's criticism about it being used mainly against women and also against those who deviate from society's norms. Operations on children with behaviour disorders were carried out in the USA, India and Japan.

16. This claim is based on an open follow-up study of 9 patients, two of whom appeared to have responded to the operation. The other seven continued to have repeated hypomanic episodes and required drug treatment. One patient developed schizophrenia, one epilepsy and a stroke, one died.

era in which the Soviet Union was rejecting much of "bourgeois" Western science, which included genetics and cybernetics. Physical methods of treatment were seen as part of the Western bourgeois system of values, based on lack of respect for the material substance of the brain and also on simplistic notions of localization. According to Babayan (1985) lobotomy and leucotomy were used in the Soviet Union in the same way as in the West in the early days. He writes that various "in depth" studies, including those of Giliarovsky, Snezhnevsky and himself, proved that there was no practical benefit to the treatment. There were no encouraging results and at the same time they inflicted "tremendous damage". He uses rather strong language for the treatment, saying that it is "brutal" and "lacks scientific substantiation."

The current position is that the legal ban remains, but there is some interest in some of the techniques [17]. The conventional position remains that psychosurgery, including the newer techniques, is harmful and ineffective. Sluchevsky and Petsevitch (1988) from Leningrad review the progress of 15 cases who had psychosurgery before the 1954 ban, reporting poor outcome and neurological damage. They consider that the newer techniques (including stereotactic methods) that are in use in the West are based on the same principles as classical leucotomy and essentially do no more than disrupt the function of the brain. They conclude their article: "From the perspective of contemporary psychiatry this kind of interference is not tolerable neither from the point of view of therapeutic efficacy nor from that of medical ethics."

ECT

The "shock therapies" were introduced in Hungary by Von Meduna and were based on his incorrect view that there was some kind of mutual antagonism between schizophrenia and epilepsy. He induced convulsions chemically, firstly with camphor and then metrazol (cardiozol). In 1935 he published an account of his successful treatment of a number of schizophrenic patients by these means. The treatment was used in both Europe and the USA (Meduna emigrated to the USA in 1939), but was soon supplanted by electrically induced convulsions. In 1938 Cerletti and Bini in Rome had induced fits by passing an electric current through the brain. The treatment rapidly came into use in the USA and much of Europe and was being extensively used from the early 1940s onwards. Whether it is the convulsion that is important for the effect or the quantity of electric current passed is still not resolved. The accepted line seems to be that the convulsion is critical, although the case is far from proven (eg Robin and DeTissra, 1982 and Sackeim et al, 1987).

ECT still generates controversy and is not viewed in a particularly favourable light by the general public. As Clare (1980) put it: "there is scarcely a more controversial or a more widely used treatment in contemporary British psychiatry than electroconvulsive treatment". ECT is condemned by most anti-psychiatry groups and is a particular target of the Scientology movement [18]. The result, as one might expect, is that equal passion is generated in its defence, and this

17. Bekhtereva, director of the Leningrad Institute of Experimental Medicine, has developed techniques involving the use of electrical stimulation of parts of the brain via implanted electrodes. This has mainly been in patients with epilepsy. Their work is largely experimental, but they claim good results in some patients with severe, chronic disorders.

sometimes leaves the realms of the strictly scientific. This is partly because politics has entered into the arena, for instance with the use of ECT being restricted in certain American states [19]. In many European countries, including Holland, Switzerland and Germany, the treatment is used rarely, with a complete ban in some areas.

ECT is still widely used in Britain and the third world, especially in those countries where there has been a "Western" psychiatric influence. Cohen (1988) reports that unmodified ECT (ie with no anaesthetic or muscle relaxant) is used in Egypt and in India. He also reports on one private hospital in India, where conditions were reasonably good on the whole, where up to a quarter of the 300 patients were receiving unmodified ECT every day. There is no doubt that ECT is sometimes used unnecessarily, often given to patients who would have improved anyway [20].

Another recent trend has been the increase in its usage in the USA for economic rather than clinical reasons. This is related to the developments in diagnosis related groups and case management (which aim to set standards in psychiatric care - generally looking to reducing inpatient stay). The use of ECT had been steadily dropping during the 1970s (Thompson and Blaire, 1987), but from the early 1980s onwards began to increase again [21]. An article in the American Journal of Psychiatry suggested that use of ECT led to substantial cost savings in the treatment of depression in that it led to faster recovery and shorter admissions (Markowitz et al, 1987). The authors report a projected saving of $6402 per patient. A similar claim was made by Small (1988) for the use of ECT in mania. These issues are discussed in more detail on page 247.

As discussed above, the treatment is used less frequently in the Soviet Union. An American psychiatrist, Holland (1977), reporting from a year spent on a psychiatric attachment in Moscow, writes that ECT is seldom used. My own experience confirmed this and indeed there were some psychiatrists who never used it. Figures are not published, but one account of the treatment of patients with severe depressive illness showed that only 3 out of 112 patients received ECT (Sinitsky et al 1988). Although most Soviet psychiatrists regard ECT as a useful adjunct to treatment they are critical of some aspects of its use in the West. In particular there is concern about its use in vulnerable groups, including children, the aged and patients with organic complications. By contrast, in the West, it is considered to be safer than drugs in many instances and age is not a contraindication. Despite restrictive legislation, ECT is widely used in children in the USA (Winslade et al, 1984). In Britain it is less used in children, although a report in the British Journal of Psychiatry (Powell et al, 1988) describes the case of a 13 year-old boy with depressive stupor. He was given three courses of ECT

18. An issue of its journal "Freedom" (Spring 1987), which was handed out to psychiatrists at a Royal College of Psychiatry meeting, carried the lead "Psychiatrist recommends electric shock for nursery tots". Underneath is a picture of a group of children playing happily together with the caption "Britain's Children - in for a shock?"

19. As well as the legal status there has also been fear of litigation. Dongier and Wittkower (1981) discuss some of the controversial issues, giving a number of references for its damaging effects on the brain. Recent studies, using newer scanning techniques, suggest that many of the earlier claims might have been exaggerated.

20. Dodwell and Goldberg (1989) report on the use of ECT in 17 patients with schizophrenia, finding that good outcome was associated with short duration of illness and fewer pre-morbid schizoid personality traits (classic features of good outcome in schizophrenia).

21. 100,000 patients per year received ECT treatment and the number was increasing each year (Science, 1985).

despite the fact that during the first episode he responded to drugs and on another occasion recovered from the stupor by himself after four days (his condition eventually resolved after his parents divorced).

Some Soviet psychiatrists are puzzled by the wide and increasing use of ECT within English-speaking psychiatry (as compared to mainland Europe). A peculiar devotion to ECT, together with lip-service to the social model, is seen as the trademark of British psychiatry. It is thought that there is too much emphasis on sociology and psychodynamics at the expense of psychopathology and psychopharmacology. Because of this psychiatrists are not taught how to use drugs properly and therefore have to resort to ECT if their attempts at social work are unsuccessful. Another view is that the cross-sectional, disease-oriented approach leads psychiatrists to expect cures and that when these expectations are frustrated they tend to resort to drastic measures.

Drug treatment

The main differences in drug usage are discussed in the section above. There is more specific, symptom-directed treatment, in the Soviet Union and also more polypharmacy. Some differences relate to particular drugs, for instance the nootropes, and different antidepressants and tranquillisers such as fenazepam. Benzodiazepines are widely used in the Soviet Union, the commonest indications being anxiety and insomnia. In the West, by contrast, the "benzodiazepine backlash" has almost led to the view that it is bad practice to prescribe this group of drugs, despite the fact that they have a well-tried and valuable place in the alleviation of distress and the treatment of psychiatric disorders. Tyrer and Murphy (1987) write that "a dark shadow has been cast over the benzodiazepines by the spectre of dependence." They argue that this group of drugs still has a valuable role in the treatment of psychiatric disorders. However, some psychiatrists argue that they have no place in clinical practice, perhaps reflecting the fact that doctors become wary if patients get too fond of their medicine. One suspects the legacy of the nursery, the view that it can't be doing you any good if you like it. In 1983 the State of Victoria, in Australia, changed the law so that chemists could sell up to ten tablets of nitrazepam or temazepam without prescription. This did not presents problems and the practice was also adopted in New South Wales.

To some extent all this was simply part of a marketing exercise for a new generation of drugs. It is similar to the publicity given to the dangers of the barbiturates when the benzodiazepines came onto the market. Now it is the turn of the benzodiazepines. The old products, which are no longer under patent and are therefore not profitable to the drug industry, are criticized at the expense of new products under patent.

The long-acting depot neuroleptics are used more widely in the West than in the Soviet Union. This is partly the result of the reduction in the number of hospital beds and the move into the community. This puts pressure on psychiatrists to cut down on admissions and so avoid the risk of relapse. This may result in keeping patients on depot neuroleptics longer than they would have been in the past. There is also an unfortunate trend, inevitably encouraged by the pharmaceutical industry, to over-emphasize the place of these drugs in the treatment of schizophrenia.

Many patients are told that they may need to be on the drugs for life and some psychiatrists come to believe this. In many Western countries psychiatrists are not necessarily the people prescribing these drugs. With the developments of community care in Britain there is a trend for General Practitioners, perhaps working with Community Psychiatric Nurses (CPNs), to look after chronic psychiatric patients in the community. The results is that patients may be on depot neuroleptics for long periods without seeing a psychiatrist. Many patients are maintained on depot neuroleptics for decades (eg Curson et al, 1985).

The control of violent behaviour
One of the most difficult problems facing psychiatry and, more particularly, psychiatric nursing, is the control of aggressive and violent patients. Physical restraint measures are used less than in the past. In the West the advent of smaller units with fewer numbers of skilled nursing staff on site has meant that simple physical restraint is less used. This has led to greater reliance on the use of psychotropic medication, and, at times, ECT. Soviet psychiatry shares these problems, but it is claimed that because of good staff ratios there is less need to rely upon drugs to control violent behaviour and that ECT should never be used in this way. There are reports of crude restraint measures being used in Soviet psychiatric hospitals, for instance wrapping patients in wet blankets and giving injections of sulphazin as "punishment". Such approaches were condemned by the Soviet psychiatrists that I met. Strait-jackets are also used in the Soviet Union, although it is rare and is said to be mainly to control self-harm [22]. Straight-jackets are widely used in the USA for violent patients, less so in Europe.

The use of the "cold wet sheet pack" procedure in the USA is described by Ross et al (1988). They say that their purpose is to "raise new questions about an old treatment". They describe the procedure: "The cold wet sheet pack is a procedure in which the patient is wrapped in cold wet sheets so that he or she is comfortable but immobilized...a table is prepared with two sheets that have been immersed in cold water and wrung out; a blanket is placed underneath the sheets. The patient is placed on top of the wet sheets and wrapped with arms and legs placed within the coverings. A top blanket is used for insulation, a pillow is placed under the patient's head, and a hot water bottle may be used to provide warmth for the feet. The patient initially experiences cold, but warming is rapid due to vasomotor changes. A nursing staff member sits with the patient while he or she is in the pack. The patient is monitored medically (pulse and color and condition of skin) and is allowed to ventilate whatever is on his or her mind. The procedure may last up to two hours." They report on the use of this treatment in 46 patients, six of whom had more than 20 treatments. Most of the patients had a diagnosis of personality disorder and it was used mostly for disruptive behaviour. They argue that the treatment has "interesting and useful effects", citing the fact that some patients were able to bring up repressed memories. They claim that the advantages are that it is a non-chemical, and safe method of restraint.

The management of the small proportion of psychiatric patients who are violent continues to pose a considerable problem and it seems inevitable that for some time there will be reports of the abuse of treatment measures and of the use of undue

22. I saw one in use with a young woman who was mentally handicapped who had been mutilating herself.

restraint.

Rehabilitation

In general Soviet psychiatrists are complementary about Western psychiatry, recognizing the progress on the biological front. When it comes to the psychosocial side, however, they maintain that there are short-comings, in particular with regards to rehabilitation. They claim that rehabilitation has never really been a major part of Western psychiatry and that the current interest in it has been forced upon psychiatrists by the closure of psychiatric hospitals. Because it has come about for political reasons it is being done half-heartedly: the purpose is not to return patients to society, but to get patients out of hospitals. According to Zharikov (1983) foreign psychiatrists are interested in rehabilitation, although perhaps with too much emphasis on the psychotherapeutic aspects.

Soviet psychiatrists consider that rehabilitation is difficult within the context of a laissez-faire economy, firstly because of the problems of unemployment and secondly because private industry does not consistently provide for disabled groups. It is argued that a socialist economy and lack of unemployment allow for broad opportunities for rational vocational placement (Zharikov, 1983; Babayan, 1985). There is concern that the economic changes under way in the Soviet Union might endanger this. Warner (1985) argues that there are important social influences on the medical management and course of schizophrenia, and argues that this may be closely related to the level of unemployment. He states that the worst period for recovery from schizophrenia was in the 1930s during the period of high unemployment due to the great depression. The situation was better before that and also improved in the 1950s when there was low unemployment and a need for labour [23].

Rehabilitation also depends upon the availability of housing and the problems of homelessness contribute considerably to the difficulties experienced by psychiatric patients in the community. The plight of the homeless mentally ill in Western countries has recently been widely discussed in the media. In the Soviet Union it is relatively easy to find housing for a someone with a mental illness. Indeed, it used to be said that it was considerably easier than for someone without a mental illness.

---

23. He does not refer to the introduction of the phenothiazines in the 1950s.

Chapter Seven

PSYCHOTHERAPY

Psychoanalysis can be said to have hijacked psychotherapy to the extent that for many people the distinction between the two terms has become blurred. Indeed, the terms are sometimes considered synonymous. However, especially when considering psychotherapy within the Soviet Union, it is important to distinguish psychotherapy, the treatment of mental illness by psychological means (also defined as a treatment involving the interaction, mainly verbal, between patient and therapist), from psychoanalysis which is one specific form of psychotherapy bound to a particular theoretical framework. It should be added that there is also some confusion in the general population about the distinction between psychiatry and psychoanalysis. Psychotherapeutic techniques are used in psychiatry, but very few psychiatric patients are treated with psychoanalysis. Even in the USA psychoanalysis reaches only a tiny minority of psychiatric patients, mainly those in the private sector with less severe disorders.

The development of psychotherapy in the Soviet Union
Rozhnov (1985) is unhappy with what he sees as the Western view that there is no psychotherapy in the Soviet Union, an understandable concern for the director of the All-Union psychotherapy centre in Moscow. He writes that this has come about because of the Soviet criticism of Freudianism. He writes that there are no grounds for linking psychotherapy to psychoanalysis and that the basic principles of psychotherapy have a long history. The main Soviet criticism of Western psychotherapy, psychoanalysis, cognitive and behaviour therapy, is that they are too concerned with "intra-psychic" and individualistic aspects of man and do not take enough account of environmental and social factors. He writes that Soviet psychotherapy continued in the tradition of the nineteenth century Russian psychiatrist, Korsakoff, who founded Russian psychiatry on psychotherapeutic principles.

There were two early trends in Soviet psychotherapy: the physiological/Pavlovian and the social/Marxist. Pavlovian theory provides the basis for suggestion and hypnosis. These techniques developed from the 1950s onwards and were mainly used in the treatment of neurotic disorders although they also had a wide application in general medicine. The second trend in psychotherapy developed from the theory that social processes and activity determine mental processes (Segal, 1975). This is characterized by Vygotsky's view that "..all higher mental functions are internalized social relationships" (Kozulin, 1984). In the early post-revolutionary period Giliarovsky introduced group psychotherapy based on these principles.

Rational Therapy, based on the work of Dubois, was developed by Bekhterev who emphasized the need to pay close attention to the personality and life circumstances of the patient. He established the triad of explanation, hypnosis and auto-suggestion. Pathogenetic psychotherapy (see below) evolved from this.

Psychoanalysis in the Soviet Union
During the early Soviet years there was a small psychoanalytic movement, based mainly in Moscow. The works of Freud were published in Russian translation in 1923 and up until the late 1920s there was a Moscow section of the International Psychoanalytic Association. The movement began to die out after the Russian Psychoanalytic Society was disbanded in 1933. It is generally held that Soviet psychology gradually moved away from psychoanalysis because it fell out of favour on ideological grounds. It is worth bearing in mind, however, that psychoanalysis did not stand still and did some moving of its own. In its early years it was seen as a system of thought which attempted to explain human behaviour on a materialist basis, breaking with the dualist psychology of the nineteenth century. However, although Freud considered the mechanisms that he described had a neural basis, the psychoanalytic movement began to view mind as separate from the brain [1].

In the Handbook of Psychiatry, Smulevitch (1983) describes psychoanalysis as a form of psychotherapy based on the theories of Freud which ascribe a key role to the unconscious in explaining behaviour and to unconscious conflicts, especially sexual conflicts, in the genesis of neuroses and other disorders. Although he is sceptical about what he calls some "fantastic interpretations" [2], he is kinder to psychoanalysis than many Western critics. Thus, he writes that treatment may remove symptoms in some cases, but that this does not prove the underlying theory. Other mechanisms may account for the improvement, not least the fact that treatment tends to happen over many months or years, allowing for spontaneous remissions. According to Zachepitsky (1986) personality develops as a result of real situations within the family and outside it and does not "follow the mythological scheme of the Oedipus triangle".

1. Gellner (1985) attempts to account for the dramatic rise of psychoanalysis in the Western world and suggests a number of reasons. It filled a gap left by religion by providing a doctrine acceptable to post-Darwinian man who could accept his place in the natural world. Psychoanalysis did that, and, unlike Marxism, also had the component of pastoral care. By trying to account for what he calls the "dark, lower forces" in man it also filled the need that some people have for a religious or superstitious element. He compares free association and dreams with the omens and portents of religion. Gellner also argues that the actual process of psychoanalysis has been a powerful reason for its success. Central to this is the real phenomenon of transference, a process which can, of course, be understood within the framework of many different theoretical positions, and is, as has been discussed, accepted by Soviet psychiatry. Gellner argues that in going to an analyst a patient suspends his belief system, and that doubts about the process are interpreted from within the doctrine. Thus, doubts about Oedipal fantasies might be seen as resistance to unacceptable interpretations. Many hours of analysis, which combines confession, authority and closely applied attention, inevitably develops a strong bond of loyalty towards the analyst, strengthening the belief system. This process also helps to ensure the "monopolistic-apostolic succession" rather like Christian bishops and their links back to Christ. Everyone being analysed today could probably able to trace his analyst or his analyst's analyst back to Freud or one of the early group of trustees appointed by him.

2. One of the foundations of psychoanalysis is that the latent content of dreams can be understood in terms of symbolism. This is the world of towers and tunnels, much beloved by the public.

Despite the criticism of psychoanalysis, Soviet psychiatrists are less dismissive of psychoanalysis than is commonly thought. The general attitude is that Freud was an important figure in the development of psychology and psychiatry and that he introduced some important concepts.

Current practice

Psychotherapy in the Soviet Union has traditionally been short-term and directive. It is thought to cover most interactions between patients and doctors. Babayan (1985) defines psychotherapy as a system of healing based on the influence of language and says that it is an indivisible part of medicine, in that the doctor-patient relationship is built on psychotherapeutic principles. In the broadest sense Soviet psychotherapy also covers a wide range of activities such as exercise, gymnastics, sports, art, psychodrama, games, music, discussions based on watching films or reading newspapers and books. Smulevitch (1983), in the psychotherapy section in the Handbook, quotes early Soviet psychiatrists like Gannushkin and Yudin as stressing the importance of the interview and the ability to pay close attention to everything that the patient tells you. He considers that the goals of psychotherapy depend upon the clinical picture and the stage of the disorder, also the content of the conflict-producing situation. In the acute stage it should encourage calming and relaxation and reduce anxiety. Later stages are directed towards the reconstruction of the disturbed relationship between the person and his environment, aiming for resocialization and a return to work. He considers that early drug treatment facilitates psychotherapy and also makes the point that it may be necessary to change the patient's environment if that is part of the conflict.

The notion that it might be appropriate in the context of psychotherapeutic treatment for altering the environment differences is one of the major differences between the Soviet and Western approaches. Most Western psychotherapy is geared towards the resolution of internal conflicts and changing the attitude towards the external environment, not changing the external environment. Soviet psychotherapy does, of course, incorporate this, but, because of the concept of a dynamic relationship between personality and environment, allows for changing the environment within the context of therapy. Western psychotherapy, especially Freudian and cognitive therapy, is criticized because they simply expect a change in the way the patient looks at reality. In some ways this is similar to some radical criticisms of psychotherapy, especially of cognitive therapy, that it is simply a way of adapting people to the deficiencies in society.

Rational Therapy

Rational Psychotherapy (RT) was developed by Bekhterev and later generations of Soviet psychiatrists on the basis of the work of Dubois [3], which was translated into Russian in 1912. Smulevitch (1983) writes that it is a form of psychotherapy which employs logic, reason and explanation, but may also use indirect suggestions and emotional influence. It is a dialogue between the patient and doctor which requires the active participation of the patient. Because it relies upon the doctor-patient relationship the personality of the doctor is critical. The disorder is

---

3. He believed that false reasoning was the cause of neurosis and that this could be treated by logically demonstrating the patient's false ideas.

explained and various measures are used in order to try and remove false ideas.

Lauterbach (1984) writes that the psychiatrist attempts to give patients a scientific explanation of his disorder and the purpose of treatment. There is also a rational examination of the patient's attitudes and memories and an attempt, using logic and reasoning, to change attitudes and to resolve the underlying conflict in the context of the environmental circumstances. As well as explanation and analysis there may also be suggestions and instructions. Each session begins with a recapitulation of the previous session and of the homework. This usually consists of the patient working alone on some of his questions, for instance using a notebook to record symptoms and test aetiological theories. There may be practical exercises, for instance setting a patient to walk upstairs to demonstrate that the pulse rate goes up ie that it is a physiological mechanism rather than a sign of an impending heart attack.

A structured approach to RT might consist of the following phases:
1. A relaxation phase in which patients are encouraged to rest, sleep, possibly using tranquillisers and hypnosis.
2. The clarification phase in which patients are encouraged to see the links between their symptoms and what is going on in their life (in terms of personality, conflicts and the demands of the environment).
3. The phase of reconstruction in which new behavioural patterns are developed.
4. The training phase in which these are reinforced.

Unlike the traditional psychoanalytic approaches, RT does not attempt to be neutral but appeals to the "moral" side of the patient [4]. The general drive towards improvement in moral standards and increased knowledge is illustrated by the discussion of "bibliopsychotherapy" (which may be used as part of RT) which involves reading followed by group discussion of the material (Zavilianskaya, 1987). She writes that the choice of material depends upon the educational level of the patient and the nature of the problems, especially of the conflict-producing experiences.

Some Soviet psychiatrists are critical of Rational Therapy, arguing that the patient's problem is not that they have the wrong information, but that they are not able to integrate new information properly. Therefore the attempt to persuade someone through the power of logic is inevitably doomed to failure. They claim that the successes of RT are due to the fact that other factors are playing a part - including suggestion. Lauterbach (1984) is critical of the approach in its heavy emphasis on the authority and wisdom of the doctor. He writes that there are inevitably problems in patients who are cleverer than their doctors. There is also little research into efficacy. Zachepitsky, in the commentary, stresses that RT is rarely used alone and is a general approach, only really used by those with no other background in psychotherapy.

Lezhepekova and Pervov (1977) discuss various aspects of the RT. They claim that neuroses develop as a result of a maladaptive reaction to external circumstances and/or sensations from internal organs (which in this context are

---

4. Zavilianskaya (1987) quotes the pre-Revolutionary Russian psychotherapist, Yarotsky, 1908, who stressed the importance of getting the patient to strive for some ideal. He coined the term aretotherapy (from the Greek work for prowess) as a type of psychotherapy.

also external) and that therapy must change the perception of these circumstances. In a large sample of patients with various forms of neurosis they claim to have shown that RT is more effective than hypnosis or autogenic training. Neurasthenic patients seemed to do particularly well with RT.

Suggestion and hypnosis
Karvasarsky (1980) writes that every discussion with a doctor is a form of suggestion. The words are the most important component, but gestures and expressions also play a part. Suggestions can be given to patients in full consciousness, either directly, when patients are aware of the process, or, more rarely, indirectly. Suggestions may also be given during sleep, hypnosis or under narcosis. There are also various techniques for automated suggestions. Zavilianskaya (1987) writes that suggestion is a form of mental mechanism which taps the functional reserves of the mind, mainly through unconscious mental activity [5]. It is necessary to overcome barriers to suggestion. These barriers may be logical/critical, intuitive/affective or ethical. It is easier to make effective suggestions which are closer to the patients' system of beliefs. Important factors are the affective state of the patient, the authority of the psychotherapist and the effects of previous suggestions. A certain type of mental set (*ustanovka*) predisposes people to suggestion and there have been attempts to measure suggestibility. However, it is not thought that this is a fixed trait in people, but that it varies with age, with the stage of the illness, and, obviously, with the nature of the suggestion.

Lauterbach (1984) describes a model of information processing developed by Sviadosch. Complex information is generally processed consciously in order to test it and remove inconsistencies, but most information is processed without reaching consciousness. If information has been previously verified, and therefore fits in with the person's world view, there is greater likelihood of assimilation. Other factors that increase this are to do with the nature of the signal, for instance whether or not a message is given with conviction or is repeated by members of the group. Maturity influences the process, with greater maturity leading to a greater need for verification. Children are more likely to assimilate information without verification. Verification is also impeded in patients with altered states of consciousness and brain damage. Patients in whom reasoning is impaired, for instance alcoholics, patients with atherosclerosis, psychopaths with high emotional arousal are more suggestible [6]. Suggestion and hypnosis rely upon the fact that suggested information is not processed critically by the patient, but has an immediate effect on the organism. Ideas and emotions can be influenced without involving the patient's personality or without information being logically processed.

Suggestions can be made when patients are alert in individual and group sessions. The conditions under which the procedure takes place are important. Patients should be quiet and comfortable. The doctor generally takes an authoritative line, and, in contrast to RT, the patients are encouraged to relinquish their critical faculties and become passive. However, the passivity is only a feature

5. Pavlovian theory explains the efficacy in terms of partial inhibition (during the near-sleep hypnotic state) which allows a suggestion to exert its maximal influence.
6. It is sometimes suggested that this is why some alcoholics turn to religion.

of the actual session, not of the treatment as a whole. There is normal interaction outside the sessions, and it is generally considered necessary to use RT to convince the patient of the value and sense of the suggestions which are being given.

Hypnotherapy
Rozhnov (1985) claims that Pavlov dispelled the "fog of mystery" about hypnosis and put it onto a scientific basis by showing that the hypnotic trance was a stage of cortical inhibition. Hypnosis is a state of somnolence or near-sleep, but with an alert "monitoring point" in the cortex which allows rapport to be maintained and suggestions made. EEG studies suggest that the hypnotic trance represents a state of altered consciousness similar to that achieved in deep relaxation, drowsiness or near-sleep. Smulevitch (1983) gives some techniques for inducing a state of relaxation and writes that it is then necessary to make verbal contact and give the suggestions. The whole technique must be explained to the patient. Sessions last for 35-40 minutes and generally 10-15 sessions are used. It may be done on an individual basis, or, more commonly, in groups, a technique again introduced by Bekhterev.

Karvasarsky (1980) writes that hypnosis has a more powerful effect than suggestion. It is helpful with most neurotic symptoms, but is most useful in the hysterical neuroses and least in the obsessive-compulsive. The technique is especially useful in sleep disorders, but   longer sessions may be required. Medication, generally barbiturates, can be used in patients who are difficult to hypnotize [7]. Rozhnov (1985) describes the technique of hypnocathartic suggestion as one of the more promising methods. This is given at the deepest stage of hypnosis, which is established by the recording of super-slow waves on the EEG. He considers that there is a special relationship between the conscious and unconscious in hypnosis which allows meaningful conceptual suggestions to affect the patient. Poliakov and Kokhanov (1988) review hypnotherapy for the Korsakoff journal. They describe it as a useful, but non-specific treatment, and say that more research is required.

Narcopsychotherapy.
In this technique patients go through various stages of consciousness by use of intravenous barbiturates, also, more rarely, nitrous oxide. It can be used to give suggestions in patients who are difficult to hypnotize. Its main use is in the neurotic disorders.

Autosuggestion
Autosuggestion is usually done after preliminary treatment with RT and suggestion. The patient concentrates his thoughts on some therapeutic content. It might involve repeating to himself, about twenty or thirty times, a simple phrase like "I can cross the street" or "Every day I feel better and better" (Lauterbach, 1984). This can be done 1-3 times a day for just 2-3 minutes. Bekhterev suggested that the best times were on waking and just before sleep [8].

---

7. Tokarsky, towards the end of the nineteenth century, used chloroform to facilitate hypnosis.

8. It has been pointed out to me that this bears some similarity to the Jesus prayer of the Eastern Orthodox Church, an incantation repeated many times over.

Uses of suggestion techniques

The various suggestion techniques are used in neurotic disorders, insomnia and also psychosomatic and organic disorders such as hypertension, duodenal ulcers, asthma. They are also considered to have a place in the treatment of addictions. Rozhnov (1985) mentions that they are particularly helpful in dermatology, where intractable skin diseases such as eczema, warts, psoriasis can be successfully treated by hypnotic suggestion. Endocrine, gynaecological and obstetric disorders, for instance the vomiting of pregnancy, can also be helped. They may be used the in major psychoses along with drugs, but their main value is in the borderline conditions. As discussed above they are generally combined with RT and, sometimes, drug treatment. Depending upon the setting there may be a wide variety of different treatments combined, including, for instance, measures to stimulate activity such as work, sport or various types of exercise and baths. The combined use of tranquillisers and hypnosis might be followed by a spell of occupational therapy and music therapy, possibly accompanied by psychotherapy.

Lauterbach (1984) describes suggestion techniques involving the use of recording equipment, telephones and televisions. These tend to be used on the fringes of psychiatry, for instance in health resorts and sanatoria. These are generally situated on the Black Sea or Baltic coast and deal with minor neurotic disorders, tired managers, actors and workers. There are beds with earphones which can tune into different channels: eg soothing wave noises, suggestions accompanied by music, hypnosis. Also the therapist can talk directly to the patient. Suggestions are also broadcast on a regular basis. He writes that there is some research to suggest that resorts with these devices are more beneficial than those without. However, he quotes some of the criticisms of these methods, for instance by Velvovsky, the former Professor of psychotherapy at Kharkov, who argues against the mystification and commercialisation of psychotherapy, claiming that some of the newer methods are no more than a form of fairground entertainment.

Autogenous training

According to Karvarsarsky (1980), autogenous training is a technique which aims to achieve relaxation and normalization of vegetative (autonomic) function by creating new conditioned reflex links. It was developed by the German psychiatrist J.H.Schultz (1932) who demonstrated that it was possible to bring about physical effects, for instance changes in pulse rate, by suggestion. The techniques were first used in the Soviet Union at the end of the 1950s and early 1960s. The efficacy of the technique is thought to be related to the relaxation induced and the self-suggestion. It is carried out on an individual, or, more commonly, group basis with sessions lasting for 20-90 minutes and taking place once or twice a week. It is considered most useful in anxiety, sleep disorders and the syndrome of neurasthenia, especially for the somatic symptoms. It is less effective in patients with asthenia, hypochondriasis, obsessive-compulsive syndromes and hysteria.

Pathogenetic psychotherapy

Pathogenetic psychotherapy is a form of exploratory psychotherapy based upon Miasishchev's theory of relationships or *otnoshenia* [9]. Lauterbach (1984) writes that pathogenetic psychotherapy is the only dynamically oriented psychotherapeutic approach within the Soviet Union [10]. Zachepitsky's commentary to Lauterbach (1984) stresses the fact that Miasishchev's psychology was based upon the tenets of Marxism. He writes that Miasishchev considered that the most important aspect of the personality was the system of otnoshenia, especially the social relationships, but this was not independent of the functioning of the brain or Pavlovian physiological principles.

Karvasarsky (1980 and 1986), a psychiatrist at the Bekhterev Institute in Leningrad and the leading advocate of the treatment, writes that the aim of pathogenetic psychotherapy is reconstruction of a disturbed system of otnoshenia (relationships/attitudes). Incompatibilities between the personality and particular life situations produce pathogenic conflicts which result in neuroses. The personality in this context is the system of interactions between the individual and the social environment. It is made up of all his attitudes and relationships, both to people, the world, and also to abstract concepts. Neurosis is produced by the conflict between two different sets of otnoshenia which are of significance to a particular individual. The disruption of the otnoshenia should normally be resolved, either by satisfying a need, resolving a contradiction or changing the otnoshenia. Failure of resolution produces a state of tension and excitability in which thought processes become subjective and behaviour lacks clear direction so that it is no longer adaptive. These conditions promote the development of the neurosis. Thus, the conflict is critical in producing the neurosis, but, as expected from the theory, the duration and severity of a conflict is less important than the significance of the conflict to that individual. Moreover, particular types of conflict produce particular neuroses. The theory attempts to explain the psychogenesis of the three forms of neurosis: hysterical, obsessional and neurasthenic.

The first stage of psychotherapy is the exploration of the patient's emotional reactions, motivations and attitude systems. The second stage is the identification of the pathogenetic circumstances that led to the onset and development of the neurotic reaction. The third stage is to achieve insight, making the patient aware of pathogenic links. The final stage is to attempt to resolve the situation and/or conflicts. The method can be used individually or in groups. He suggests that moving from individual to group is most appropriate for the final stage when the aim is to resolve the situation or the conflict.

The hysterical conflict is essentially one between desire and reality. The individual overestimates his abilities and often strives for unrealistic goals. There are increased expectations of the world, and he finds it hard to modify his wishes to the needs of society. The symptoms are the result of the way in which the patient tries to overcome this contradiction in an irrational manner. There is poor insight. The main feature of the upbringing is the lack of boundaries. Thus, there may be a history of being "spoilt" and pampered, with parents giving way to the child's whims and fancies. There may be a history of a deprived upbringing, although a feature of this would be that clear boundaries were not set. Thus, attention might have been gained by certain types of behaviour such as tantrums or inappropriately adult behaviour.

---

9. The term otnoshenia can be translated as relationships, links or relations (usually the latter). This can cause some confusion because the psychology of obshchenia is also translated as relationships. However, the term obshchenia is concerned with social processes rather than intra-psychic processes. By contrast, the term otnoshenia could almost be translated as attitudes in that it incorporates the person's mental attitudes as well as his "links" or relationships.

10. The method has been assessed from a psychoanalytic perspective by Ziferstein (1964).

The obsessive-psychasthenic conflict is between two different sets of inner demands or tendencies. Thus, it might be a struggle between desire and duty or between a natural drive and an ethical principle. This could be a conflict between love and obligation or between a personal inclination and a sense of social responsibility. If one or other of the conflicting attitudes became dominant it would meet resistance and lead to hesitancy and indecision. This creates the circumstances in which an obsessional neurosis may arise. The feature of the upbringing is excess care and caution. In attempting to avoid possible dangers the parents allow no room for independence and initiative to develop in the child.

An example is given of a 40 year-old woman who had a strict upbringing out in the rural areas. After leaving school she went to work on a State Farm and then married "without love", although she was fond of her husband. Her obtrusive neurosis, with a marked dirt phobia, began after she started to have an affair with another man. Lauterbach (1984) gives another example, describing the case of a woman with typical hysterical symptoms but who, on the face of it, seemed to have a conflict more typical of obtrusive neurosis. She was torn between her husband and lover and the conflict seemed to lie between desire and duty, a typical obsessional type of conflict. On closer analysis, however, it turned out the real conflict centred around the fact that she would have nowhere to live if she left her husband. Thus it turned out to fit the theory in that it was actually a conflict between desire and external reality, the kind of conflict one would expect to see in hysteria.

The neurasthenic conflict is between basic ability and the attempt to meet the demands of the environment. There is a mismatch between one's own abilities (which, in contrast to the hysterical conflict, are recognized as limited) and the persons own expectations or those from the outside world. This leads firstly to overexcitation and then to exhaustion. This is thought to be especially related to the increased demands of modern life. The main feature of the upbringing is that parents tend to have expectations of the child which are beyond him and do not take into account his real abilities.

An example is given of a 42 year-old man who came from a family in which success and position in society were all important. Although he had limited abilities, he was pushed hard by his parents and he managed to graduate from his institute and get a good job, eventually becoming head of his section. Unfortunately, at this point he began to find it difficult to cope with the job, and the performance of the collective suffered, leading to criticism of him. At this stage he began to develop headaches, insomnia and irritability.

An important component in the structure of the neurotic conflict is what is referred to as the compensatory mechanism. Some types of compensation just deal with the particular problem and don't touch the real conflict. Others, however, might solve the conflict fully. Changing behaviour to meet the demands of a situation and simple denial are types of compensatory mechanism. A longitudinal study of 200 neurasthenics was able to show the development of the disorder from rational adaptation to neurotic symptomatology. The first stage was characterized by an attempt to adopt an active strategy in dealing with the psychotraumatic situation. If this did not work, for instance because the situation became worse or was prolonged, the second stage saw the development of a new position relative to the situation: firstly a passive attitude, with an attempt to accommodate or adapt, and, subsequently, attempts to avoid the situation, using more pathological mechanisms, closer to neurotic defences. This second stage is shorter than the first and soon leads into the stage of neurotic adaptation and the "flight into illness".

It might seem that in many ways the concept of neurosis derived from this theory is close to a traditional Freudian concept. A fundamental difference, however, concerns the role of the unconscious. A second major difference concerns the nature of the underlying conflicts, especially the emphasis on innate drives, sex or aggression. Soviet psychiatrists are sceptical about these and about the traditional conflicts that derive from them, especially more exotic notions such as that of castration anxiety and penis envy. The concepts were scathingly dismissed by Miasishchev as "pseudo-scientific fantasies concerning the inner world."

Lauterbach (1984), who worked with Karvarsarsky and his colleagues at the Bekhterev Institute, gives examples of the methods and stages of pathogenetic psychotherapy. The psychology of otnoshenia is becoming increasingly used in Soviet psychotherapy, for instance being taught at the All-Union psychotherapy centre in Moscow.

Collective or group therapy
Smulevitch (1983 and 1985) writes that collective or group psychotherapy has been used since the second half of the nineteenth century. Soviet psychiatrists, including Bekhterev and Giliarovsky, took up the method. The goals include activating patients and explanation of the disorders. The groups are run by a psychotherapist (usually a doctor or psychologist), but allow for the influence of members of the group on each other. The groups may be large (25-30 people), medium (10-15) or small (6-8) and may be open or closed. They should be heterogeneous with regard to age, sex, and, when possible, diagnosis, but all patients should have disorders thought to have a psychogenic aetiology. There should be no more than two to three patients in a group who have either hysterical or obsessional character traits. He stresses that in some groups, especially those for alcoholics and psychopaths (personality disorders), it must be used in combination with other social methods like work or culture therapy. Lauterbach (1984) quotes a Soviet author, Libikh, as writing that the contraindications are drug addiction, various somatic hysterical symptoms, some physical disorders. Caution should be applied in the young and in acting-out psychopaths.

The sessions are of ninety minutes and can be once a week or once a day for various periods of time. The relationships within the group are important and it is necessary to have an atmosphere of mutual trust, openness and respect for others. There are various types of activity:

1. Discussion. This may be biographical (the life history of one member of group) or thematic (discussing general problems) or interactive (looking at the relationships within the group)
2. Acting situations and role-play. This produces extra material for discussion. It is especially useful when it is difficult to verbalize emotions and there is excess "intellectualization". Members may change roles to experience the feelings of others and see themselves through other eyes.
3. There are also non-verbal activities such as psychogymnastics, miming, pantomimes.

Ponomareff (1986) describes a session of group therapy on his visit to an acute admission ward. Transference issues were not discussed and the psychotherapist was seen more in the light of a caring friend. However, unconscious processes were looked at and he notes that there were attempts at giving insight to patients with delusions.

Family therapy

Family therapy, as one of the forms of collective or group therapy, has a long history in the Soviet Union. It is used particularly in child and adolescent psychiatry [11]. Smulevitch (1983 and 1985) writes that family psychotherapy is one type of collective psychotherapy. It examines family relationships and aims to improve or reconstruct relationships within family members. It is used in treatment-resistant neurotic disorders, but also in the rehabilitation of psychotic patients in order to create a better emotional atmosphere in the family of the patient.

Karvarsarsky (1980) writes that family therapy has an important place in foreign literature, with a theoretical basis which covers a wide spectrum of concepts from the psychoanalytic to the existential. He argues that it can be done as a type of pathogenetic group therapy to look at the interpersonal relationships within the family and to work on emotional disturbances. Conflicts are investigated by analysis of the history of the family and of the previous experiences of the family members. The reconstruction of the family relationships is especially important in the rehabilitation and prophylaxis of neurotic patients. The treatment is carried out in in-patients and out-patients by one or two therapists and with one or more families.

Behaviour therapy

Behaviour therapy, generally referred to as conditioned reflex psychotherapy is used in the Soviet Union, although not widely. The theoretical and practical objections to the treatment are discussed below. Karvasarsky (1980) describes typical regimes, including desensitization and flooding, based on the work of Wolpe. He writes that this might be used in patients with isolated phobias and general obsessive-compulsive disorders, but should be combined with pathogenetic psychotherapy. The behaviour modification includes techniques familiar in the West: keeping a diary, planning strategies, in-vivo exposure. "Functional training" is an earlier form of Soviet behaviour therapy, essentially a form of desensitization.

Lauterbach (1984) describes a number of "behaviour therapy" techniques that are used, although not particularly widely. These include aversive conditioning in alcoholism, with the use of apomorphine to produce nausea. It is thought that there are better results if the treatment is used in groups, with some patients having the apomorphine, and others not. Insomnia may be treated with "conditioned sleep" in which a stimulus, for instance the ticking of a metronome, is paired with sleep after a hypnotic drug.

Lauterbach (1984) describes the work of Pokrass, a psychotherapist working at the Bekhterev when he was there. He considers that Pokrass, who has a traditional background in Soviet psychotherapy, seems to have independently developed a

---

11. According to a standard Czechoslovakian text-book, in use in the Soviet Union, it is "...not always the most disturbed member of the family who breaks down, more often the one with least resistance."

form of behaviour therapy based on operant conditioning ie a system of rewards and punishments. It is used mainly in the treatment of obsessive-compulsive disorders.

The availability of psychotherapy
Psychotherapy in the broadest sense is widely practised in the Soviet Union, mainly because of the dispensary system which means that the sector psychiatrists and nurses form long-standing, often close, relationships with the patients on their lists. This tends to be supportive, rather didactic psychotherapy, essentially based on the principles of Rational Therapy. The "symptomatic" types of formal, structured psychotherapy discussed above are also available to many in-patients and out-patients. Exploratory psychotherapy has only been available in a few specialist centres in the past, but, with the spread of the psychology of otnoshenia and the gradual increase in the number of psychologists, this is also developing. This momentum for this has come from a number of centres, perhaps with the Bekhterev Institute in Leningrad taking the lead.

The Bekhterev runs in-patient pathogenetic psychotherapy for patients with borderline disorders. Admissions are generally planned and an attempt is made to admit patients together, generally in a group of ten or so. Admissions last for two months and there are four ninety-minute sessions per week run by psychiatrist and/or psychologists. Nurses carry out behaviour therapy, for instance taking patients out of the hospital. Drugs are used sparingly.

Kabanov (1986) reports that group psychotherapy for psychotic patients has also been introduced at the Bekhterev Institute. One aim of the group is to provide emotional support to other members. There is also work on improving social behaviour and work on relationship skills. At a research meeting at the Bekhterev in 1988, Vid, the psychiatrist involved, argued that psychotherapy in schizophrenia was insufficiently used in the Soviet Union, maintaining that his work on group in-patient psychotherapy showed that re-admissions are reduced by 20%. There was a heated debate about this approach at the meeting that I attended, and a number of psychiatrists were rather dismissive about it. One psychiatrist argued that psychotherapy could not affect an endogenous process, a view which is not in keeping with the Soviet concept of disease and did not seem to be shared by others. Others argued that the patients in the group were not really schizophrenic but fell more into affective or borderline categories.

One feature of psychotherapy in the Soviet Union is its relatively wide usage in general medicine in the treatment of somatic disorders. Psychotherapy is carried out in general hospitals and polyclinics and there are plans to increase this. According to Babayan (1985) the Ministry of Health attaches importance to the development of psychotherapy rooms within general hospitals. Psychotherapy is considered to have a particularly important role in certain types of illness, especially dermatological, endocrine and gynaecological disorders. There are also plans to increase the availability of sex therapy. There is also psychotherapy in some of the sanatoria which are run by trade unions and other organizations [12].

According to Lichko, most adolescents in Leningrad with psychiatric disorders will get some form of psychotherapy. All will receive individual psychotherapy,

12. Lauterbach (1984) writes that psychotherapy is available in 300 or more sanatoria.

119

generally carried out by a psychiatrist. Most will also receive family therapy. About 10% have some form of behaviour therapy and collective therapy for this group is used very little.

There are clearly marked regional differences with regards to the availability of psychotherapy. However, it is claimed that usage is not confined to the major centres. Some areas, for instance the Ukraine, have more of a tradition of psychotherapy than, say, the Asian republics.

Comparative aspects

Some of the Soviet literature seems to suggest that psychoanalytic psychotherapy is widely available to psychiatric patients in the West, a view that is far removed from the reality of day-to-day psychiatry. In Britain a range of psychotherapeutic techniques, mainly behavioural and socially-oriented, are available to patients within the National Health Service. Exploratory psychotherapy, on the other hand, is available only to a limited number of selected patients. In the USA exploratory or psychoanalytic psychotherapy is mainly used in the private sector. A patient might be seen once or twice a week for two to three years. This is more intense individual input than a patient would receive in the Soviet Union. Patients with adequate insurance are still able to get a reasonable number of psychotherapy sessions, although the recent trend has been to limit these to perhaps thirty or forty [13]. Centres which cover "Medicaid" patients generally offer a small number of half hour sessions. Exploratory psychotherapy, albeit limited in duration, is therefore available to a fairly wide section of the population and the accusation that this treatment is the preserve of the rich is perhaps unfair.

The picture is different for patients in the public sector who generally have little or no opportunity to have psychotherapy. This covers the majority of patients with severe, chronic psychiatric disorders, in that even patients who started out in the private sector will eventually tend to drift into the public sector because of the high cost of treatment. In the Soviet Union, by contrast, a limited range of psychotherapeutic interventions is available to the majority of patients, including those with severe and chronic disorders [14]. Most of these would be seen as behavioural or social in the West, and viewed with suspicion as being too directive by psychoanalytically-oriented psychiatrists.

---

13. In the USA, especially on the West Coast, there is a remarkably wide choice of psychotherapeutic techniques, and some authors have managed to count up to 400. They range from traditional lengthy Freudian analysis through to the briefest of encounters with the most unusual of therapists. What they have in common is that they tend to be expensive, with rates of up to $200 per hour. What they do not have in common is their acceptability to insurance companies. Non-medical therapists have recently had a minor victory in getting certain types of treatment by psychologists accepted for insurance purposes.

14. Most Western visitors have made favourable comments about the wide usage of psychotherapy in the Soviet Union, although it is generally described as being brief, superficial and more directive. Salzman (1963) reported on the availability of different forms of psychotherapy in Moscow, for in-patients as well as out-patients, writing that this was in marked contrast to the USA. He writes: "During my visits to the mental hospitals I noted that psychotherapy is widely practiced in the Soviet Union and practically every hospitalized patient receives some form of it. Patients are seen at least once a week for regular psychotherapy sessions..". By contrast, other visitors such as Allen (1973) and Holland (1975) comment on the relative lack of psychotherapy, although they are referring to psychodynamic psychotherapy. Ziferstein (1966) spent a year observing the practice of psychotherapy at the Bekhterev Institute in Leningrad. He considered Soviet psychotherapy to be more active, directive and superficial, with much less emphasis on the transference. Rollin (1972) also comments on the more directive approach and the greater use of suggestion rather than insight in psychotherapy as applied to children and adolescents.

Chapter Eight

SCHIZOPHRENIA

The first point to be made about the Soviet concept of schizophrenia is that it is not very different to that of many Western psychiatrists. The symptoms making up the diagnosis are familiar enough, although there is greater emphasis on the course and development of the disorder. This has led to a classification of schizophrenia developed by Snezhnevsky according to the "forms" of the illness, based upon the course that the disorder takes, rather than the cross-sectional symptom profile. The three main forms are continuous schizophrenia, recurrent schizophrenia and an intermediate form, episodic-progressive. The traditional syndromes (eg paranoid, hebephrenic and catatonic) may occur at different stages in the development of the illness, and thus may be found in any of the three basic forms. It is this longitudinal approach that is perhaps the most distinctive feature of Snezhnevsky's classification and what has provoked much of the controversy about the Soviet concept of mental illness [1].

Snezhnevsky (1983), writing in the Handbook, defines schizophrenia as a progressive mental illness in which there is dissociation of mental function, that is a loss of unity of mental processes, and personality changes of a particular type which may develop rapidly or slowly. The features of the personality change are emotional impoverishment, lowering of energy potential and progressive introversion. "Productive psychopathological features", that is positive symptoms such as delusions and hallucinations, vary. The progressive nature of the illness differentiates schizophrenia from manic-depressive psychosis and the borderline mental disorders (neuroses and personality disorders).

Snezhnevksy (1983) writes that the clinical features in schizophrenia are determined, not just by the illness itself, but also by age, sex, social and cultural factors and sometimes by organic brain changes due to other disorders. This approach has something in common with the Bleulerian concept of schizophrenia: the notion of a basic underlying process in which many of the clinical features are actually determined by secondary factors, factors which may be psychological, social or biological [2].

An interesting view is that some of the features of the mental state may be related not to the disease itself but to processes that reflect the vulnerability to

---

1. A moving account of the development of schizophrenia from early childhood and its effects on the parents is given by Nabakov, an emigre Russian, in "Signs and Symbols" (Nabakov's Dozen, Penguin, 1960).

developing the disease. This notion is based upon the fact that similar abnormal mental states may be found in the healthy relatives of schizophrenics. Thus, some of the features of the mental state in schizophrenia, perhaps those that distinguish it from disorders such as manic-depression, may be the ones which have a genetic basis, whereas the features responsible for the disease itself may be more determined by environmental factors, possibly a physical agent.

One aspect of the Soviet concept of schizophrenia is that it includes the existence of intermediate forms, so that schizophrenia does not necessarily imply a poor prognosis, even though it might be thought of as a chronic disorder. Vartanian (1983) writes that genetic and clinical studies indicate the existence of transitional forms, and suggests two different continua, one running from normal health through personality disorder of the schizothymic or schizoid type and on to continuous schizophrenia. The second continuum runs through cyclothymia to recurrent schizophrenia or the affective psychoses. There may also be a third continuum for the intermediate form, episodic-progressive schizophrenia.

Development of the concept
In the nineteenth century Kandinsky, probably influenced by the French psychiatrist, de Clerambault, described a psychotic syndrome whose features included the passivity phenomena - essentially describing patients who would now be diagnosed as schizophrenic. Korsakoff introduced into Russian psychiatry a similar concept to Kraepelin's Dementia Praecox. Bleulerian and psychoanalytic concepts had an impact, leading to a greater emphasis on features such as thought disorder and the affective changes and the description of relatively benign forms, both acute and chronic. In contrast to this, in the 1920s and 1930s there were also attempts to explain schizophrenia in terms of the infectious psychoses that were being investigated at the time. At the Second All-Union Congress of Neuropathologists and Psychiatrists in 1936 a clearer definition of schizophrenia was called for and the concept was narrowed down. This is said to have been in contrast to trends in the USA and some European countries where psychological processes were being seen as features of schizophrenia (Galachian, 1968). However, as there was a narrowing down of the concept along symptom lines, there was a parallel development to broaden the concept along a different axis. Leading psychiatrists like Osipov, Krasnushkin and Giliarovsky argued for the retention of the concept of mild schizophrenia as defined by the course of the disorder rather than by symptomatology or the psychological content of thinking.

Over the past few decades the concepts have been developed further by Snezhnevsky, Nadjharov and a number of their colleagues based at the Institute of Psychiatry in Moscow (Snezhnevsky, 1972 and 1983). Their classification has been based on the historical trends described above and, despite the limited

---

2. Bleuler (1911) distinguished between fundamental symptoms, which he considered to be directly related to the underlying pathological process, and accessory symptoms which are influenced by personality, environment and psychological factors. The fundamental symptoms are related to thinking and emotions. There is a disruption in normal associations, for instance between ideas and emotions, and this results in changes in the way the world is perceived and understood. The other fundamental changes are ambivalence, autism (withdrawal into ones own inner world) and changes in affect, including the split between affect and cognition. Accessory symptoms are reactions of the personality to these primary changes and are particular to the patient rather than the disease. Although accessory symptoms such as hallucinations and delusions are often more prominent, Bleuler did not consider these to be related to the actual pathological process in that they could occur in other illnesses. He thought that they were related to psychological factors and might prove to be understandable in terms of Freudian psychology.

122

contacts, some developments in European psychiatry. In discussing the development of the concept of schizophrenia, Snezhnevsky (1983) emphasizes the contributions of Kraepelin and Bleuler. He also mentions various psychological approaches and the Schneiderian emphasis on phenomenology, but stresses the importance of what he describes as more objective approaches, for instance investigations into the defect state. He refers to the work of Kleist and Leonard who divided schizophrenia into different forms, based on the course of the disorder[3].

Descriptions of the longitudinal course are not unique to Soviet psychiatry. There have been similar descriptions by Western psychiatrists such as Arnold, Huber and Kohlmeyer. Snezhnevsky quotes the work of Arnold (1955) who followed up 500 schizophrenic patients for a period of 3-30 years. He reported that about 20% of patients had a phasic course with a good outcome, 40% showed a gradual deterioration and 40% had what he described as a "shift-like" course - episodes with changing symptomatology and partial recovery.

Classification

Snezhnevsky's classification is based on three main forms of schizophrenia: the continuous form, the recurrent form (which describes discrete episodes of illness with return to normality between episodes) and the episodic-progressive form (which describes episodes of illness but with steady deterioration).
The detailed systematization is given in the Table 6.

Table 6: Classification of schizophrenia (Snezhnevsky, 1983)

Continuous	malignant	
	progressive	- delusional variant
		- hallucinatory variant
Episodic-progressive [4]	malignant	
	progressive	
	schizo-affective	
Recurrent		
Special forms	febrile	
	paranoid	
	sluggish or slow-flow	

NB Slow-flow schizophrenia is sometimes placed as a variant of the continuous and episodic-progressive forms.

---

3. Kleist (1953) and Leonhard (1961) divided schizophrenia into the progressive (systematic) forms, marked by poor prognosis and deteriorating course, and the episodic or non-systematic psychoses, with good outcome and return to normality between episodes. There was a third "episodic-progressive" group which had a course between the two.
4. Episodic-progressive schizophrenia is sometimes referred to as *shuboobraznii*, which means shift-like (schub-like), that is developing with sudden shifts (schubs) or in fits and starts.

Although this classification has had a wide influence in the Soviet Union, particularly in research work, there are different approaches and there is no single concept, as is sometimes thought in the West. Even in Moscow there are schools of psychiatry which adhere to the traditional syndromal approach, essentially relying on ICD-9 for classification. Both systems may also be used together, the ICD-9 for administrative purposes and the Moscow system for clinical work, prognosis and research.

Korkina, the head of psychiatry at the Patrice Lumumba Medical School, places more emphasis on Schneiderian symptomatology in diagnosis, although she also stresses the disintegration of personality (Korkina et al, 1980). She writes that there is no agreed view about classification, but her approach is closer to most Western concepts in that she describes six basic types of schizophrenia which incorporate the traditional syndromes. The importance of the course is accepted as is the conventional division into the three basic forms. Moreover, she accepts that syndromes can change during the course. She describes paranoid, hebephrenic and catatonic types, and also simple schizophrenia. In simple schizophrenia there is marked change in personality which distinguishes it from ordinary pubertal crises, and there may be fragmentary psychotic features. In addition to these four classic syndromes she also mentions two syndromes related to the recurrent form of schizophrenia. Circulatory schizophrenia is similar to manic-depression but is distinguished by the fact that there is personality change between episodes. "Febrile" schizophrenia has a very acute onset; there are psychotic features with hyperthermia and somatic symptoms. She also makes the point that the use of neuroleptics has meant that schizophrenia often takes a forme fruste. There may be poorly developed forms, in which, although there is a progressive change, this is patchy and there are symptoms more suggestive of affective disorders, neurosis or psychopathy.

Bacherikov et al (1989) and the Handbook (1990), both published in the Ukraine, do not use the Snezhnevsky classification, giving the syndromal forms instead, although the Handbook (1990) also describes slow-flow as a variant of paranoid schizophrenia.

Clinical features
In this section the clinical features of the forms described by Snezhnevsky (1983 and 1985) will be described, in places with direct translations from these texts. Individual symptoms and syndromes have already been briefly described in chapter 2.

Symptoms
Symptoms may be considered as positive or negative. The positive symptoms include delusions, hallucinations, pseudohallucinations, depersonalization and oneiric symptoms. Negative symptoms include autism, lowering of energy potential, changes in emotionality, interests and attachments. Many of the negative symptoms may be reflected in a changed pattern of relationships, and, as with all of the above symptoms, they are not specific to schizophrenia. These symptoms combine to make up the different syndromes.

Syndromes
Nine basic syndromes were described in patients with schizophrenia in a large

study of 5000 patients followed up over the period 1951 to 1966 at the Institute of Psychiatry in Moscow. These were: asthenic, affective, pseudo-neurotic, paranoiac[5], hallucinatory, hallucinatory-paranoid, the syndrome of Kandinsky-Clerambault (a syndrome characterized by passivity phenomena: see page 25), paraphrenic and catatonic. The ninth was a terminal, polymorphic state, which seemed to be a relatively stable state.

Syndromes tend to change rapidly from one to another in episodic-progressive schizophrenia and more slowly in continuous schizophrenia. They usually change from the less serious to the more serious (eg from paranoiac to the syndrome of Kandinsky-Clerambault) and also within operational systems (eg obsessional to delusional thinking). The syndrome profiles have been modified over recent years with the advent of newer drugs, and this particularly applies to catatonia. The marked changes in syndrome patterns reinforce the view that diagnosis should be based on the forms, not on the presenting syndrome, which would tend to result in a changing and confusing picture.

Forms

CONTINUOUS SCHIZOPHRENIA
The main feature of this form of schizophrenia is the chronic, unremitting course. The speed of progression varies, as do the symptoms and the degree of personality change, but the fluctuation that is generally considered to be typical of schizophrenia is only manifested by a series of acute episodes with gradually worsening symptoms and fewer periods of remission. A bad outcome, with serious personality damage, is not inevitable, but even in the best cases the process of the illness never approaches total remission, so that some features always remain evident, the most characteristic one being the "stamp of inertia".

*Malignant continuous schizophreni*a, the variant with the worst prognosis, is characterized by early onset, generally in adolescence, and is commoner in males. It accounts for 4-5% of all cases. Onset is gradual, and the early stages show three basic components. There is loss of mental productivity ("energy potential"), which is most marked in the worst cases. There are rudimentary delusions and hallucinations. There are emotional manifestations consisting of atypical changes at the pubertal stage with bizarre preoccupations and behaviour, marked instability, aggression and difficulties with family relationships. Subsequently there are fundamental changes in the structure of the personality and a halt to further development. Inner life gradually becomes less rich and there is a decline in earlier interests and a decrease in activity. There is a profound change in the emotional sphere, with loss of drive and the ability to make relationships or maintain existing relationships. Patients may be calm and passive outside the home but aggressive within the family, and sometimes selectively eg cold and hostile with one parent and affectionate, sometimes rather tyrannically, with the other - usually the mother. Mental activity is reduced, so that new knowledge is poorly assimilated, despite the fact that the patient might spend many hours on a particular task, for instance in making bizarre collections of things. There may be "metaphysical intoxication" as shown by a preoccupation with particular aspects of philosophy. Activities like

5. See footnote 8 on page 25.

these may begin to dominate the patient's life, but are carried out in a solitary, unproductive way. There tends to be a fanciful approach to the subjects with loss of contact with reality. In this stage there may be depersonalisation and dysmorphophobia, but patients are not usually brought to the attention of doctors as parents tend to judge this stage to be due to laziness, lack of drive, general adolescent bad behaviour. It is important to note that these symptoms are not specific, and that they do not lead to a diagnosis of schizophrenia, but that they are more likely to be present in patients who subsequently develop this form of schizophrenia.

The development of the major psychosis is characterized by a polymorphic picture with affective, delusional, hallucinatory and pseudohallucinatory symptoms, mental automatism (passivity phenomena) and catatonic features. Before the era of pharmacotherapy there may also have been prolonged stuporous episodes or prolonged catatonic excitement, but they now tend to be rudimentary, with episodes of motor retardation or odd behaviour or catatonic excitement. The syndrome picture generally develops from the affective to the delusional to the catatonic, although there are no clear boundaries between these. The earlier that catatonic features appear the worse will be the final prognosis. A chronic catatonic-paranoid syndrome is often the final outcome. In this there are features of catatonia combined with mental automatism and non-systematized delusions which may be persecutory or fantastic. There may be remission in the early stages of the development of the psychosis, generally related to treatment. Stabilization in the catatonic-paranoid state occurs anything from 1 to 15 years after the major psychosis.

The premorbid personality is often characteristic and patients are often described as having been extremely compliant, even model children. They appear not to experience difficulties in adapting to family, kindergarten or school. With age, however, emotional responses become impoverished, and there is absence of creativity and originality. In up to a half of the patients there may have been some developmental abnormalities in childhood, either in mental development or motor skill.

Progressive continuous schizophrenia usually begins after the age of 25 and most cases develop in people in their thirties. Prognosis is worse in younger onset cases. One of most characteristic features of schizophrenia, the presence of delusions, dominates the picture in this form, which is sometimes called delusional (paranoid) schizophrenia. It is recognized that the major problem in diagnosis is defining the borderline between delusional and non-delusional thinking. The basic features of this disorder are that the delusional features dominate the picture and that there is a characteristic development with no phasic course.

In the early stages there may be obsessional and/or hypochondriacal features. Delusional ideas, usually of persecution or jealousy, are episodic and fluctuating at first, but they gradually systematize. There are usually some changes in personality at this stage. There may be rigidity, loss of affective flexibility, a narrowed range of emotional reactions and a gradually diminishing circle of interests and acquaintances. Patients become mistrustful, often gloomy. They may voice their suspicions at this stage, perhaps just when drunk, and often the changes are only noted by those who are closest to them. This opening phase can last anything from 5 to 20 years and over this time patients do not usually present to psychiatrists.

The obvious psychosis develops late and is characterized by delusions and hallucinations. Usually one or other predominates so that there are two variants: the delusional variant and the hallucinatory or hallucinatory-paranoid variant.

In the *delusional variant* there is a predominance of delusional thinking at all stages of the disorder. A typical progression might be from the paranoid syndrome with systematized delusions, but with no hallucinations or passivity phenomena, on to the syndrome of Kandinsky-Clerambault, in which there are paranoid delusions with passivity phenomena, and then on to a paraphrenic syndrome, in which fantastic delusions predominate. This course is only seen in severe cases and the condition may stabilise at an early stage either spontaneously or because of treatment. Patients with the worst prognosis, those who go on to develop the end-stage most quickly, are those in whom there are serious changes in personality, with psychopathic-like features, early in the course. This happens before the manifest psychosis, and there is loss of social adaptation, with anti-social acts, alcoholism, break-up of the family. On this background polymorphic, often non-systematized delusional ideas may develop. Poor outcome is associated with the presence of secondary catatonia and of fantastic (paraphrenic) delusions, for instance with megalomania. The end stage is characterized by a gross defect in emotional life, with thought disorder and disrupted speech, often with schizophasia. There may be mannerisms, catatonia, poorly systematized delusions and, commonly, pseudohallucinations. In the most serious cases there may be delusional confabulation. Deterioration does not always take place, and the disorder can stop at the paranoid phase. There are some patients in whom the symptoms are confined to the paranoid syndrome, and this may be thought of as an independent variant, paranoid schizophrenia. In this there are ideas of reference, hypochondriacal features and persecutory delusions, often with early systematization.

In the *hallucinatory variant* of progressive schizophrenia there are marked perceptual abnormalities, at first verbal illusions combined with delusional interpretations, and also elementary hallucinations (noises, whistles, calls, single words). Soon after this stage verbal hallucinations develop. These may consist of monologues, dialogues or commands. The content is generally hostile and unpleasant for the patient. There may be a background of unsystematized delusions of jealousy and persecution, ideas of reference and neurosis-like symptoms. This stage has a varying length, but rarely exceeds a year. The experience of hearing voices commenting on the thoughts and actions of the patient is the forerunner of change from hallucinations to pseudohallucinations. From that stage there is a rapid development into the syndrome of Kandinsky-Clerambault, in which pseudohallucinations are dominant. There are passivity phenomena: thought withdrawal and insertion, made images, memories, sensations and acts. At the peak of the syndrome there may be the phenomenon of delusional depersonalization in which there is a feeling of complete alienation. Although the syndrome of Kandinsky-Clerambault may occur in other forms of illness, it is most characteristic of the hallucinatory variant of progressive schizophrenia. Despite the passivity phenomena the key symptom is still the pseudohallucination. This stage usually last from 6 to 10 years. In the final stages there may be a paraphrenic syndrome with fantastic delusions.

EPISODIC-PROGRESSIVE SCHIZOPHRENIA

The feature of this form is a continuous course during which there are episodes which often have a marked affective component, either manic or depressive.

Malignant episodic-progressive schizophrenia has an early onset, and some features may manifest themselves before adolescence. There may be evidence of developmental disorder in children before any manifest psychosis. There is early reduction in mental activity and poor progress with loss of previous interests, secrecy, lack of activity, alienation. The manifest psychosis tends to develop early, usually at adolescence. There are affective, delusional and catatonic features, all of which tend to be rudimentary and unformed. Affective features are atypical, so that there may be hypomania without the raised mood. Depression tends to be accompanied by asthenic symptoms, irritability, malice, self-pity rather than self-blame. Dysmorphophobia and depersonalization are common. Delusional features include rudimentary ideas of grandiosity, persecution or reform. There may be psychopathic-like features as shown by problems with relationships, a tendency to sadistic acts, outbursts of irritation, abuse of drugs and alcohol. There may be hebephrenic crises consisting of episodes of excitement with silly movements and fatuous behaviour. The catatonic features vary so that retardation may suddenly change to impulsive aggression. Poses are adopted and there may also be other catatonic symptoms such as stereotypies, grimacing, pointless laughter. Pseudohallucinations are common.

Soon after the first episode the signs of schizophrenic defect becomes apparent. Remissions tend to be short, and there may be some catatonic symptoms during these periods. The features of later episodes are similar to the early ones, but with more of a tendency towards catatonic stupor, with pseudohallucinations. Affective features persist but are even more atypical with dysphoria rather than real depression. After a few episodes there is a severe deterioration in the level of mental activity and social functioning. In some cases the progression halts at an early stage and there is a period of relatively stable remission.

Many of the features are similar to the malignant variant of the continuous form and in many ways, especially after several episodes, it would be hard to differentiate between them. There are differences in the emotional sphere, however, and there is not the complete loss of affectivity that is typical of the continuous form. Thus, the ability to relate to people and show affection, especially to closer family members, is retained to a greater extent.

Progressive episodic-progressive schizophrenia is characterized by episodes of delusional disorder with affective features. On a syndromological classification it would correspond to paranoid schizophrenia with a remitting course. Thus, the predominant feature of the clinical picture is the presence of delusions. There may be fleeting catatonic features at the height of an episode, but they generally disappear quickly with treatment. Onset can be from childhood to middle age, and this may be preceded by personality changes such as autism, emotional impoverishment, unreliability, rigidity. There may be atypical affective changes. There are various different types of outcome after a manifest episode. There may be just one episode followed by a minor defect state. There may be progression with gradually worsening episodes and more of a defect state during the periods of remission. There may also be a more or less continuous type of paranoid schizophrenia.

Several types of episode are described: paranoiac, paranoid, paraphrenic and hallucinatory. Acute paranoiac episodes are characterized by a gradual development of interpretive delusions, generally with a concrete content, often hypochondriacal or persecutory or of jealousy. They may arise from a background of general suspicion and tension. The delusional ideas are often linked to aspects of the past life and they slowly develop to include a wide circle of suspected people. Signs of delusional behaviour might develop at this stage, but in situations unconnected with the delusional system they might carry on as normal. This stage might last from two months to two years, after which there is generally an onset of more acute symptoms such as marked anxiety, worry, premonitions of death. Afterwards there may be some depressive affect combined with limited insight and there is usually some defect state from the first remission onwards. Acute paranoid episodes are more like an acute variant of the Kandinsky-Clerambault syndrome and there are delusions, hallucinations, passivity phenomena and atypical affective changes. In acute paraphrenic episodes the delusions are more rudimentary and generally of a bizarre and fantastic nature.

In the acute hallucinatory episodes the key feature is the presence of interpretive delusional ideas, usually persecutory or of jealousy, but the episodes are also characterized by auditory hallucinations. These might begin as auditory illusions before developing into true hallucinations, the content of which generally matches the plot of the delusional system. In serious cases pseudohallucinations develop. In the early stages there are often affective symptoms, with anxiety, tension and depressed mood, the mood usually related to the delusional ideation. During remissions there is partial insight.

Schizoaffective episodic-progressive schizophrenia has also been referred to as polymorphic episodic-progressive schizophrenia. The clinical picture is similar to that described above, but there are more pronounced affective features, and, in some patients, psychopathic-like features. The attacks are more acute and polymorphic. The content of both delusions and hallucinations generally depends on the affect and do not generally become fully systematized. Just as the progressive variant is closer to continuous schizophrenia so this variant is closer to recurrent schizophrenia.

There tends to be a long stage before the psychosis becomes manifest during which time there may be mild character changes. There may be autism, alienation from family and friends and atypical, mild depression. Preoccupation with various themes is characteristic. These may be hypochondriacal or they may involve grand world schemes, often with a philosophical bent. There may be a depressive phase, usually with dysmorphophobia, hypochondriasis, jealousy and obsessional symptoms. There may be one episode or several. If the episodes get longer the disorder may become progressive. Many patients, however, remit and are left with cyclothymic personalities. In general there is no defect state (no decline in mental activity or social adaptation) despite the personality changes.

There is a subdivision into *affective-paranoid* and *affective-hallucinatory types*. In the former delusional ideas are found in the context of either depression or mania. In depression these tend to be either persecutory or delusions of jealousy. In mania they are often delusions of reform or invention. There is often rapid onset with demands for instant recognition and appreciation for the ideas. Patients are often agitated and irritable, and may progress into a melancholic or dream-like state of acute paraphrenia. The affective-hallucinatory type usually presents with depression and hallucinations. There may be symptoms of worry and anxiety/fear. There are verbal hallucinations with a depressive content, often of a rather dramatic nature and with a rather fantastic content. There are changes in personality with some withdrawal and a general loss of drive.

RECURRENT SCHIZOPHRENIA

This form, which is more common in women, carries the best prognosis. Onset is usually early and, as with manic-depressive psychosis, it has a phasic course, but various psychotic symptoms (delusions, hallucinations and pseudohallucinations) differentiate it from typical affective disorder. The important feature of this form is that however florid the symptoms might be during the acute episode the outcome is good, and there is usually full adaptation to work and life in general. The clinical picture varies during attacks and individual patients may present with the same picture during each attack or present with marked variations ranging from simple affective episodes to catatonia with clouded consciousness. Early development is generally normal, but the premorbid personality is often abnormal, with the prevailing feature being immaturity.

This form often begins with vague somatic symptoms which develop into affective swings. Mood may be increased with hyperactivity, increased self-confidence, an overestimation of one's worth, feelings of joy and/or exaltation. This may suddenly swing into a lowering of mood with absent-mindedness, feebleness, overestimation of dangers and difficulties. Genuine difficulties and conflicts can produce an over-reaction. The mood swings are intense and may be very brief, often lasting just a few hours. There are unusual bodily sensations and vegetative symptoms, with changes in blood pressure, palpitations, sweating, disturbance of appetite and sleep. This initial stage may be of very brief duration, weeks or months, and several years may elapse before the next stage.

The next stage usually begins with more marked affective symptoms, especially worry and anxiety/fear. There may be vague, non-specific, near-delusional fears about the self or the surroundings. These may fix into a particular delusional system, possibly with manifestations of delusional behaviour. This fluctuates and insight might be regained only to be lost again when a new set of circumstances produces more delusions. Subsequently an affective-delusional stage develops in which there is depersonalization and derealization, often with dramatic delusions, and passivity phenomena. This may develop into an acute paraphrenic episode (with fantastic delusions). There may be motor disorders and catatonic symptoms, in which there may be periods of excitement on a background of substupor. These were more prevalent before the era of pharmacological treatment. Oneroid states, in which there is dream-like and changed consciousness, may also occur.

Before the onset of the manifest psychosis most patients will have had fluctuations of affective tone which are subclinical and endogenous. The cycle of these swings tends to be shorter in patients going on to get catatonic-oneroid type symptoms and longer in those going on to develop a mainly affective picture. There may be more definitely cyclothymic picture before the onset of the psychosis and the phasic affective swings might be seasonal. During remission cyclothymic swings tend to continue.

The personality changes in this form usually date from the first years of the psychosis. They tend to be fairly mild, perhaps with some impairment of basic cognitive function (memory problems are often complained of) and also loss of interests, loss of drive and initiative. There may be excessive passivity, dependence on others, even rather childlike behaviour. In some cases there are compensatory personality changes, so that patients pay increased attention to their mental and physical health, possibly adopting their own regimes of work, rest and treatment. There may be marked rigidity and touchiness. Sometimes there are more profound changes with schizoid or psychopathic-like traits and definite lowering of mental productivity. On the other hand there may be no change in the personality structure. A significant number of people have only one attack in their lives.

An example of a patient with this diagnosis is given by Holland and Pavlova-Shakhmatova (1977).

The patient was a 35 year-old junior scientific worker at the Institute of Atomic Energy, who finished middle school (high school) with a "brilliant record", graduated from the physics faculty of Moscow University, and was asked to join the Institute of Atomic Energy where she was highly regarded as a good worker. She married at the age of 24, got along well with her husband, but had no children. She was always reserved and self-contained in her manner. At the age of 28 she had a psychotic episode in which she was depressed, deluded and experienced auditory hallucinations. She felt that she should be killed because she was so bad. She was in a catatonic stupor for six weeks, although there were also periods of excitement. She responded to treatment with trifluoperazine in high doses (80mgm per day). There were similar episodes when she was 33 and 35, and on both occasions she was again treated with trifluoperazine, and had long admissions to hospital, the last one being for five months. After her first admission she wrote up her dissertation for her Candidate of Science degree. During periods of remission, she was quite normal and functioned well at work. She was interviewed after the third episode had resolved and she was ready to return to work.

SPECIAL FORMS OF SCHIZOPHRENIA

Febrile schizophrenia is a rare form which has also been referred to as hypertoxic or fatal schizophrenia in that before the advent of neuroleptics it sometimes led to death. It may start like typical recurrent or episodic-progressive schizophrenia before the onset of the febrile attack. At this stage there is usually a change from catatonic excitement, with or without oneroid features, to an amentia-like state, possibly with more hyperkinetic excitement. Excitement is usually worse towards the evening. There is confusion and incoherence. There may be fantastic and disjointed delusions. Temperature tends to be higher during the periods of hyperkinesis and the amentia-like states. There may be disorders of movement with choreiform movements and lack of coordination.

Some authors have suggested that this is the natural progression of episodic-progressive schizophrenia, but Nadjharov (1972) argues that it is an atypical form of schizophrenia. There may be one attack followed by a series of non-febrile episodes or there may be several febrile attacks and then a return to a typical episodic-progressive course. It may occur at any age and is not linked to any particular somatic disorder. There is no consistent pattern to the fever. The raised temperature can occur from the beginning or at the onset of catatonia or only at the height of an attack. There may or may not be the general features of a febrile illness. Changes in the haematological picture include a raised white count, with lymphopenia, and a raised ESR. There may be changes in the proteins and raised bilirubin levels. The disorder is rarely lethal these days. Occasionally it progresses into coma or heart failure can occur during the amentia-like or hyperkinetic states.

SLUGGISH OR SLOW-FLOW SCHIZOPHRENIA *(vialotekushaya shizophrenie)* is discussed on page 149.

Diagnosis
Because schizophrenia may "wear other clothes" it is sometimes diagnosed provisionally, although Snezhnevsky (1983) maintains that the endogenous nature should always emerge over time and clarify the diagnosis. Thus, in the early stages, symptoms characteristic of neurotic disorders or personality disorders are common [6]. Smulevitch (1985) describes some of the prodromal features typically found in patients before developing schizophrenia and writes that they may resemble those found in patients with personality disorders except that they are not fixed or stable as they would be in a patient with a personality disorder. There may be schizoid traits, often with hysterical features, vegetative symptoms or with hyperthermia. Reactive lability is a feature of all these. By contrast, the personality changes after an endogenous psychosis tend to be more fixed, often with exaggerations of premorbid personality traits such as paranoia or hyperthymia.

Comparative aspects: concepts, classification, clinical features
The Bleulerian concept of schizophrenia had a major impact in the USA, and considerable influence in several European countries. Bleuler broadened the concept of schizophrenia in that his concept implied that the diagnosis did not rely upon the presence of delusions and hallucinations, but on his fundamental symptoms. These are related to changes in thinking and emotion and are more difficult to quantify and obviously more open to wide interpretation. After the Second World War attempts were made to define schizophrenia on the basis of more clear-cut symptoms. Schneider (1950) described a list of "first rank symptoms", consisting of certain types of delusions, auditory hallucinations and passivity feelings. Unlike Bleuler's fundamental symptoms, which were considered to be related to aetiology, these "first rank symptoms" have no theoretical significance, but are a pragmatic attempt to standardize the concept of schizophrenia. These symptoms have become the mainstay of diagnosis in several countries, especially Britain.

The British concept of schizophrenia, however, does not rely solely upon use of

---

6. It is, of course, recognized in the West that schizophrenia may present with neurotic episodes before the diagnosis manifests itself. Cancro (1985), in the Comprehensive Textbook of Psychiatry, writes that there are often brief, transient neurotic-like episodes in the past histories of patients with schizophrenia. Berrios and Bulbena (1987) report that subsequent admissions after a first admission with schizophrenia are often not for psychosis, but for variety of symptoms, including anxiety, depression, phobias, obsessional thoughts.

the first rank symptoms alone. The Oxford textbook adopts a pragmatic approach and divides schizophrenia into acute and chronic syndromes. The former is characterized by delusions, hallucinations and interference with thinking, whereas the features of the latter are "..apathy, lack of drive, slowness, and social withdrawal....often called "negative" symptoms." Thus, the acute syndrome is based on the presence of Schneiderian first-rank symptoms and the chronic on a vaguer picture, which takes into account the course of the disorder over time. In the Handbook of Psychiatry (1982) the European tradition is invoked, and indeed several of the authors are from mainland Europe. Discussing the concept, Stromgren emphasizes the importance that Bleuler placed upon the symptoms of autism and splitting and also mentions the "feel" of schizophrenia, described by the Dutch psychiatrist Rumke. Leff distinguishes between acute and chronic schizophrenia. The predominant features of acute schizophrenia, which may arise spontaneously or be preceded by neurotic symptoms, are said to be delusions and/or hallucinations with disturbed behaviour. Schizophrenia may be diagnosed in the absence of first rank symptoms if there are delusions with inappropriate affect. The chronic syndromes include the defect states and also schizophrenia of insidious onset in which there is a breakdown in relationships and social functioning.

German psychiatry places less emphasis on Schneiderian first rank symptoms and the importance of the longitudinal picture is increasingly recognized. Gross (1989) discusses Huber's work on the "basic" symptoms of schizophrenia which concern drive, energy, sensation, autonomic and cognitive changes. It is argued that these are the primary abnormalities in schizophrenia rather than the traditional psychotic symptoms. In longitudinal studies it is found that schizophrenics often have no psychotic features; in many patients pre-psychotic syndromes precede a first psychotic episode by ten years on average.

The American concept of schizophrenia was influenced by Bleuler, mainly through the teaching of Adolf Meyer, who described the schizophrenias as a set of behavioural patterns, essentially exaggerations of normal behaviour. There has also been a strong influence from psychoanalysis, despite the fact that Freud wrote little about the disorder. However, a number of psychoanalysts, most notably Harry Stack Sullivan, brought psychodynamic concepts to the study of schizophrenia, emphasizing the importance of the disturbance in interpersonal relationships from a dynamic perspective. Despite recent developments in nosology there remains a psychoanalytic tradition in which accessory symptoms (hallucinations and delusions) are considered to be understandable psychologically, thus requiring treatment by analytically-oriented psychotherapy. Cancro (1985), in describing schizophrenia as "an effort to adapt to a highly altered experience of both inner and outer reality", leaves room for the traditional psychoanalytic understanding of schizophrenia.

With the introduction of DSM-III, however, the concept of schizophrenia has moved closer to Europe (Andreasen, 1989). However, although DSM-III incorporates Schneiderian criteria, it still allows diagnosis on the basis of Bleulerian criteria alone. According to DSM-III criteria, the diagnosis of schizophrenia is based on evidence of deterioration in social functioning and the presence of one or more specific symptoms. These may be relatively short-lasting, and may be either delusions and/or hallucination or a combination of symptoms of the "Bleulerian" sort eg thought disorder and flat affect. An important aspect of DSM-III is that it brings in duration of symptoms as a diagnostic criterion. Symptoms must be present for at least six months, thus distinguishing schizophrenia from other brief psychoses, or temporary diagnoses eg schizophreniform psychosis (where the same symptoms may be present but for less than six months). It is important to note, however, that the "psychotic" symptoms may be of brief duration; all that is required for the diagnosis is evidence of social deterioration and poor functioning for six months - before or after the time of the acute symptoms. They give examples of possible combinations eg someone with six months of prodromal symptoms (deterioration in the level of social functioning or peculiar behaviour) followed by acute symptoms for a week.

There is resistence to the check-list approach of DSM-III. Lehman and Cancro (1985), for instance, argue that in some patients it is necessary to infer symptoms, also that patients might try to deceive the interviewer. They are also doubtful about the use of check-lists on the grounds that symptoms change over time and thus a diagnosis based upon check-lists changes over time [7]. They maintain that thought disorder, reflecting Bleulerian loss of associations, is the best guide to the disorder (although this may be present in one sentence and not the next) and conclude that there is no substitute for clinical judgement. Another key feature, "blunting of emotional response or a strikingly inappropriate emotional response", also favours a diagnosis of schizophrenia, and recognition of this requires clinical experience, for instance to differentiate it from an adolescent's "sheepish or defying smile". Thus, despite the introduction of diagnostic criteria, something of an intuitive approach lingers on. Cancro and Lehman (1985) also mention the "feel" of schizophrenia which has also been referred to as a Precox feeling. This is said to be "an intuitive experience by the examiner that determines whether it is possible to empathize with the patient." They quote a study in which 54% of 1000 European psychiatrists said that this Precox feeling was a reliable criterion for the diagnosis of schizophrenia.

We are left with a number of different views of schizophrenia, all based on different historical developments, but all carried through into various current concepts. The "Kraepelinian" emphasizes disintegration of the personality and the course and outcome, and tends to concentrate on the disease rather than the person. The "Bleulerian" makes a hypothetical division of symptoms into fundamental, which are disease-related (or process-related) and the accessory, which are psychological (complex-related), and provides a broad set of diagnostic criteria. The "Schneiderian" adopts a number of symptoms on pragmatic grounds for making the diagnosis. These are assessed at a particular point in time, and there is no emphasis on the course. There is no theoretical construct, except, perhaps, for the idea of permeability of ego boundaries ie a breakdown in the barrier between the individual and the environment.

Although the "Schneiderian" view is widely held it is also widely criticized. Hoenig (1983) quotes Kety's view of this. He writes of Schneiderian schizophrenia that it "..may be more prevalent, have a more favourable outcome, and be more responsive to a wide variety of treatments, but it is not schizophrenia." This

7. This is very similar to Snezhnevsky's view.

view reflects the attempts to isolate the core schizophrenia from other syndromes which present in a similar way, but which have a better outcome and possibly represent different disorders. Langfeldt (1937, 1956) distinguished this core group, true or process schizophrenia, from what he referred to as schizophreniform psychoses (patients with more acute onset, often precipitated by stress and having a better prognosis).

Soviet criticisms of Western concepts
Earlier Soviet criticism of psychological and phenomenological approaches was that they produced vague, broad concepts of schizophrenia and that attempts to find a simple psychological explanation for the disorder resulted in the neglect of the "clinico-pathological approach". Snezhnevsky (1983) criticizes the Schneiderian emphasis on phenomenology, writing: "...enthusiasm for the phenomenological approach led to a widening, not always clinically warranted, of the diagnosis. This is significantly linked with a subjective approach to the evaluation of the individual features in each different person." A further criticism is that diagnostic criteria tend to favour a static (cross-sectional) picture and fail to take into account the development, course and the different manifestations of the forms. His criticisms of the traditional psychoanalytic approach are that it proved fruitless to try to understand psychosis by drawing analogies with the psychoanalytic processes of normal mental life. He does not suggest that psychological processes should be ignored in schizophrenic patients, but makes the point that such processes apply to different groups of patients, also to non-patients, that they cut across nosological boundaries. Thus, they are not in any way fundamental to schizophrenia and cannot predict which treatment might be helpful or what the outcome might be.

There is some basis for these criticisms, even in relatively recent American texts. Thus, Lehman and Cancro (1985), in the Comprehensive textbook of Psychiatry, describe a number of core features of schizophrenia. They say that one of the most characteristic features is the "pronounced symbolism in the patient's often bizarre behaviour, ideation and speech" and that this is generally incomprehensible to others. Other key features include social withdrawal and loss of ego boundaries. They do not consider the first rank symptoms to be specific. They place particular emphasis on thought disorder, and refer to over-inclusion and concrete thinking, but also include false syllogisms and mystical-magical thinking (which some people would consider to be disorders of the content of speech rather than the form). "The one common factor running through the schizophrenic's preoccupation with invisible forces, radiation, witchcraft, religion, philosophy, and psychology is the leaning towards the esoteric, the abstract, the symbolic." Affective changes, with reduced emotional responses, are typical, but they stress the importance of cultural factors, and point out that what might be considered normal in an Anglo-Saxon culture might be thought of as a reduction of emotional response in a Mediterranean culture.

Snezhnevsky (1983) questions various sociological (sociogenetic) models which postulate factors in the macro (society) or micro (family) environments as possible aetiological agents. He claims that adherents of this view tried to establish a simple sociogenesis for schizophrenia, divorcing it from its essential biological nature. He argues that it was the claims of the more radical supporters of the sociogenetic school that provided the basis for the development of the "notorious" anti- psychiatry movement which maintained that schizophrenia was a myth or artefact and a product of society. He argues that such views are the inevitable consequence of vague, poorly defined concepts of mental illness.

Soviet and Western differences
Holland (1977) attempted to draw up a table to compare the different forms of schizophrenia with the syndromal classification. She suggested that the malignant subgroup of continuous schizophrenia might be equivalent to hebephrenic, catatonic, simple or undifferentiated schizophrenia, and that the moderate (progressive) subgroup was generally equivalent to paranoid schizophrenia. Recurrent schizophrenia is described as being equivalent to manic-depressive psychosis, psychotic depression or schizo-affective disorder. Severe episodic-progressive schizophrenia is equivalent to catatonic or undifferentiated schizophrenia, moderately severe to paranoid schizophrenia and the mild to paranoid states, neurotic disorders, latent schizophrenia and adolescent adjustment reactions. Slow-flow schizophrenia would also be equivalent to paranoid states, neurotic disorders, latent schizophrenia, adolescent adjustment reactions.

The classificatory system has changed somewhat since Holland's paper was published and episodic-progressive schizophrenia is now divided into malignant, progressive and schizo-affective types. Moreover, it is unlikely that the overlap between psychotic depression and recurrent schizophrenia would be found now. There is a logical problem in trying to compare a system based upon the course of the illness with one based upon the presenting symptoms. This explains the considerable overlap. Indeed, it is fundamental to the Soviet classificatory system that the different syndromal presentations cut across the main forms[8]. Comparisons with DSM-III are difficult for the same reason. Although DSM-III criteria require a six month period of social decline this is not the same as taking a longitudinal approach to diagnosis. The six month period will often relate to one episode of illness.

Although it is not possible to make direct comparisons between disorders defined on the basis of a cross-sectional picture of symptoms and one based on a longitudinal history, some of the forms are close to Western equivalents and in others the clinical profile allows direct comparison. Snezhnevsky (1983) writes that recurrent schizophrenia is similar to the DSM-III concept of schizoaffective disorder.

In order to examine the influence of the different concepts of schizophrenia upon classification it is worth at this stage attempting to summarize the main ways of conceptualizing schizophrenia. These are:

1. The traditional syndromal approach. This gives the main syndromes: paranoid, catatonic, hebephrenic, simple.
2. The Kraepelinian approach. This puts emphasis on the course of the illness and also on personality disintegration. Kraepelin considered that the

---

8. Several Western authors who write about the Soviet concept of schizophrenia have misunderstood this point and end up confusing the forms and syndromes. Cutting (1985) writes that the Snezhnevsky/Moscow school describes nine types of schizophrenia including asthenic, affective, paranoid types. However, he appears to have misunderstood the article that he quotes (Snezhnevsky, 1968). The article, which is in English, mentions that the nine syndromes do occur in patients with schizophrenia, but that they change and vary over time and may, moreover, occur in other conditions. They are not considered to be different forms of schizophrenia.

traditional syndromes were not fixed, but varied during the course of the illness.

3. The Bleulerian concept relies upon evidence for disturbance of intrapsychic processes: loosening of associations, autism, ambivalence and blunting of affect. The acute episode of florid psychosis, with "accessory" symptoms (delusions and hallucinations) is seen as being a response to psychological stress. However, even when these accessory symptoms are not present, the pathological process continues as a latent illness, although the person might appear to be relatively well.

4. The Schneiderian approach is a pragmatic attempt to achieve consensus about the diagnosis, basing this on certain "first rank symptoms" (certain types of delusions and hallucinations, also passivity phenomena). This is based on a cross-sectional picture of the patient.

5. The Psychoanalytic tradition generally regards the central process as being related to a break-down of ego barriers, with consequent difficulty in distinguishing self from the outside world. A wide variety of symptoms, mainly to do with relationships, can be considered as diagnostic.

Table 7 suggests the way in which these approaches have influenced current classificatory systems.

Table 7: Classification schemes in schizophrenia:
impact of different concepts of the disorder.

ICD-9:	Syndromal/Kraepelinian with Bleulerian influence
Britain:	Schneiderian and syndromal
USA:	
Traditional	Bleulerian and psychoanalytic
DSM-III	Bleulerian and Schneiderian
USSR:	
Snezhnevsky	Bleulerian and Kraepelinian
ICD-9	
Leningrad tradition	See page 12

Who is right?
There is still little consensus amongst Western psychiatrists about the concept of schizophrenia. The DSM-III criteria are criticized by the British school on the grounds that the definitions of the symptoms are unclear, thus increasing the variability of patients included under the category of schizophrenia (Wing, 1987). On the other hand, Linn (1985), in the Comprehensive Textbook, makes the point that first rank symptoms, the basis of the British approach, do not represent schizophrenia. He reminds his readers that in the IPSS 43% of those with schizophrenia did not have first rank symptoms [9]. In his view the two fundamental symptoms of schizophrenia are an irrational fear of human relationships, leading to

137

social withdrawal, and the loneliness that is secondary to this. This leads to the need-fear dilemma, which is the root of the schizophrenic reaction, the rest being secondary to this. This intensely Bleulerian/psychodynamic approach is now less popular amongst American psychiatrists. It is ironic that this psychoanalytic approach is in some ways similar to the Soviet position with regard to the diagnostic importance of the ability to make relationships and to participate in collective life. It differs in that the American position sees this in terms of intra-psychic activity rather than social processes.

An obvious point of divergence between Soviet and Western psychiatry is with regards to the relationship between manic-depressive psychosis and schizophrenia. There are different views about the issue within the Soviet Union. Many centres make a clear distinction between schizophrenia and manic-depressive psychosis and usually use ICD-9 criteria for diagnostic purposes. Some psychiatrists argue that many patients with recurrent schizophrenia, even if there are personality changes between episodes, should be classified as manic-depressive psychosis. Snezhnevsky's view was that there was no clear distinction between manic-depressive psychosis and schizophrenia. He stated that schizophrenia could present with a single episode, that there might be a good outcome with no change in personality. In patients with recurrent schizophrenia in whom there are no personality changes it is only the clinical picture during the actual episodes that distinguishes the disorder from manic-depressive psychosis. Moreover, there are patients with typical manic-depressive psychosis who develop defect states. The term endogenous psychosis is used to include both of the groupings.

In the West, by contrast, the distinction between the two disorders is becoming more entrenched. There are implications with regards to aetiology in that this assumes that the underlying pathology in a patient with manic-depressive psychosis (possibly with delusions and hallucinations) has more in common with that of a patient with a mild depressive episode than it has with a patient with paranoid schizophrenia (with delusions and hallucinations). The evidence in support of this position is flimsy. Some studies suggest that it is not possible to make a clear distinction between the two functional psychoses, that there are mixed forms and that a dimensional approach might be more useful than the categorisation into schizophrenia and manic-depressive psychosis (eg Kendell and Gourlay, 1970; Kendell and Brockington, 1980; Johnstone et al, 1988)

It is clear that the shoreline of schizophrenia is still tidal, and that regular ebb and flow in diagnostic practice continues to obscure just where terra firma begins. The criticisms of the Soviet concept of schizophrenia for being too broad are scarcely justified in view of the lack of consensus in the West about the nature of the disorder. Most Western concepts are also broad, with the exception of the strict Schneiderian concept, and this is criticized for not reflecting clinical reality or predicting outcome. Moreover, the consequences of the different systems of diagnosis are not necessarily different. Patients with the diagnosis of personality

---

9. The International Pilot Study of Schizophrenia (WHO, 1973) showed that 58% of acute patients with a hospital diagnosis of schizophrenia had a first rank symptom. Radhakrishnan et al (1983) reported that only one third of patients had first rank symptoms out of a group of schizophrenics that met both the ICD-9 criteria and the research criteria of Feighner et al (1972). Marneros (1988), reporting from the University Clinic in Bonn (located in Sigmund-Freud-Strasse) on a massive population of patients (1,208 with schizophrenia and 1,698 with organic psychoses), found that first-rank symptoms were present in 47% of schizophrenic patients and 7% of patients with organic disorders.

disorder may be detained compulsorily in hospital and treated with the same drugs that are used in schizophrenia (eg Goldberg et al, 1986; Davis, 1987). It seems unlikely that there will be any significant progress on this issue until there is some external validation for the diagnostic criteria.

Epidemiology
Epidemiological evidence is mixed with regards to the prevalence of schizophrenia in the Soviet Union as compared to the West. Epidemiological studies are relatively easy to carry out within the Soviet Union, mainly because of the organization of psychiatric services, in particular the dispensary system. There have been several large Soviet studies, and figures for prevalence are generally comparable with those in the West. In one of the biggest studies in the Soviet Union Rotstein (1977), from the Institute of Psychiatry in Moscow, reports the results of a large study from four towns and one rural area. A prevalence of schizophrenia was found to be 3.8 per 1000. Fuller Torrey (1987) quotes three Soviet studies giving prevalence rates of 2.6, 3.1 and 3.6 per 1000. However, one particular study which was carried out at the Institute of Psychiatry by Shmaunova and Lieberman (1979) found much higher rates of schizophrenia. They looked at the populations of various regions of the city of Moscow and reported an overall prevalence of schizophrenia of 9.59 per 1000 population. Broken down according to the form of schizophrenia the prevalence rates were 0.49 per 1000 for the malignant variant of continuous, 3.32 for episodic-progressive schizophrenia, 1.81 for paranoid schizophrenia (taking this as a separate type), 1.05 for recurrent, 2.87 for slow-flow schizophrenia and 0.06 for undifferentiated. There was also a high incidence (the number of new cases per year) in one city region. The figure reported was 1.91 per 1000, with no significant difference between men and women. The continuous form, however, both malignant and slow-flow, was commoner in men (1.4 to 0.03 for malignant and 0.78 to 0.44 for slow-flow) whereas episodic-progressive and recurrent forms were commoner in women (0.26 to 0.16 and 0.34 to 0.20). Incidence was highest in the teens and also in the 20-29 year band and dropped with increasing age.

Apart from the study of Shmaunova and Lieberman (1979), quoted above, most prevalence studies suggest higher rates in the USA than in the Soviet Union, and the Soviet Union tends to have only slightly higher rates than the UK. The figures quoted by Fuller Torrey (1987) for three studies in the Soviet Union (2.6, 3.1 and 3.6 per 1000) compare with two studies in the USA giving figures of 3.6 and 4.1 per 1000 and Scandinavia, which seems to have the highest rates, with a rate of 5.8 per 1000 for Norway and of 3.3, 6.3, 6.7 and 4.6 for Sweden. The Book studies in the far north of Sweden gave prevalence rates of 9.4 and 17 per 1000. The figures for three British studies are 2.1 per 1000, 2.8 and 3.4 per thousand.

Jablensky (1986), reviewing epidemiological studies in Europe, claims that, with the exception of certain isolated areas such as Northern Sweden, the rates of schizophrenia are similar in most countries. The incidence varies between 0.17 and 0.57 per 1000 population. The lowest figure was recorded in London and is probably related to the strict diagnostic criteria; the highest was in Dublin. Similarly, prevalence ranged from 2.5 to 5.3 per 1000 population. He reviewed various Soviet studies and found comparable rates, although some studies suggested higher rates. It is clear that diagnostic criteria and variations in what might be considered a case will account for most of the differences in prevalence between these studies. A case can range from someone with active, productive symptoms such as delusions or hallucinations to someone with slight personality changes who had productive symptoms in the past.

Aetiology
Zharikov and Sokolova (1989) write that the interaction of biological and social factors determines the level of morbidity, even in disorders such as schizophrenia which are in the main biologically determined. They describe a lower prevalence of schizophrenia in the extreme North-Eastern regions of the Soviet Union as compared to the cities. They discuss migration effects but also regard social and cultural effects as explaining some of the differences. A related study by Vul et al (1988) showed that schizophrenia and alcoholism are more prevalent in the newly developing cities of the remote Northern Tyumen region in comparison to the old cities of the region.

Genetic studies
Western studies are mainly quoted with regards to genetic predisposition and the usual figures are given, a ten to fifteen percent likelihood of schizophrenia in first degree relatives of probands. Several Soviet studies show differences between the different forms of schizophrenia, adding to the picture of clinical heterogeneity. On the whole it appears that there is more psychopathy in the first degree relatives of patients with continuous forms of schizophrenia as compared to patients with recurrent schizophrenia. It is argued that this is evidence that there are different genotypes in these disorders. As in the West, there have been attempts to link the clinical picture of schizophrenia to the HLA type. Genetic studies are also quoted as supporting the continuum theory. Shakmatova-Pavlova et al (1975) studied the families of 346 patients with schizophrenia, reporting on 818 first degree relatives. They found that the majority of relatives of patients with schizophrenia had some personality abnormality, although these were often no more than accentuations (an emphasis on one or more personality traits which does not affect the whole personality or have any impact upon social adaptation). Thus, relatives of patients with continuous schizophrenia tended to have abnormal personalities of the "emotional blunting" type along with schizoid traits. Smulevitch (1987) reports that in families with a proband with paranoid schizophrenia 41.8% of the relatives have some form of psychopathy, 22% having paranoid personality and 15% schizoid. This compared with 5% in the general population.

Viral/immune hypotheses
This is perhaps the most widely held aetiological theory in schizophrenia. It is thought that viral infection of the brain or an immune process, possibly triggered off by viral infections, are important in the pathophysiology. There may be a critical age for this to happen, possibly early childhood or even in utero. It is argued that this theory is consistent with what is known about the genetic component and the recent findings in molecular biology [10]. Vartanian (1983) writes that infection might have a pathogenetic role in schizophrenia but that this

might be non-specific, possibly responsible for some of the negative symptoms (which also occur in dementia and in late stages of affective disorders) whereas other factors cause the positive symptoms. He also considers that infection could be non-specific in the sense that it might be a trigger for other biological processes, for instance by affecting the immune system. There has been speculation about the nature of the infectious agent, with viruses and prions being the main suspects. Avrutsky et al (1988) give evidence for the role of neurotropic viruses in febrile schizophrenia. Nevidimova et al (1988) from Tomsk suggest that the Herpes Simplex may produce aetiologically significant herpes-induced immune responses. They claim to have shown that this is associated with the psychopathological signs in schizophrenia. They point out that the immunomodulatory effect of the psychotropic drugs (demonstrated by several investigators, for instance Potapova (1985)) may be the reason for their efficacy in schizophrenia.

There are many studies on immune function in schizophrenia. As yet it is difficult to integrate the various findings into a coherent picture. Vartanian (1983) quotes a number of studies, including some in the West, which report the presence of a variety of antibodies in the blood and CSF of patients with schizophrenia, but notes that many have methodological weaknesses. There has been some correlation between immunological disturbances and various clinical stages of the illness. Lymphocytes in some schizophrenic patients have an atypical morphology and show similar changes to those found in autoimmune disorders, although it is also argued that these changes may be secondary to whatever pathological process is taking place. Various indices of T-cell function are reported as being abnormal. It has also been shown that there are thymus antibodies in patients with schizophrenia and manic-depressive psychosis. However, the serum of a high proportion of controls also has antithymic activity. There is no correlation between antithymic activity and clinical picture although there is with duration of illness. Patients with a duration of schizophrenia of less than five years have greater antithymic activity. By contrast, there are more antibodies to brain cells in patients with duration of more than five years. One theory is that thymus antibodies cause permeability of brain cell membranes, because of cross reactivity, causing leakage of brain antigens which results in the production of antibodies to brain tissue.

Many of these changes have also been found in some relatives of schizophrenics, and thus might represent a hereditary predisposition rather than something pathogenetic. Vartanian (1983) is cautious about the findings, arguing that they may be spurious associations and that experimental models are necessary to establish aetiological links. Clinico-biological correlations should also be demonstrated along with positive results from relevant interventions. Some researchers argue that this latter requirement has been partly fulfilled in that neuroleptics and lithium have immunomodulatory properties.

Potapova and Trubnikov (1987) report increased immune activity in the acute phase of schizophrenia, although this is with regard to the level and activity of B lymphocytes. Vilkov et al (1987) report on the neurotropic activity of the serum of patients with schizophrenia, both in remission and during acute episodes. They write that cytotoxic anticerebral antibodies increase lipid peroxidation in

---

10. There is a strong genetic component in many infectious diseases. Twin studies carried out when tuberculosis was common in the population showed similar MZ/DZ concordance rates to schizophrenia.

homogenated rat brains. This neurotropic activity is significantly greater in psychotic patients as compared to controls and those with borderline disorders. The activity is greater during acute episodes than during remissions. The paper does not state whether patients were on medication. Vetlugina et al (1989) report decreased in-vitro phagocytic activity of leucocytes from patients with schizophrenia. They argue that this might be a primary defect or due to overload of biologically active substances. Sekerina et al (1989) report decreased levels of interleukin-2 in drug-free schizophrenics as compared to controls. The lowest levels were found in patients with the least progression of the disorder, that is patients with episodic schizophrenia. Patients with slow-flow schizophrenia also had reduced levels, but those with the malignant form had normal levels.

Biochemical theories
Biochemical theories are similar to those put forward in the West. Abnormalities of amines and enzymes are discussed, but the methodological limitations of many of the studies are stressed. The dopamine hypothesis is viewed with some suspicion and it is argued that changes in dopaminergic function may be secondary to some other process. There has been interest in the role of the opioid peptides, the endorphins and enkephalins, and a relationship has been shown between the level of beta-endorphin and the severity of schizophrenic symptoms.

Aliev (1985) attempts to integrate the immune and neurotransmitter/receptor hypotheses. He demonstrates a link between immune function and neurotransmitter systems in patients with paranoid schizophrenia, suggesting that the dopaminergic system intensifies the immune system and that cholinergic, serotoninergic, GABA-ergic systems inhibit it. Changes in endocrine function are reported, although the role of environmental factors is seen as critical in this.

The autointoxication theory is less popular than formerly. There have been Western and Soviet findings of various "toxic factors" in the blood and other biological fluids. Neurotoxic factors appear to have been identified as have substances in the blood with membranotropic effect on nerve cells. These substances either have a suppressing effect on various biological systems, or appear to have an effect on neuronal activity. The presence of the substances is established, but it is unclear as to whether there is any specific mechanism in schizophrenia. It is thought that the findings could be secondary to neuronal damage due to other causes. That said, however, there are also studies suggesting that these changes are found in a proportion of the relatives of schizophrenic patients.

The results of enzyme studies seem to be inconclusive and non-specific. Enzymes studied include MAO and creatinephosphokinase. The four isoenzymes of lactate dehydrogenase have been shown to have different profiles in schizophrenia, Pick's disease and epilepsy, all of which differ from control subjects. In schizophrenia there are changes in the level of various cytoplasmic enzymes. Many of these changes are thought to reflect disturbances in the function of cell membranes, probably with increased permeability. It may be that these are important in the pathogenesis of the psychoses. Another possible explanation is that the changes are non-specific. Thus, damage to nerve cells may increase cell membrane permeability, resulting in increased level of enzymes due to leakage.

This would fit with the viral hypothesis or the various immunological hypotheses.

Morphology
Vartanian (1983) describes the results of autopsy studies in some detail. He reports that post-mortem studies of patients with schizophrenia often show evidence of encephalopathy, characterized by diffuse, dystrophic processes of a toxic or hypoxic type, possibly the result of metabolic changes in the nervous system. There are no macroscopic changes and the microscopic changes are polymorphic. Neurones are reduced in number and tend to be atrophied, wrinkled and loaded with lipofuscin. There are other general changes such as degeneration, oedema and the presence of karyocytes, and these are not simply related to age or chronicity.

Lukacher et al (1989) from the Serbsky Institute carried out neurological examination on 111 schizophrenic patients. Investigations included fundoscopy, echoencephalography and spinal puncture. They found that 53% of the patients had raised intracranial pressure. This was twice as likely to occur in the episodic forms of schizophrenia than in the continuous forms. It was also more likely to be found during psychotic episodes. All nine patients with the catatonic syndrome had raised intracranial pressure and it occurred in 61% of patients with affective-delusional episodes as compared to 28% of those with paranoid syndrome (unless there was secondary catatonia).

Neurophysiology
Many psychiatrists adhere to Pavlovian concepts and discuss the activity of the brain in terms of zones of inhibition and excitation. Babayan (1985) writes that Pavlov's neurophysiological concepts about the higher nervous system should be used to investigate schizophrenia. Although these views are less prevalent, the legacy is the large number of neurophysiological studies, for instance those investigating the relationship between mental state and various parameters such as EEG activity. Functional links in different areas of the brain, reflecting the functional system of complex sets of conditioned reflexes, are thought to be disrupted in schizophrenia. These are especially diminished over the frontal lobes. It is accepted that this might be a spurious result, reflecting the underlying process. There are also attempts to describe the neurophysiological profiles of the different forms of schizophrenia.

Treatment
Some aspects of treatment are discussed in chapter 6. As with all psychiatric disorders, the combined use of psychotherapy, social therapy and work therapy along with physical treatments is emphasized. Snezhnevsky (1983), who has written widely on the biological treatment of schizophrenia, stresses the importance of social therapy and work therapy. The necessity of favourable environmental conditions, especially with regards to working conditions, is particularly emphasized. Many factors, including age, background and physical state, determine the different components of treatment. Many Soviet psychiatrists, particularly those of the "Leningrad school" would say that this is a more recent view and that the traditional Moscow line was to concentrate almost exclusively on biological treatments or work therapy. Certainly in-patient treatment consists

mainly of these two approaches, although there does tend to be some involvement with the family.

It is generally felt to be desirable that all patients with a diagnosis of schizophrenia should be on a dispensary list, although it is recognized that many patients with milder forms do not actually see psychiatrists. Most patients are managed as out-patients, and admission is only considered necessary when there are active symptoms. Out-patient treatment is generally considered optimum for patients in remission and those with milder forms of the disorder such as slow-flow schizophrenia. There is debate about the benefits of early treatment, but some authors consider that particularly in episodic-progressive schizophrenia it is important to have early admission as delayed treatment has an adverse effect on prognosis (Snezhnevsky, 1983). It is thought desirable that patients should move as quickly as possible to open wards, followed by periods of leave and discharge and either day hospital or dispensary follow-up. In slow-flow schizophrenia, acute episodes require day hospital or sanatorium type of treatment rather than admission to hospital. Some patients with severe defect states or fixed psychoses may have long-term in-patient treatment, although this comprises a tiny proportion of the patients seen.

Physical treatment

A wide range of drugs are used in the treatment of schizophrenia. This includes the regular use of antidepressants and minor tranquillisers as well as neuroleptics. Dosages are similar to those used in the West. Examples given are: chlorpromazine 300-600 mgm over a twenty-four hour period; trifluoperazine, usually 10-20 mgm, but up to 50-80 mgm; haloperidol 10-40 mgm (Snezhnevsky, 1983; Korkina et al, 1980). Drugs less familiar in the West are: thioproperazine (majeptil) 50-70mgm; etaperazin 150-200mgm per day. Reserpine (serpasil) 9-12mgm is also used at times. As might be expected, dosage and duration of use depend largely upon the clinical state. Blood and urine levels of drugs may be measured.

Drug treatment tends to be more specific in its targeting of particular symptoms and syndromes. Snezhnevsky (1983) stresses that the choice of drug should be determined by the stage of the disorder. In the stable phase the aim of treatment should be to lower emotional tone and to treat any vegetative symptoms, also symptoms such as tension, anxiety, obsessional or hysterical features. Minor tranquillisers, possibly with small doses of neuroleptics and antidepressants may be used. Major tranquillisers are primarily indicated for the active phase when there are productive symptoms. Thus, there is less use of prophylactic neuroleptics such as depot preparations during periods of remission. Lithium, however, may be used when there are affective features. Chlorpromazine is considered to be more sedative, and the piperazines more effective in patients with fixed delusions. Thus, trifluoperazine may be used in doses of 40-80mgm per day for up to two months, after which the dose is reduced. Haloperidol may also be used. Haloperidol or etaperazin are used when hallucinations are a prominent feature. The same drug might be used in different dosages for different syndromes. Thus in lower dosages trifluoperazine is useful when there is an affective component and in higher dosages when there is a fixed delusional system. Chlorpromazine, thioridazine and clozapine are considered more useful for positive symptoms and fluphenazine, pimozide, majeptil for negative symptoms. Haloperidol is useful for paranoia when there is elevated mood and trifluoperazine for paranoia with lowered mood.

Continuous schizophrenia, especially the malignant variant, tends to be resistant to treatment. Catatonic features are treated with the more active psychotropics such as majeptil or clozapine and also higher doses of chlorpromazine, haloperidol or trifluoperazine. This usually succeeds in treating the more serious manifestations of the condition, either stupor or excitement. Sudden cessation of all drug treatment can be tried in resistant cases. Other physical treatments such as ECT are also occasionally used.

Drugs are the mainstay of treatment in *episodic-progressive schizophrenia*. Antidepressants may be given when there is an affective component and stimulating drugs, such as indopan or melipramine, in patients with anergy and adynamic features. This may be combined with the nootrope, piriditol. If a neuroleptic is necessary the more "activating" drugs such as trifluoperazine and pimozide are used. Various combinations of major and minor tranquillisers and antidepressants are used to treat the different syndromes that arise during the course of the disorder. Hypochondriacal features are seen as difficult to treat, and tranquillisers like diazepam are often used. In more severe cases, for instance when there are marked hysterical features, tranquillisers with more psychotropic action are used, for instance fenazepam, lorazepam, sometimes intravenously. These may be combined with neuroleptics. The hysterical syndromes might also be treated with intravenous drugs, particularly in the acute stages or in hysterical psychosis with disassociation. Fenazepam or lorazepam may be used, or, in resistant cases, these combined with small doses of neuroleptics.

Depersonalisation may be treated with a combination of antidepressants, usually of the sedative type such as amitriptyline, clomipramine or maprotiline, and also neuroleptics such as teralen, etaperazin or trifluoperazine. In cases of severe depersonalization intravenous antidepressants and tranquillizers, diazepam or chlordiazepoxide, might be used, or even intravenous neuroleptics. When depersonalization is combined with cognitive impairment stimulants and nootropes might also be used eg sidnocarb, aminolon, indopan.

Obsessional features may be treated with various combinations of drugs, including neuroleptics and lithium. Intravenous antidepressants and neuroleptics may be used in cases with fixed obsessional features. Depot neuroleptics, such as modecate 12.5mgm to 50mgm weekly to monthly, might also be used when there are fixed, treatment-resistant obsessional features.

In depressed-paranoid states sedative antidepressants such as amitriptyline or clomipramine might be used. Snezhnevsky (1983) urges caution in the use of neuroleptics in these episodic-progressive states with affective features. He argues that they may "fix" states of prolonged depression. Chlorpromazine should be avoided and use made of the piperazines eg trifluoperazine or "soft" neuroleptics such as thioridazine or chlorprotiksen. In manic-like states chlorpromazine and haloperidol are used. When there psychopathic-like features in the presentation, possibly with fatuous, wild behaviour, the most effective drug is considered to be pericyazine. Occasionally lithium alone may be used.

In febrile schizophrenia it is considered vital to treat the basic physical state, and this might involve corticosteroids, intravenous feeding, possibly diuretics and vitamins. Chlorpromazine is used and occasionally ECT.

Carbemazepine has been used more recently in the endogenous psychoses, having been reported as more useful in schizophrenia than in manic-depression (Vovin, 1987).

There is serious concern in the Soviet Union as well as in the West about the side-effects of neuroleptics, in particular tardive dyskinesia and the neuroleptic malignant syndrome. Avrutsky et al (1987) argue that the features of the neuroleptic malignant syndrome are similar to the "extrapyramidal-psychotic" side effects of neuroleptics. They argue that there is probably a continuum of side-effects and that there are many variants of hyperthermia from mild, transitory states right through to the neuroleptic malignant syndrome.

Psychosocial approaches
There has been a long-standing tradition of rehabilitation in Soviet psychiatry, and considerable emphasis on work as a form of treatment, especially in schizophrenia. This is discussed in chapter 6. All Soviet authors stress the importance of psychosocial treatment in schizophrenia. Korkina et al (1980) stress that rehabilitation and social integration are not possible without adequate psychotherapy and ergotherapy (work therapy).

Psychotherapy is mainly carried out in groups, and is generally based on RT, but there is also emphasis on social skills and inter-personal relationships. Family therapy is less commonly used, but there has been some work which is similar to the Western family work on expressed emotion. In the 1960s there were studies to assess the efficacy of rehabilitation measures by looking at the improvement in family relationships and of family roles using various scales and "sociograms" to measure the quality and quantity of relationships (Lauterbach, 1984).

Snezhnevsky (1983) advises caution about expecting people to return to work before a remission is fully established. The nature of the remission determines the ability to work, and residual symptoms are considered to be grounds for some form of invalidity, although it is stressed that capability is more important than the actual symptoms or defect state. Grade 3 invalidity [11] is considered appropriate for those in the early or late stages of progressive schizophrenia when there is partial ability to work. This might also be granted on a more long-term basis for patients with fixed paranoid states who find it difficult to work. Grade 2 invalidity would be appropriate for more established, chronic cases where a defect state is present, and would apply particularly to patients with continuous schizophrenia. Patients with psychotic symptoms which did not respond to treatment would also be entitled to grade 2 or 3 invalidity.

Comparative aspects: treatment
Holland (1977) reported that drug treatment in schizophrenia was similar to that in the USA and that the same range of drugs was being used. This is true with regard to the neuroleptics such as chlorpromazine, haloperidol, perphenazine and thioridazine, but, as discussed above, a range of other types of treatment is also used in the Soviet Union. One difference between Soviet and American/British approach is the greater use of intramuscular or intravenous drugs in the early

11. See page 98.

146

stages. My own experience was that drugs are used in a fairly similar way, although there is a general tendency to use lower doses of neuroleptics.

Another important difference between the Soviet and American/British approaches is the specific targeting of drugs to particular symptoms and syndromes and the tendency to treat these irrespective of the nosological grouping. Smulevitch (1987) makes the point that one should move away from the simplistic approach of equating particular groups of drugs to particular diagnoses. He argues that the split between drugs for psychoses (neuroleptics, major thymoleptics) and those for borderline conditions (tranquillizers, nootropes, minor thymoleptics) is arbitrary and unhelpful. In the West drugs are generally linked to particular nosological entities rather than to symptoms. Schizophrenia is treated with the major neuroleptics, which are usually thought of as specific treatments (linked to the dopamine hypothesis). Standard practice is to persevere with neuroleptics both in the acute and chronic stages, irrespective of the clinical picture.

Long-term treatment with depot neuroleptics has now become the cornerstone of treatment in the West [12]. This is partly due to the current emphasis on prevention of relapses. One reason for this is the belief that each relapse or acute exacerbation progressively damages personality and worsens the long-term outcome of the disorder, although there is little evidence to support this view as yet (Curson et al, 1986). It is self-evident that patients with a bad prognosis will suffer more relapses. However, it has not been clearly established that it is possible to prevent long-term deterioration by reducing the number of individual episodes of psychosis by drug treatment or psychosocial intervention. A pragmatic reason for the policy of preventing relapses is the policy of community care itself. With the closure of the large psychiatric hospitals and the move into the community there are fewer hospital beds available. Thus there is greater pressure on the reduced number of beds so that it is necessary to keep admissions to a minimum. It is therefore desirable to keep patients in the community and relapse-free.

In the Soviet Union, partly because of problems with availability, depot neuroleptics are less used. There is, moreover, a theoretical reason for the more limited usage. The concept that schizophrenia is a progressive disorder with a particular course suggests that treatment should be directed towards the different syndromes when they arise. The concomitant to this is that no treatment is necessary when there is no syndromal presentation.

The wider range of Soviet treatments (generally theory-based eg linked to the toxin, viral or immune hypotheses) including insulin coma therapy, hyperbaric oxygen, and various immunomodulators are rarely used in the West. However, ECT, which is generally not used in the treatment of schizophrenia in the Soviet Union, is being used more frequently in the West [13].

One thing to emerge from the comparison is that there is probably more emphasis in Soviet psychiatry on psychological and social aspects of treatment.

12. A large study, carried out in nine centres, followed 120 schizophrenics who were put on a randomised controlled trial of neuroleptics (Crow et al., 1986). The two year follow-up showed that 46% of patients on the active compound (ie the depot neuroleptic) and 62% on the placebo relapsed. The main predictor of relapse was the duration of the illness before admission. As with many studies it is shown that the longer the period of follow-up the less the difference in outcome between active drug and placebo.

13. Simpson and May (1985) give the American Psychiatric Association recommendations, but suggest that the treatment should also be used in resistant schizophrenia, in acute catatonia and acute paranoid states. They write that multiple ECT or "regressive" ECT is of interest, but that there are no well-controlled studies.

This is related to the patient's system of relationships in society. It is considered important to restore his social standing, both at work and within the family, and to attempt to minimize the damage to personality. Recent Western approaches concentrate on the biological aspects, although there has been a long tradition of social rehabilitation in Britain. American psychiatry has paid relatively little attention to social treatment. One reason for this is that most chronic patients end up in the public sector which has limited facilities beyond the state hospitals.

Prophylaxis

There are different views within the Soviet Union about the value of early diagnosis. One volume of the Korsakoff journal (1986 volume 10) is devoted to the outcome in childhood schizophrenia, and suggests that early diagnosis does have predictive value. However, it is recognized that the implications for prevention are still far from clear. It is thought that secondary prevention, essentially giving treatment early, does have an impact, but as yet there is little empirical evidence to support this. Primary prevention presents major difficulties. Vrono (1988) discusses some of the ethical issues to do with genetic counselling. He stresses that any counselling to families must be done on the basis of decisions taken by the patients themselves who must be given adequate information. Vartanian (1983) writes that it is difficult to attempt to eliminate the genotype in the population in a disorder with multifactorial aetiology. It is hard to make any recommendations to families with a genetic predisposition to mental illness. Tables of empirical risk can be used, but great caution is necessary and doctors must be aware of the current state of genetic knowledge. He stresses the fact that there are important moral, legal and psychological aspects to the question as well as the purely medical ones. There are no significant differences between Soviet and Western approaches with regards to genetic counselling, although, because of the emphasis on environmental factors in the Soviet Union, there more scepticism about its value. The question as to whether there would actually be some harm from trying to eliminate or reduce a particular genotype is also raised, but, again, without any answer.

Prognosis

Snezhnevsky (1983) writes that prognosis is better than was previously thought. There are personality changes in schizophrenia, but these may be adaptive and they tend to stabilize out with time. Long-term follow-up indicates that a significant proportion of patients make an almost complete clinical recovery with full social rehabilitation. He writes that outcome is likely to be better with early detection and treatment, although no evidence is cited to support this view. The Institute of Psychiatry study on 3,500 patients with recurrent and episodic-progressive schizophrenia showed that 30% of patients had only one episode in their lives, 25% had two episodes, 25% had three or four and 20% had more than four.

All the continuous forms of schizophrenia share a tendency to show a "reverse development" in the late stages of the course when there is some stabilization and improvement. Slow-flow schizophrenia has the best clinical and social prognosis, and there may be improvement in the negative as well as the productive symptoms. The progressive variant has an intermediate outcome and the malignant variant has the worst prognosis. A long-term follow-up study showed that in the twentieth year of illness 60% of patients with slow-flow schizophrenia, 25% of patients with progressive and virtually no patients with the malignant variant were still working.

The prognosis of a disorder depends upon the original criteria used in making the diagnosis and also on the criteria used to determine outcome. In the West, and especially in Britain, schizophrenia is generally considered to have a bad prognosis. In clinical practice, therefore, the diagnosis tends to be avoided whenever possible, resulting in a tightening of the concept down to a core group with a poor prognosis. There is, however, some inconsistency in the position overall in that the criteria used in most research instruments, including the PSE, produce a group which includes patients who do not necessarily have this poor prognosis.

The Soviet view of prognosis is more optimistic. Clearly, the continuum model and the broader concept of schizophrenia will produce a better overall prognosis by including milder forms. The wider the concept the more heterogeneous the population, and, therefore, the higher the proportion of successful people (in terms of work, relationships, long-term outcome) who fall into the category. It is perhaps optimistic to hope that this might eventually have a destigmatizing effect. This effect, however, is partly counterbalanced by a somewhat more stringent way of evaluating outcome. Soviet criteria include factors such as personality change and social withdrawal which are tougher measures of outcome than simply looking at the presence of absence of positive symptoms. Thus, Harding et al (1987) reported on a cohort of patients discharged from the "back wards" of the Vermont State Hospital. 68% of those patients who had met DSM-III criteria for schizophrenia on admission had no features of schizophrenia at follow-up and 45% of the patients had no symptoms. However, the majority of patients were single, unemployed and living restricted lives.

SLOW-FLOW ("SLUGGISH") SCHIZOPHRENIA

In view of the controversy about the concept of slow-flow schizophrenia *(vialotekushaya shizophrenie)*, sometimes referred to as sluggish schizophrenia, this form will be discussed in some detail. *Vialotekushaya* translates literally as flowing sluggishly or listlessly *(vialo* = inertly, listlessly, languidly). The term is sometimes translated as torpid schizophrenia or sluggish schizophrenia, but this is misleading in that it suggests a judgement about personality or about the syndromal presentation, whereas vialo actually refers to the course that the disorder takes. A better translation, therefore, might be slowly-flowing or slowly-progressive, but the term used here is slow-flow for brevity [14].

The concept of a slowly developing psychosis with relatively favourable outcome was described in the literature before Kraepelin's nosology. Various terms have been applied in the twentieth century European literature. Snezhnevsky (1983) and Smulevitch (1987) quote several terms which describe these disorders.

14. Soviet translators use different terms. The abstract in an article by Gorchakova (1988), from the Institute of Psychiatry, uses the term slowly-progressive whereas that of Prokopochky et al (1988), from the Serbsky, uses sluggish for the same Russian term.

These include latent schizophrenia (Bleuler, 1911), "soft" schizophrenia (Kronfeldt, 1928), non-psychotic (Rosenshtein, 1933) and pseudoneurotic schizophrenia (Hoch and Polatin, 1949), and, more recently, ambulatory, subclinical and borderline schizophrenia. The term *vialoprotekushaya* (similar to *vialotekushaya*) is attributed to Melikhov (1963)[15] by Snezhnevsky and Smulevitch, although Holland and Shakhmatova-Pavlova (1977) write that in the 1930s Sukhareva, a child psychiatrist, described different forms of schizophrenia in children, including a "sluggish" form.

There is debate as to whether the disorder should be considered as a variant of schizophrenia or as a borderline condition (psychopathy), with Snezhnevsky (1983) arguing the former case. Smulevitch (1987), however, writes that it has much in common with the borderline conditions and that genetic studies support this association. Psychopathy is commonly present in the families of patients with slow-flow schizophrenia, most commonly the schizoid type of psychopathy with emotional coldness, lack of friends, egocentricity, and "oddness". There may also be some association with the type of psychopathy and the type of slow-flow schizophrenia. Thus, paranoid psychopathy is found in patients with the paranoid type of slow-flow schizophrenia. Moreover, he considers that the whole question of the overlap between the functional psychoses and borderline states is still unclear. There is evidence that schizophrenia occurs in the families of patients with neurosis[16]. Thus, he argues that there is some overlap anyway between schizophrenia and the borderline conditions, with a greater overlap in slow-flow schizophrenia.

Whether it is a form of schizophrenia or psychopathy it is agreed that slow-flow schizophrenia should be considered as a separate type of disorder and not simply an "aborted" form of schizophrenia (one that has failed to develop into a full-blown endogenous psychosis), or an atypical form with a prolonged course or the precursor of some more serious form of schizophrenia. It is considered an independent entity, with its own course and development with a latent phase, active phase and period of stabilization. The general agreement about this means that the debate about whether it should be classified under schizophrenia or personality disorder is somewhat less critical with regards to treatment, prognosis or research.

The condition is said to be characterized by a slow course with gradual changes in personality. The initial onset is usually before the age of twenty. Symptoms fluctuate and they usually start out as vague and undifferentiated before becoming more specific and, possibly, showing psychotic features, often later in life. The profound emotional damage typical of other forms of schizophrenia is not found, but the core feature is the change that takes place in manner, behaviour, motivation and the circle of interests. There is a distortion in the essence of the personality (Snezhnevsky, 1987). Long periods of stabilisation with compensatory mechanisms are characteristic of the disorder.

There may be a long latent stage with no signs of progression, and, unlike other forms, no signs of intellectual or social impairment. There are usually no psychotic symptoms at this stage and patients may continue to function well at work. There

---

15. The reference is to a book by Melikhov (1963) on the assessment of work capability in schizophrenia.
16. He quotes a Japanese author, Mitsuda, who reports that a family history of schizophrenia is least common in patients with hysteria and neurasthenia and most common in those with obsessional states and anxiety.

are affective symptoms which are generally mild and there is often marked lability with somatic symptoms. They may present like a response to a period of strain or overwork. The affective component tends to be reactive, but in later stages becomes more autonomous. There are often seasonal fluctuations and, possibly, premenstrual symptoms. There may be long hypothymic periods with pessimism, self-pity and irritability, a strong tendency to engage in self-doubt and self-analysis. Anxiety symptoms are often predominant in these subdepressive phases. There may be some mild hypomania, generally with a fixed and monotonous affect. Patients have increased energy levels, a characteristic "tireless activity", excess optimism and a high opinion of themselves. In this background of chronic hypomania there may be rudimentary obsessions, tics, fixed rituals. There tends to be a sudden switch into depression.

There are also features which are similar to those found in the psychopathies and neuroses. The terms pseudoneurosis and pseudopsychopathy are used to distinguish the syndromes (clinically similar to the neuroses and psychopathies) that arise during the course of an endogenous psychosis from the true neuroses and psychopathies. The pseudopsychopathies are usually of the schizoid type. Autism, withdrawal, profound egotism and difficulty in making contact with people are all seen. There is often a mixed picture, so that the schizoid features might occur along with hysterical traits, with demonstrative behaviour and hysterical manifestations. There may be psychasthenia, with anxiety, self-doubt, pedantry and rigidity of mental activity, and also paranoid traits. Neurotic symptoms are varied, commonly with obsessional and phobic syndromes, but also vegetative and hysterical.

Smulevitch (1987) describes the case of a patient with the pseudopsychopathic type of slow-flow schizophrenia.

The patient is a fifty year-old man with a facility for languages who lives with his mother. He is described as having been a quiet, intelligent child who was given the nick-name "The Professor" at school. He was successful academically, and was ahead of his class in most subjects. When he was six years old he gained a step-father who is described as "coarse and mocking". When he was ten years old he missed school for a few weeks because there was a teacher there who reminded him of the step-father. At fifteen he was described as having been excessively shy and secretive, but continued to do very well at his studies. At the age of nineteen he gained a place at an institute where he was unable to form relationships with his fellow students. At that time he had an episode of illness with some paranoid and depressive symptoms, and there was a suicide attempt. He spent two months in hospital and is reported as having made a good recovery. He did not, however, continue with the institute, but took up evening classes and began a job in a library. He took up a new way of life with many "artistic" acquaintances, although he did not have close friends. He married because his girl-friend became pregnant, but this relationship soon ended. At the age of 50 he lives an isolated life, having no real friends. He has a mundane job and helps his mother, with whom he is living, much of the time. He is most happy working at his languages and spends eight hours a day at his writing desk reading English and Spanish. His only other interest is his son, who lives with his ex-wife. He considers that any difficulties he had were because of women. He likes to go to the doctor regularly, although there is no real need for him to be seen.

In some cases an unusual reaction to life events may be the only clinical manifestation of the disorder during the latent period. The reactions may be depressive, often combined with hysterical or hypochondriacal features, or, more rarely, delusional. Acute anxious-phobic, anxious-depressive and obsessive-phobic states may present as raptoid states in which there is sudden fear, panic, confusion, often insomnia, a feeling of impending doom and the strong sense of being left without any guidance. These are generally in response to some minimal stimulus, usually events which require some action or an independent decision. These are different from schizophrenic reactions, described below, which persist longer than raptoid states.

There is also a distinction between this reactive lability in slow-flow schizophrenia and the reactive component in psychopathy. In psychopathy the reactive state is closely related to the nature of the "over-valued complexes" that are a feature of the psychopathy. Mood change is precipitated when these are impinged upon or when there is loss of an overvalued object. In slow-flow schizophrenia, however, there is no formation of overvalued complexes, and the psychogenesis is related to everyday experiences. The tendency towards introspection and retrospection means that gradually a wide circle of events and associations can provide the psychogenic traumas which can trigger off the affective changes. Thus, even neutral events acquire a special sense and trigger off memories of the source of grief. There may be obsessional memories, and vivid imagery, also rudimentary ideas of reference, so that patients think that their neighbours are taking pleasure in their misfortune and that they are on the receiving end of hostile glances from all around.

The active stage of the disorder may consist of a series of episodes or take a more continuous form. The most likely presentation, however, is of repeated episodes on the background of a gradually developing course. The episodes may present with more marked exacerbations of pseudoneurosis or pseudopsychopathy, and there may be affective or paranoid features. Younger patients are more likely to have episodes with hypochondriasis and depersonalization. Older patients present with affective and paranoid features, often with overvalued ideas and delusional ideas of jealousy or litigiousness.

There are different presentations during the active stage, and the main features of the clinical picture define the variants of slow-flow schizophrenia.

In the *obsessional* variant a short, rudimentary phobic episode is often noted some ten to fifteen years before the actual onset. This might have been a fear of heights, a fear of blushing, a fear of going into certain places and the use of various magical rituals for protection. The disorder presents with fixed obsessional symptoms, usually at the end of the second decade. There are prolonged episodes, often lasting from months to years, often without proper remissions. Depressive features are common. There are marked obsessional features with all kinds of preoccupations and doubts. The obsessional thoughts are often concerned with abstract matters, perhaps metaphysical speculations or blasphemous thoughts. There may be acute paroxysms of phobic fear. Progression is characterized by "systematization" when all kinds of secondary obsessions develop around the primary ones. The contents become sillier and less psychologically understandable. Rituals develop and there are very gradual changes in personality. Negative symptoms are found only in the late stages. These can be thought of as exaggerations of the changes found in obsessional personality disorder and consist of emotional impoverishment, rigidity, helplessness and excess dependence.

The *depersonalization* variant is more common in men, and the onset is early, often in adolescence. It is a disorder of the awareness of the self and of relationships with others. The personality is often schizoid. In the early stages patients themselves complain about a loss of sharpness and flexibility, a change in the precision of their impressions, a loss of interests. A key feature is isolation and a breakdown of contact with people. During the active stage the depersonalization is more marked, often becoming total with a complete loss of the sense of self. This can be to the extent that the patient's own biography does not seem to apply to him. There is also derealization so that the world around is changed and empty. There may be anxious depression with "psychic anaesthesia" and complete loss of emotional resonance. Music does not sound the same and nuances of feeling are lost. Stabilization usually takes place in the mid twenties with improvement in affective symptoms and depersonalization. There are, however, some negative symptoms of schizophrenia. There is loss of earlier sharpness and of spontaneous and natural emotional reactions. The full sense of the self does not return and along with this there is alienation, egotism and emotional aloofness from those closest to them. Patients are often preoccupied with their own condition, and actively seek out treatment to try and help them to get back to their former level of mental functioning. Most return to work and may be able to undertake further education, and this contrasts with their continuous complaints about their mental activity and their attempts to find a cure.

The *hypochondriacal* variant is characterized by unusual hypochondriacal features. It is distinguished from other hypochondriacal syndromes by the fact that the symptoms complained about are often bizarre, with bizarre explanations suggested by the patient. Thus, patients might think that their difficulty in breathing is due to an insufficiency of oxygen in the atmosphere or a dysfunctional piece of lung. There is a fear of illness, with, for instance cardiophobia, cancerophobia or fear of dementia, and patients may go from specialist to specialist and call out ambulances. Patients read medical books and keep records of their various sensations and symptoms. They develop extensive systems for trying to improve their health and may embark on eccentric dietary regimes. The outside world tends to be divided up into things which are good or bad for the health.

The *senestopathic* variant differs from the above in that the main feature is the experience of odd sensations from all over the body. The personality is often marked by extreme rigidity, with limited views and interests and no sense of humour. The sensations are commonly from the head, so that a persisting headache is complained of, but may also come from other organs such as the gut or the genitals. The sensations are often described in bizarre language eg the sensation of crushed bones or brains, a hardening of the stomach. There may be a fantastic colouring to them, and yet patients often refer to them with indifference. This is more a disorder of sensation than mentation; thus, unlike the hypochondriacal variant, there is not the same anxious self-monitoring and concern.

Patients with the *hysterical* variant are described as being "unbalanced", impulsive and capricious. They are often artistically talented. However, some of the expectations are often unrealistic, so that fantasies abound and they consider themselves to be great artists, scientists and unusual people. In childhood they may have formed odd attachments, perhaps deifying a teacher or acquaintance. This might take on inappropriate proportions so that they try to meet them out of school, give flowers, telephone them at home and write letters, perhaps with a sexual nuance developing irrespective of the age or sex of the person concerned. There may be mystical visions and voices, magical thinking, strong intuitions, fatalism, ideas about sorcery, a beliefs in their ability to foretell the future.

Another variant, the *simple* variant, is rarely described and its course is characterized by purely negative symptoms. Patients are secretive, lacking in drive or initiative and show no emotional attachments. In the latent period there may be some diminution in the level of mental functioning, but there are no behaviour disorders. The definite signs of illness arise in youth, usually from about fourteen to twenty. In this active period the negative changes develop and it gradually becomes clear that there is some mental insufficiency in the patient. Patients may, for instance, feel that they cannot continue with their studies. The few positive symptoms arise only after a long period of decline; there may be affective symptoms, often a picture of adynamic depression with hypochondriacal ideas and rudimentary senestopathic features. There may be a substuporous condition with awkwardness, hypokinesis, odd movements etc, akin to the "soft catatonia" of Kahlbaum. These positive symptoms tend to be fleeting. The third or fourth decade of life sees the period of stabilization, with a fixed asthenic defect with intellectual and emotional impoverishment and an ill-defined disturbance of thoughts. There is a lowering of the circle of interests, but patients do not have any signs of regression of behaviour. Outwardly they often seem to be fully normal, and may retain practical and uncomplicated professional skills.

Latent schizophrenia differs from the above variants in not having an active stage, although sometimes there is progression much later in life. The course is, therefore, particularly favourable. The clinical significance is unclear, and the term is rarely used in practice, mainly because such people are unlikely to come to the attention of doctors.

Differential diagnosis

Smulevitch (1987) devotes much of his monograph on slow-flow schizophrenia to the question of differentiating it from the borderline states. The conditions that may develop during the course of slow-flow schizophrenia (the pseudoneuroses, pseudopsychopathies and reactive psychoses) may present in a similar way to the borderline states when considered from a cross-sectional perspective. Although it is only the longitudinal picture that allows a final diagnosis there are a number of features which differentiate the disorders. The psychogenic episodes in the borderline states are easier to treat, generally with simple psychosocial intervention and minimal medication. The short-term outcome is better. Psychogenic episodes in the context of an endogenous process are more resistant to treatment. There are more likely to be psychotic features, for instance reactive paranoia. Reactive affective episodes (reactive depression, mania or anxiety) are often bizarre or atypical, so that, in comparison to true borderline states, they may be caused by very minor events or family conflicts.

He describes a case of a young man with an apparently normal and uneventful upbringing. At the age of fifteen he had a fracture of the ankle which generated an unreasonable amount of anxiety which went on for about two years. After this he settled down, but became somewhat isolated from his family and friends. At the age of twenty-three he had another episode of marked anxiety when he suddenly came across his "girl-friend" with a group of her colleagues. He ran home and for some time had anxiety symptoms in response to all kinds of things such as the telephone ringing. When followed-up at the age of 29 he was living at home, not working and believed that he was helping his mother, having a somewhat "infantile attitude" towards her. He rarely left his room, avoided the neighbours, tried to dress in a modish fashion and was pre-occupied with his former girl-friend. He tries to live a quiet life, free of any stress. He avoids a street where he saw a dog run over by a car because might it provoke a "nervous change".

Lichko (1986) writes that differential diagnosis is particularly difficult in adolescents. He suggests that a greater degree of "schizoidness" is the most discriminating feature. This manifests itself in various ways depending upon the personality traits. Thus, people with schizoid personalities often have rather bizarre hobbies. However, in differentiating pseudopsychopathic schizophrenia from schizoid personality disorder, the degree of bizarreness may help to differentiate. He gives an example of a patient with slow-flow schizophrenia who pursued with great intensity the hobby of collecting the excrement of various animals. With regards to delinquent behaviour he writes that, in contrast to someone with an unstable personality, the schizophrenic might be a member of a delinquent group but is always seen as an outsider.

Schizophrenia or personality disorder?

Smulevitch (1987) writes that slow-flow schizophrenia should not be thought of as a variant of schizophrenia, but as an independent form. He suggests that clinically and genetically it is closer to the personality disorders than it is to schizophrenia. There is also the view that it should be considered as an independent form of psychosis. Snezhnevsky (1987), in the introduction to the above work, maintains that the disorder should be classified with schizophrenia, arguing that the processes are similar, especially the personality changes, though these are less marked in slow-flow schizophrenia. There are also similarities with regards to the course and outcome, and there are also some genetic links with the psychoses. However, he does appear to acknowledge that Smulevitch makes a reasonable case for placing it with psychopathy.

Outcome studies have not resolved the problems of classification. A follow-up of 100 teenagers given a diagnosis of pseudopsychopathic schizophrenia showed that one third were improved after 5-10 years, one third fell into the psychopathy group and one third had developed clear psychoses (Lichko, 1986). Kazanetz (1989), writing in the British Journal of Psychiatry, argues against the concept of slow-flow schizophrenia on the grounds that patients with the diagnosis are either suffering from borderline disorders or from "manifestly typical cases of schizophrenia". He writes: "There is no reason to subdivide verified cases of schizophrenia into rapidly developing and "sluggish" forms. According to the follow-up data (in his study), most cases of schizophrenia originally classified by the physicians as "sluggish" later proved to be manifestly typical cases of schizophrenia with prominent deterioration."

Treatment

Psychosocial approaches are considered to be of prime importance in the treatment of slow-flow schizophrenia irrespective of whether it is considered to be a form of schizophrenia or nearer to the borderline conditions. Snezhnevsky (1983) writes that psychotherapy has an important role along with other social rehabilitation measures. Different types of psychotherapy might be used, including hypnosis, rational therapy or collective/group therapy, depending on the condition and on other factors such as the family structure. Psychotherapy is considered most effective when there are no severe personality changes and with symptoms of anxiety, obsessional doubts, loss of activity and poor socialization. The aim is to stimulate activity, build on patients' own strengths and to improve social contacts. It is thought that psychotherapy or hypnosis should only be carried out during periods of stability as they might worsen the condition during psychotic states. Psychotherapy is essentially supportive rather than interpretive. Drugs may also be used, and, as with any other disorder, usage depends on the phase and the nature of the syndromes. Thus, in the stable phase, the emphasis is on reducing vegetative tone. Lithium prophylaxis may be indicated if there are clear periodic affective phases with somatic, neurotic or hypomanic symptoms.

Smulevitch (1987) writes that treatment should be similar to that for the borderline conditions. Admission is rarely indicated, but might be necessary in some patients in the acute phases. Indications include cases where more active therapy is planned, treatment-resistant cases and for some paranoid patients who refuse to attend the out-patient department. He lays much emphasis on complex combinations of various types of treatment such as psychotherapy with physiotherapy. The aim of the social measures is to deal with conflicts at work and within the family. He does, however, also stress the need for biological treatments when appropriate. Drugs and treatment in general should interfere with the normal daily rhythm as little as possible.

Neurosis-like cases of slow-flow schizophrenia are rarely seen by psychiatrists. They generally require psychotherapy, mild pharmacotherapy and other treatments such as vitamins, physiculture, physiotherapy and trips to sanatoria or resorts. In neurotic hypochondria and also in the asthenic states tranquillisers are mainly used, sometimes, in the acute stages, intravenously. Nootropes and stimulants might also be helpful. In asthenic depression antidepressants and possibly stimulants may be used. Acute anxious-phobic, anxious-depressive and obsessive-phobic states presenting as raptoid states or schizophrenic reactions are also treated with tranquillisers, with neuroleptics and antidepressants often being necessary in the latter. Neuroleptics might be used if there are marked obsessional, phobic or hypochondriacal features. The thymoleptics, especially the sedative ones such as amitriptyline or clomipramine, are indicated when depersonalization is a major feature.

Smulevitch (1987) makes the point that one cannot be sure of a long remission even when there has been a good response to treatment. Sometimes it is necessary to combine intense pharmacotherapy with other forms of treatment such as insulin coma or atropine coma. There are also various regimes of more intensive therapy. He gives two examples:

1: A combination of depot neuroleptic and large doses of a benzodiazepine. Modecate is given every two weeks in doses of 12.5mgm to 25mgm. At the same time, over a 6 week period, a gradually increasing daily dose of intravenous diazepam is used. This is increased to a peak dose of about 150 mgm day at the fourth week and then gradually decreased to nothing.

2: A regime of 50mgm diazepam in the mornings and 3-5mgm trifluoperazine in the evenings along with a small dose of clozapine at night.

He suggests that the first approach is better for simpler disorders and the second for those with more complex clinical features. He emphasizes that both would have to be combined with other approaches.

Comparative aspects

The concept of sluggish schizophrenia has been criticized in the West, and the term has acquired a certain notoriety. The main criticism for its diagnosis is that the criteria are so vague as to be meaningless [17]. This criticism, however, has been made of many psychiatric entities in the West. It can be applied to the Bleulerian concept of schizophrenia and, therefore, to DSM-III criteria in which a diagnosis of schizophrenia can be made on the basis of flat affect, loosening of associations and a decline in social functioning. These require judgements which are potentially just as subjective, and open to wide interpretation, as those required for making a diagnosis of slow-flow schizophrenia. Moreover, concepts similar to slow-flow schizophrenia are still a feature of in American psychiatry, although rarely used in clinical practice. Cancro and Lehman (1985) write that latent schizophrenia, also known as borderline schizophrenia, may be diagnosed "in those patients who may have a marked schizoid personality and who show occasional behavioural peculiarities or thought disorders, without consistently manifesting any clearly psychotic pathology." Residual schizophrenia is considered to be similar to latent schizophrenia, except that it is found after a clear schizophrenic episode rather than being a possible precursor of one. These terms, latent, borderline and residual, are sometimes known as ambulatory schizophrenia. The terms pseudo-neurotic and pseudo-psychopathic schizophrenia still appear in some American literature to describe disorders characterized by non-psychotic symptomatology of the neurotic or psychopathic type, in which there might be brief psychotic episodes. In pseudoneurotic schizophrenia patients have mainly neurotic symptoms, but, on closer examination, have abnormalities of thinking and emotion more typical of schizophrenia. Anxiety tends to be diffuse and generalized, and phobias are vague and unfocussed.

Patients with a diagnosis of slow-flow schizophrenia in the Soviet Union would receive a variety of diagnoses in the West. Kazanetz (1989) argues that on follow-up most of them turn out to be schizophrenia (see page 32). Other patients would be considered to have some form of affective disorder, neurosis or personality disorder. In Britain more would receive a personality disorder diagnoses than in

---

17. Mersky and Shafran (1986) discuss some of the Soviet literature on slow-flow schizophrenia, quoting a number of articles in the Korsakoff journal which concentrate mainly on various clinical descriptions. The article is mainly concerned with how poor diagnostic criteria can lead to the potential for psychiatric abuse.

America, where the proportion would vary according to whether traditional concepts or DSM-III were being used. It is also possible that some of these patients would simply be regarded as being eccentric, although this would usually require some particular circumstances - generally strong family or financial support to shield the person from the consequences of their disability/personality. In theory, however, anyone with a diagnosis of slow-flow schizophrenia in the Soviet Union would have enough symptoms to meet one or, more usually, several of the categories of personality disorder in the DSM-III. Certainly the DSM-III categories of schizotypal, schizoid, paranoid and borderline personality disorder [18] would account for many of these patients.

McGlashan (1987) discusses borderline and schizotypal personality disorders. The core features of the borderline personality are impulsivity, self-damaging acts and difficulties in relationships. More equivocal are the affective instability, problems with identity and complaints of emptiness and boredom. The key features of schizotypal personality disorder are social isolation, odd patterns of communication, suspicious or paranoid ideation, and, more equivocally, ideas of reference, magical thinking, poor rapport and social anxiety. Transient psychotic episodes and depression may occur in both. On follow-up, about 20% of borderline patients and about 55% of schizotypal patients go on to develop schizophrenia. The level of social functioning tends to lie somewhere between that of patients with affective disorder and those with schizophrenia (McGlashan, 1983 and 1986).

The next question that should be addressed is how the diagnosis affects treatment. What happens to the group of people called slow-flow schizophrenia in the Soviet Union as compared to the group with schizotypal or borderline personality disorders in the USA? The brief answer is that there are greater similarities than differences. For both groups treatment is on an outpatient basis in the majority of cases. In general the treatment relies on psychosocial measures and the milder range of drugs. However, neuroleptic drugs are used in some cases and patients may be admitted to hospital. Thus, in a study on fifty in-patients with Borderline Personality Disorder and Schizotypal Personality Disorder it was shown that there was an improvement in various symptoms with a neuroleptic, thiothixene (Goldberg et al 1986). Cowdry and Gardner (1988) describe various drug treatments, including trifluoperazine and carbemazepine, for patients with borderline personality disorder. Davis (1987) quotes other treatment studies and argues that many patients with DSM-III diagnosis of personality disorder should be treated with low-dose neuroleptics.

Compulsory admission and treatment may be used with both groups [19], although it must be emphasized that the majority of people with personality disorders are not seen by psychiatrists, and, similarly, the majority of patients with slow-flow schizophrenia have no contact with the psychiatric services (eg Rotstein, 1977; Smulevitch, 1987). Some form of social disruption, however, may call attention to the symptoms, and, with either diagnosis, compulsory detention and

---

18. This must be distinguished from the Soviet usage of the term. Borderline here refers to a specific type of personality disorder, based upon psychoanalytic theory. The criteria are flexible: lack of a stable identity, the use of primitive defence mechanisms (splitting and projective identification) and partial insight. The definitions are somewhat tighter in DSM-III and in the Diagnostic Interview for Borderlines (Gunderson et al, 1981). Smulevitch (1987) criticizes the concept because of its derivation from psychoanalysis, ego psychology and "biometrics", also commenting that the criteria are too ill-defined.

treatment could be used.

As yet it is not possible to say which line is more correct or even more useful. There are implications for research into aetiology and mechanisms, especially with regard to the concept of the schizophrenia spectrum. A number of studies provide support for this concept, for instance studies which suggest that the relatives, including twins, of schizophrenics have more "schizophrenic equivalents" eg antisocial behaviour, poor school achievement, particular personality traits. The strongest case has been made for the concept of the schizophrenia spectrum as it relates to schizotypal personality disorder. Although twin studies are equivocal, family studies indicate a strong association with schizophrenia and follow-up studies also show the overlap with schizophrenia (eg Kendler et al, 1985). Rutter (1987) argues that schizotypal personality disorder differs strikingly from the other subtypes of DSM-III personality disorder with its emphasis on odd and eccentric behaviour, the abnormalities of cognition and perception, suspiciousness, ideas of reference and paranoid ideation. He argues that they should be grouped with schizophrenia rather than personality disorder (this is planned for ICD-10). Studies in molecular biology may help to resolve some of the issues. The evidence suggests that the same genotype abnormality may predispose to schizophrenia and a range of other non-psychotic disorders and personality disorders (Mullan and Murray, 1989). Moreover, the findings of molecular genetics appear to support the notion of a schizophrenia spectrum rather than a core disorder (Gill, 1988).

Chapter Nine

MANIC-DEPRESSIVE PSYCHOSIS

In the Handbook of Psychiatry (1983), manic-depressive psychosis is described as an illness which develops with affective phases (which may be manic, depressive or mixed) with intermissions characterized by a return to normal functioning and the absence of any defect state (Papadopolous and Shakhmatova-Pavlova, 1983) . The clinical features are characterized by changes in mood and in the level of motor function and mental activity. There may be associated features which are not directly related to mood. For instance, vegetative and obsessional syndromes may occur during the affective phases. There is a severe form of the disorder, cyclophrenia, and a mild form, cyclothymia. As with other disorders, the distinction is made between the cross-sectional syndromal presentation and the course of the illness. The typical progression is from somato-vegetative disturbances (with sleep disturbance often a key feature) through to simple, depression, delusional depression and then melancholia. The development is usually arrested at the phase of simple depression or delusional depression.

The features of the depressed phase are reduced mood, reduced intellectual and motor function and general lowering of vital functions. The syndromal presentation may be simple or complex and a variety of syndromes are described by different authors. The syndromes are: anxiety depression, agitated depression, adynamic (anergic) depression, asthenic depression and ironic (smiling) depression. Milder forms are tearful depression, sullen depression and whining depression. Sonnick (1984) refers to some of the above and also depressive-paranoid and depressive-hysterical syndromes. In their book on depression, Nuller and Mikhalenko (1988) describe four main affective syndromes: anergic depression, the melancholic syndrome, the anxiety-depressive syndrome and depersonalization-depression.

The manic phase is characterized by raised mood with speeding up of mental processes and motor excitement. There are different degrees: mild hypomania, hypomania, mania, mania with delusions of greatness or mania with confusion. Mixed affective states and atypical and special forms of depression are also described [1].

---

1. The atypical forms include senesto-hypochondriacal depression and depression with obsessional manifestations. The special forms are: masked depression, in which patients have mainly somatic and vegetative disorders, and "endo-reactive dysthymia".

The section on affective disorders in the Handbook (1983) does not discuss neurotic depression as this is considered to have more in common with the neurotic disorders than with manic-depressive psychosis and the related endogenous disorders. However, in his textbook of neurotic disorders, Karvarsarsky (1980) writes that there is a wide range of depressive manifestations from simple psychological reactions within the normal range through to neurotic depression and reactive depression and on to cyclothymia and manic-depressive psychosis. The symptoms of neurotic depression are lowered background mood, but not reaching the degree of *toska* (the symptom of depression/melancholia found in manic-depressive psychosis). Thus, there is a different quality of mood in neurotic depression, with retention of insight and pessimism generally confined to the conflict situation. There is usually some emotional lability, often with features of asthenia and anxiety. There may be insomnia and impaired appetite, but there is no change in motor function, no diurnal variation or ideas of self-blame and no suicidal tendencies. The view of Karvasarsky (1980) is that the syndrome of neurotic depression always arises as a result of psychogenesis, although he stresses that there is no clear distinction between neurotic depression and endogenous depression.

Reactive depression is one of the reactive psychoses and is considered to be a pathological psychotic reaction to a psychogenic traumatic event or long-term unfavourable circumstances (Smulevitch, 1983). The term does not imply that the symptoms are any less severe than those in the other affective disorders. It can present with the full range of depressive symptoms found in manic-depressive psychosis. Sonnick (1984) describes the syndromal presentation in 245 patients with reactive depression as follows: asthenic-depressive in 50% of cases, depressive-paranoid in 44% and depressive-hysterical in 6%. [2].

The term masked depression is used for patients in whom the main presenting symptoms are somatic and vegetative. These overshadow the affective symptoms, which, however, must be present. Mood changes and sleep disorder, often with early morning waking, are found (Papadopolous and Shakhmatova-Pavlova, 1983; Avrutsky et al, 1987).

Aetiology
Some aspects of aetiology, in particular the genetic, are discussed in Chapter Five. Papadopolous and Shakhmatova-Pavlova (1983) write that little is known about aetiology, but that a number of factors may have a role. They give some of the evidence for genetic factors and discuss the main twin studies. The various amine hypotheses are briefly mentioned and also the reported changes in salt and water metabolism, endocrine function and circadian rhythm. The role of immunity has also been investigated. Oskolkova (1985), from the Serbsky Institute in Moscow, writes that although there has been much immunology research in psychiatry over the previous decade there has been little in the reactive disorders. In her study of 82 patients with reactive depression she reports antibodies to cerebral antigens. She writes that the following changes have been reported: the presence of heterohaemolysins (indicating an immune reaction), of S-reactive protein

2. This study is an analysis of 4,564 case histories of patients with affective psychoses in the Poltavo region of Kiev. There were 245 cases of reactive depression, 1542 cases of manic-depressive psychosis, 569 cases of recurrent schizophrenia (here classified under the affective psychoses) and 2209 cases of involutional depression.

(indicating cell destruction) and of antibodies to brain antigens and antidepressants. In her study she found that cellular immunity was not impaired but that there was evidence of humoral immunity changes. There was more S-reactive protein and more brain antibodies. This was found mostly in those with paranoid features (42.8%) and those with a prolonged course (57.8%) than in those with simple neurotic type depression (6.6%). She also gives a reference indicating that similar changes have been found in normal people under conditions of stress. Vasiljeva et al (1989) report various changes in immune function in depression including the finding of fewer T- cells.

From the more traditional Soviet perspective the genetic-biochemical aetiological theories are viewed with scepticism. It is thought that there is a more global disruption of function than one would expect to see from a genetic abnormality affecting one neurotransmitter system. The view of Golant of the Bekhterev Institute was that the affective disorders, especially the rapidly cycling, were due to infectious or inflammatory processes in the brain stem (diencephalitis). Many disorders which in the West would be considered under the remit of affective disorders (anxiety or depression) would be seen as "organic", diagnosed as vegetative disorders, diencephalitis or arachnoiditis, in the Soviet Union. Soviet texts still tend to emphasize the disorders of fat and carbohydrate metabolism and temperature regulation in the affective disorders.

Nuller (1976) describes the long-term follow-up of 340 patients with typical manic-depressive psychosis. Patients with no genetic loading were more likely to have had serious infectious diseases or severe environmental problems. Patients with bipolar illnesses, especially those whose first presenting episode was mania, had the strongest family histories. He argues for the distinction between bipolar and unipolar depression, suggesting that there are two independent pathological mechanisms. There is overlap in any individual with depression. Thus, in an individual the ratio of the two pathological mechanisms will determine when or if a manic episode develops (possibly precipitated by treatment) and how much of a manic component there will be in the course of the disorder.

Treatment
Papadopolous and Shakhmatova-Pavlova (1983) write that the treatment depends upon the phase as well as severity and syndromal presentation. Tricyclic antidepressants are the mainstay of treatment, often in combination with lithium and/or neuroleptics. Drugs may be given intravenously, especially in severe cases. In psychotic depression, for instance, intravenous antidepressants, with short drug-free periods, say for two or three days, may be used. They note that senesto-hypochondriacal depression is often resistant to treatment and a single treatment modality is rarely effective. Combinations such as antidepressants with neuroleptics or tranquillisers are often required. ECT is used mainly in patients with melancholia. The treatment of mania is with neuroleptics and lithium. Karvasarsky (1980) discuses the treatment of neurotic depression. In the asthenodepressive syndrome he recommends the MAOI nialamid, the stimulant sidnocarb and, possibly, diazepam. Amitriptyline and diazepam are suggested for anxious depression and the combination of low-dose neuroleptics with tricyclic antidepressants in depression in patients with hysterical neurosis.

162

Papadopolous and Shakhmatova-Pavlova (1983) write that there is a special role for individual, family and group psychotherapy, mainly aimed at activating "positive personal resources". In long-standing cases psychotherapy will be determined by the specific features of the disorder and the social circumstances at work or within the family. The aim is to strengthen the patient's social position and repair damage to his relationships. Psychotherapy is only carried out after the acute stage of treatment. Indeed, as will be apparent from the chapter on treatment, the treatment tends to be more structured and, possibly, more cautious than in the West. Thus, it is considered necessary to have a sufficiently long period during which the patient rests and has his acute symptoms treated before moving on to rehabilitation measures.

As discussed in Chapter Six there is an emphasis on targeting individual symptoms and syndromes. Prokhorova (1985) describes a cluster analysis study in which she tried to relate particular groups of symptoms to three treatment regimes: tricyclic antidepressants, MAOIs and "sudden withdrawal of psychotropic drugs". Nuller (1985) considers that stimulant antidepressants should be used in anergic depression, clomipramine or imipramine in the melancholic syndrome and amitriptyline in anxious depression. Nuller and Mikhalenko (1988) give a comprehensive account of the treatment of depression, discussing a wide range of drugs, including some not readily available in the Soviet Union. As well as the tricyclic antidepressants, MAOIs, "atypical" antidepressants like piradizol, they comment on the use of monoamine precursors and also alpha-adrenergic blockers such as piroxan. They suggest the use of higher doses of antidepressants than normally used in the Soviet Union, more in keeping with Western psychiatry, for instance imipramine and clomipramine in doses of up to 450mgm per day. They draw up a table showing the relative efficacy of the drugs in different syndromes: the tricyclics appearing to be most effective in endogenous depression, the MAOIs in anergic depression and the sedating tricyclics in anxious-depression. Benzodiazepines and the phenothiazines, for instance levomepromazine (tizertsin), are also shown to be effective in anxious-depression. In severe cases of anxiety-depression or agitated depression they claim that clozapine is valuable.

Their first line of treatment in severe endogenous depression is imipramine or clomipramine, and they suggest that it should be given intravenously for several days before moving on to the oral preparation. In less severe depression, or in patients in whom tricyclics are contraindicated (eg cardiovascular disorders or glaucoma) the drug of choice is piridazol. They consider that MAOIs do not usually have a place with this disorder, but in resistant cases they may be indicated and should be used in combination with anxiolytic preparations such as thioridazine or levomepromazine (tizertsin).

They find the most difficult condition to treat severe depression with depersonalization, in that ECT and stimulating antidepressants seem to make it worse. They write that "unfortunately, at the present time it is easier to say how not to treat these patients than indicate a reliable method of treatment." Their approach is to start with fenazepam or clozapine and, if this proves to be effective, add antidepressants to the regime. There is a useful section on resistant depression, with suggestions about various drug combinations.

Treatment-resistant depression

In a monograph "Prolonged Depressive Disorders" Vovin and Aksenova (1982) discuss the treatment of treatment-resistant depression. They distinguish between genuine resistance which is defined as depression which has been treated adequately but unsuccessfully for over a year and "pseudoresistance" which reflects inadequate treatment. They write that individual biochemical differences might account for the lack of effect of drugs in some patients, but that it is also important to take account of psychosocial factors. Problems with family, work, loss of social prestige, all of which are important might be hindering the effects of treatment.

Drug treatment requires finding the appropriate dosages and drug combinations. They quote Western authors on the use of tricyclics with stimulants such as methylphenidate, but warn of the danger of dependence to stimulants. They should, therefore, be used for short periods, say up to two months. They are also wary of the tricyclic and MAOI combination because of the risks of side-effects, although consider that they may be more used in the future with increased knowledge and experience. They mention the use of thyroid hormone treatment, quoting the Western work about its efficacy, especially in women. They note that T3 increases heart rate and blood pressure and suggest this may have a beneficial effect on patients with the hypotensive effects of tricyclics. Chloracyzine, a beta-adrenergic stimulant, has been used in combination with imipramine. Other combinations include the use of lithium with tricyclics or MAOIs. Other approaches are to give drugs intravenously and to use a variety of sudden cessation and restarting techniques.

As mentioned on page 89 there is more caution about the use of ECT and other physical treatments, because of their effect on the clinical picture. Even in cases of resistant depression ECT seems to be used as a last resort. It is thought to have a global, non-specific effect, which weakens the stability of the psychopathological structure and so increases sensitivity to psychotropic preparations. They do not advocate repeated courses of treatment, arguing instead for further courses of alternative treatments, for instance with intravenous drugs. They write that the current trend in treatment is to move towards treatments based on aetiological theories. They consider that sleep deprivation falls into this category in view of what is known about disrupted circadian rhythms and changes in sleep patterns in depressed patients. The use of sleep deprivation is discussed in Chapter Six.

Prognosis

Prognosis is considered good in manic-depression, as would be expected from the definition of the disorder. Indeed, those with defect states are likely to be considered to have schizophrenic or organic disorders and would therefore not fall into this category. Papadopolous and Shakhmatova-Pavlova (1983) write that patients should be able to work normally and many go on to get higher qualifications and promotions. They make the point, however, that in some cases the disorder can progress and develop into a chronic mental illness.

Gurevitch et al(1985) describe a follow-up of 329 patients admitted to hospital from the 1930s onwards. Features of good outcome were a clear diagnosis of manic-depression, and cyclothymic and somatovegetative features. Poor outcome was associated with having more than one psychotic episode early in the course of the disorder. Grigorieva and Nikiforov (1987) describe a follow-up study to determine prognosis, linking clinical features with EEG findings and giving various EEG indices indicating good or bad prognosis.

Comparative aspects

Manic-depressive disorder is diagnosed less in the Soviet Union than in Britain. This is partly due to the broader concept of schizophrenia, in that some British manic-depressives would be diagnosed as suffering from Recurrent Schizophrenia in the Soviet Union [3]. The main erosion into the concept of depression, however, is at the less severe end of the spectrum where many patients considered to be suffering from minor affective disorders in the West would be classified under the neurotic disorders, for instance neurasthenia. Organic disorders would also be diagnosed in some of these cases as well as in some patients who in the West are diagnosed as suffering from late onset endogenous depression. Overall there is a tendency to restrict the diagnosis of manic-depression cases with clear-cut affective symptoms and good preservation of personality [4].

Differences in the classification of affective disorders will be compounded by the introduction of ICD-10 and DSM-4. In lumping the affective disorders together, they imply that neurotic depression (a term which will no longer be used) has more in common with manic-depressive psychosis than it does with the other neurotic disorders. In this respect the Soviet position is closer to that of the Newcastle school (Kiloh et al, 1962 and subsequent papers) which drew a distinction between endogenous and neurotic depression. One difference between the Soviet and Newcastle position, however, is with regards to the role of precipitating environmental factors. The Soviet distinction between the two terms is only in terms of symptomatology, the difference between the quality of the mood and the biological symptoms. It does not concern the presence or absence of life events in that environmental factors might be important in both types of disorder. However, Karvasarsky (1980) argues that they are more significant in neurotic depression in that psychogenesis is required to make the diagnosis and the nature of the psychopathology is closely bound up with the underlying conflict.

Some Soviet psychiatrists are critical of what they see as excessively theory-bound approaches to treatment in the West. It is thought that the uncritical acceptance of the amine hypothesis of depression, promoted by drug companies, has led to the development of newer, cleaner drugs which are less effective than traditional approaches using the well-tried drugs, for instance the use of drug combinations and the tailoring of drugs to individual patients. One major difference between the Soviet Union and the English-speaking world is the fact that ECT is less used, and this may be related to the different approaches to drug treatment. There are regional differences, however, with ECT being more widely used in the Baltic republics and Leningrad, essentially areas with a more Western outlook.

3. As stated already there is considerable variation within the Soviet Union with regards to this. Some psychiatrists have a broader concept of manic-depression than many British and most American psychiatrists.

4. Thus, biological tests such as the dexamethasone suppression test (DST) are used to identify underlying processes and predict response to treatment rather than as markers for particular forms of depression such as melancholia or endogenous depression which has been the main approach in the West. Despite the differences in approach and also a somewhat different methodology the DST findings are similar (Lukanitsa, 1986; Nuller et al, 1986).

There are different views with regard to prognosis in that several Soviet studies suggest that there is good long-term outcome in patients with manic-depressive psychosis. This is at odds with current data in the West [5]. It might be argued that the differences are due to different approaches to treatment and rehabilitation. However, differences in the classificatory systems make any comparison difficult. Some patients who would be classified under the affective disorders in the West would be considered to be schizophrenic or suffering from organic disorders in the Soviet Union. As these tend to be the more severely ill patients this would improve the outcome figures for a group of core manic-depressives.

---

5. Recent follow-up studies suggest that the long-term outcome for patients with affective disorders is not as good as has been traditionally thought. Kiloh (1988) reports on 145 depressed patients admitted to hospital and followed-up for 15 years. 7% committed suicide and at the time of follow-up only 20% remained well. The morbidity was similar whether the patients had an original picture of endogenous or neurotic depression. Lee and Murray (1988) report on a 20 year follow-up of admissions to the Maudsley Hospital for depression. Again there was a picture of rather poor outcome in terms of morbidity and readmissions. Only 20% had remained well. This study also casts doubts on the nosological homogeneity of the group. Follow-up showed that there was a high "incidence" of other disorders, including schizophrenia, schizoaffective disorder and alcoholism. It indicates that a broader concept of MDP leads to a poorer overall outcome.

Chapter Ten

THE BORDERLINE DISORDERS

Borderline Disorders refer to the neuroses and psychopathies (personality disorders) in Soviet psychiatry. This chapter will also briefly discuss Anorexia Nervosa and a group of neuropsychiatric disorders, including "diencephalitis" and "arachnoiditis", which are generally classified along with the neuroses.

THE NEUROSES

Neuroses have had a relatively low profile in Russian and Soviet psychiatry. This is partly due to the development of a materialist school of psychology and psychiatry and the fact that Freudian psychology was not incorporated into Soviet psychiatry. Consequently, neurosis, associated as it was in the early days with the psychoanalytic movement, did not figure prominently in Soviet psychiatry. The disorders did not disappear, of course, but they were either distributed among various diagnostic categories or considered to be outside the province of psychiatry. There is disagreement within the Soviet Union about the concept and definition of neurosis, in particular over the hazy boundaries between neuroses and other disorders. This is seen as inevitable in a field with contributions from psychology, sociology and education as well as medicine and physiology, and it is recognized that it is difficult to integrate the different disciplines (Karvarsarksy, 1980). There are three main approaches.

The first approach accords with that of Schneider and the German tradition, in which neuroses are seen as variations of normal experience. They are considered as the reactions of normal personalities to severe stress or of abnormal personalities to mild or moderate stress. There is emphasis on personality and the dynamic changes in the progress of the disorder eg from the stage of a neurotic reaction to the stage where environmental factors become less important and factors to do with personality or brain damage are more significant (this is the stage of the neurotic disorder) There may be a later stage, the neurotic development, in which there are new changes quite unrelated to environmental factors. The change from a neurotic reaction to a neurotic development is facilitated when there is disorder of the personality (Smulevitch, 1983). Neurosis is seen not as a discrete disorder but as lying on a continuum intermediate between normality and more readily definable disorders such as psychoses, organic disorders or personality disorders.

A second, somewhat more recent, approach is to see neuroses as being fully determined by biological factors. Psychosocial factors have a place, but only as they would in any physical illness ie as one or more of a number of factors disturbing the homeostasis. This is the laboratory approach in that the boundaries of neurosis are gradually eroded away as more organic conditions are established and reclassified, for instance the various types of infection of the brain and meninges. Vein, a neuropathologist in Moscow, is the main proponent of this approach, and some of his work is described later. From this perspective the diagnosis of neurosis is essentially a negative one.

The third approach, perhaps the most widely held, describes neurosis as a "psychogenic, neuro-mental disturbance, generally due to some conflict, and arising as a disturbance of significant relationships, manifesting itself in specific clinical phenomena in the absence of psychotic phenomena" (Karvasarsky, 1980). The neurosis is thought to be due to a psychological trauma which produces a conflict that the individual cannot resolve because of his personality structure. There should be a direct connection between the symptoms and the system of relationships and conflicts that produces them. An important notion is the reversibility of the condition, even when it is long-standing. This concept of neurosis is based mainly on the work of Miasishchev (1960), who tried to establish a positive understanding of neurosis linked to the concept of psychogenesis. This view links neurotic processes with psychogenic factors much more firmly than most other concepts of neurosis. Thus, Karvasarsky (1980) writes:

1. Psychogenesis is closely related to personality, to the traumatic situation, to difficulty of the situation and to the inability of the patient to resolve the difficulties.
2. The course and aetiology of neurosis is connected with the pathogenetic situation and the experiences of the individual. There is a definite relationship between the neurosis and changes in the traumatic situation.
3. The content of the neurosis reflects the traumatic situation, the patient's personality and aspirations.
4. Psychotherapy is more effective than biological methods of treatment.

Genuine neuroses, therefore, are always psychogenic according to this view. It is taken for granted that there is a brain substrate for the processes, and there is emphasis on the role of personality and somatic factors, especially vegetative (autonomic nervous system). The difference between neuroses and the reactive states is that the trauma in neurosis is generally less pronounced. Because of the personality structure there is less need of a major life event. It tends to be chronic, prolonged psychogenic trauma that brings about neurosis rather than acute life events. In a sense this can be seen as a modified version of the Schneiderian view ie that of the reaction of an abnormal personality to stress. The key point, however, is that in neurosis the abnormal personality is essentially a variation of normal which, in the absence of a particular type of conflict, does not interfere with normal life.

Classification
Many of the general issues have already been discussed in Chapter 2, but it is worth recalling that the Soviet system of classification emphasizes the difference

between syndromes and forms. Syndromes are groupings of symptoms, whereas the three main forms of neuroses are defined not only by characteristic symptoms, but also by demographic features and the course that they can be expected to run; there is an implied common aetiology and underlying pathology. The three forms are:

1. Neurasthenia
2. Hysterical neurosis
3. Obtrusive neurosis

Various syndromes may be found among the three basic forms either simultaneously or at different stages of the disorder. Some of the syndromes are familiar to Western psychiatrists, and there will follow a brief description of the main ones:

Syndromes
Asthenic syndrome
The asthenic syndrome, a type of "neuro-mental weakness", is considered to be on the increase. The syndrome consists of multiple vague symptoms including fatigue, anxiety, uneasiness, tearfulness, irritability, weakness, sensitivity to loud noises and bright lights. The commonest picture is a triad of "true asthenia" (fatigue, difficulty with work, concentration and memory), sleep disturbance and vegetative symptomatology (eg tachycardia and sweating). Asthenia is subdivided into three sub-types. Hyposthenia has the essential, core features of asthenia, whereas in hypersthenia irritability and excitability are more prominent. The third sub-type, "irritable weakness", lies somewhere between these two. Asthenia is found in a third of patients with neurosis, and it may be present in almost any illness. It is also found in healthy people when they are excessively tired or overworked.

Obsessional syndrome
The main feature of the obsessional syndrome is the intrusion into the mind of sudden thoughts which have no connections with what was going on beforehand. The experience occurs in a state of clear consciousness, and, because of its alien and unpleasant quality, is resisted. The alien quality is stressed, along with the inability to rid the mind of the phenomenon, and hence the Russian term for this is better translated as "obtrusive" rather than obsessional. The obtrusive conditions have been divided into two types (Snezhnevsky, 1968):

1. The abstract type. In this there may be aimless rumination, counting (arithmomania) and naming of objects (onomatomania). This happens without a strong affective component, and there is indifference to the content of the ruminations.
2. An imagic type in which there is a strong affective component. There may be obsessional memories, fears, and doubts which may result in excessive checking. There may also be blasphemous thoughts and images.

It is also possible to subdivide the obtrusive phenomena by the spheres of activity affected: the intellectual sphere in which there are obsessional thoughts (obsessions), the emotional sphere with obsessional fears (phobias) and the motor sphere which produces the compulsive phenomena. This is considered relative, in that the different features are usually combined in any one case. Obsessional movements or actions may be independent or arise along with phobias as rituals. They may be simple or complex movements, and washing is a common example of the latter. Repetitive movements, especially of the facial muscles, may occur, and these must be differentiated from neurological disorders.

It is stressed that these symptoms are generally combined, and may be found in a wide number of disorders. In hysteria, for instance, obsessional images and movements are common, obessional thoughts less so. Indeed, obsessional thoughts by themselves are thought rarely to be a feature of the neuroses and most cases occur in psychopathy (psychasthenic or anankastic), but also in schizophrenia. Obsessional ideas are also found in the organic brain syndromes such as in encephalitis. An important clinical point here is that in organic states, in contrast to the usual rule, obsessional ideas and impulses may be acted upon, despite resistance.

Phobic syndrome
A phobia is defined as fear *(strakh)* associated with a definite situation. The fear is recognized as being irrational and is resisted. Phobias are considered to be a feature of many neurotic conditions, and there is overlap with other syndromes, although least commonly in hysteria. There is emphasis on the differential diagnosis from organic states and schizophrenia, especially slow-flow schizophrenia. In the latter condition it is thought that after a few years the phobia becomes "inert". Fixed rituals develop and the attempt to resist is gradually lost. Patients may even strive to carry out the rituals which develop an overvalued character.

Anxiety
There is no exact equivalent in Russian for the word anxiety. The word *trevoga* means worrying, which might be a normal activity or might be considered a symptom if indulged in to excess. Although it implies concern for the future it does not carry the same meaning in terms of the strength of the feeling and the somatic sensations that go along with it. It is essentially a mental activity. The word that is generally used as an equivalent to anxiety is the word for fear, *strakh*. The ICD-9 Anxiety Syndrome is actually translated as Fear Syndrome and is included with the phobias. It is not regarded as an independent syndrome. The quality of the emotion in anxiety and fear is essentially the same, the difference being that anxiety is fear directed towards the future. It can be argued that it is not necessary to make this distinction. Thus, for instance, it is not considered necessary to have an extra word for anger to describe angry feelings that are generated by potential future events as opposed to something in the present. The feeling is simply qualified. Thus, in Russian, the state of anxiety is seen as the state of being fearful. It is a morbid state in that the fear is disproportionate to the stimulus that produces the fear. The stimulus, for instance, might be the sight of a dog or even imagining the possibility of seeing a dog.

Hypochondriacal syndrome
This syndrome is characterized by an unrealistic attitude to one's own health. Anxiety (fear) and depression are commonly present in the syndrome. The syndrome may occur in all three neurotic disorders and is especially likely to occur

when somatic factors have a greater aetiological role. Once again, there are various different types: psychogenic hypochondriacal reactions; obsessive-compulsive neurosis of the hypochondriacal type; hypochondria with somatic illness; hypochondria with organic brain syndrome; hypochondria with chronic psychoses. There may also be hypochondriacal development of personality. Differential diagnosis is considered to be particularly difficult.

The syndrome of Neurotic Depression.
Depression is present in most neuroses and in many psychiatric disorders. The key feature about Neurotic Depression is that it is always psychogenic and the symptoms reflect the psychotraumatic situation. There is a lowered mood state, but this is distinguished from real depression. There is asthenia, lability of mood and general worrying. There may be appetite and sleep disturbance. The pessimism is not generalized, but limited to the area of the conflict situation, and the link between the problem and the mood state is usually recognized. There may be various combined forms such as anxiety-depression, astheno-depression and phobic-depression.

There are a number of syndromes, some of which are essentially somatic, which are considered to have a psychogenic aetiology:
Disorders of cardiac function generally occur along with cardiophobia which consists of fixed, overvalued ideas about dying from a heart lesion. Karvarsarsky (1980) comments that these patients like to spend time around hospital departments.
Respiratory disorders are less common. They include disturbance in the rate of breathing ("air hunger" or hyperventilation), neurotic hiccuping and laryngospasm.
Gastrointestinal disorders are common in all neurotic patients. They are subdivided into anorexia (which, as a symptom, occurs in many neurotic conditions but especially neurasthenia), bulimia (described as wolf-like appetite with no mention of vomiting), aerophagia, belching, gastralgia, "fear-induced diarrhoea" and vomiting. Vomiting, which may occur with anorexia, is subdivided into induced vomiting with no vegetative symptoms and no nausea, induced vomiting with nausea, vomiting of emotional genesis and periodic vomiting with nausea.
Vegetative syndromes are due to over-activity of the sympathetic nervous system, parasympathetic nervous system or both and are described more fully on page 193. There are also syndromes characterized by disorders of movement and sensation.

Forms
Neurasthenia
Karvarsarksy (1980) makes the point that in Western psychiatry the concept of neurasthenia has been gradually eroded as first anxiety neurosis and then depression were detached [1]. It ceased to be mentioned in the American literature except as an asthenic reaction. It was only in 1968, with ICD-8, that neurasthenia was brought back as a separate form of neurosis, mainly because of pressure from Soviet and French psychiatrists.

---

1. Karvarsarsky (1980) describes the 19th century as "the real epoch of nervous weakness" when the term asthenia was incorporated into Beard's concept of neurasthenia.

It is considered to be the most widespread form of neurosis. The symptoms are more or less those described under the asthenic syndrome, with insomnia, headaches, somatic symptoms, emotional lability, sexual disorders all common. There is often a depressive affect, and the hypochondriacal syndrome may be incorporated. As with the asthenic syndrome, there are three types:

Hypersthenic, with marked irritability, impatience, tearfulness and sensitivity to stimuli.

The transitional type, sometimes called excitable weakness.

Hyposthenic (or asthenic) with reduced work capability and marked fatigue.

Onset is rarely spontaneous in that there is usually a specific situation that provokes an episode, generally some kind of sudden demand on the patient. Reactive forms last for a few months and prolonged forms for several years. Even though about half the patients have a course lasting for over five years, on the whole the outcome is good and there is full recovery in over 50%, marked improvement in 25% with the rest staying the same or getting worse. The course and outcome depend on the severity and duration of symptoms. Prolonged course, depressive symptomatology and a shift from monosymptomatic to polymorphic presentation are considered unfavourable features. Personality, the psychotraumatic situation, the basic qualities of the brain and any additional somatic illnesses all influence outcome, as does inadequate treatment of the condition.

Karvarsarsky describes the following case.

A 22 year old male student developed neurasthenia soon after getting married. He had a dominant mother, who had high expectations of her son, and a passive father. His school career was not successful. He married a woman who was, apparently, stubborn and rather dominating, and who put pressure on him, for instance wanting him to arrange for a cooperative flat for the two of them (something that was unusual at the time). It was at this stage that he developed symptoms, mainly of tension and irritability. There were periods when he lost his appetite and lacked drive. In addition he was forgetful, felt tired during the day and found it hard to do any work.

Hysteria (hysterical neurosis)
This is the second commonest of the neuroses, although the incidence is said to be diminishing. Gross ("classic") manifestations such as paralysis, blepharospasm, hysterical blindness and deafness occur in only about 10% of cases and other traditional presentations such as amnesia and pseudodementia are also seen less often. There are more mixed forms such as hystero-phobic, hypochondriacal and affective states. The distinction between a neurotic form and syndrome is illustrated by the fact that other syndromes, such as the phobic or asthenic, are commonly found in this form.

There is a debate as to whether hysteria should be considered a neurosis or a form of psychopathy. Karvarsarsky says that in contrast to hysteroid psychopathy the personality abnormalities are less marked in hysteria, and they do not lead to a poor level of social or "ethical" functioning. Moreover, hysterical neuroses occur under the influence of a life experience in the context of a bad upbringing. In half the patients with hysteria the premorbid personality is quite normal and in half there is a "leaning" towards either a hysterical or asthenic type of personality.

The long-term outcomes suggests that about half of all patients improve with age, but in the rest symptoms persist, generally with more hypochondriacal or phobic symptoms. Obsessional features are a poor sign. Organic factors are important in aetiology and differential diagnosis. Karvarsarksy emphasizes that organic and hysterical features may occur together and quotes Soviet work showing that malignancies and multiple sclerosis can present like hysteria.

Some Soviet researchers believe that all hysteria is due to organic disease. Vein, a Moscow neuropathologist, argues that hypothalamic-mesencephalic pathology (most commonly due to encephalomyelitis) with the resultant limbic system damage, is responsible for the changes in emotions, needs and behaviour that are characteristic of hysteria. Sverdlov, a Leningrad psychiatrist, takes a compromise position, arguing that a weakened system, either due to genetic factors or environmental damage (eg viruses), will be more susceptible to psychogenic factors.

Obtrusive Neurosis
The Obtrusive form of neurosis combines the obsessional syndrome with the phobic syndrome and a number of other features. Because the clinical picture is often mixed it is felt that there is no justification for considering the phobias as a separate form of neurosis. This form is essentially a combination of two ICD-9 syndromes: the obsessive-compulsive and phobic. It is thought that the clinical picture has changed over time, possibly related to improved education and a greater input of information about the outside world. Phobic manifestations are becoming more prominent. Common phobias include cardiophobia, cancerophobia, madness and dirt phobias, and, perhaps the most common, agoraphobia. Persistent thoughts, memories, doubts and movements are rarer but very typical of the condition. In addition, other neurotic syndromes are present. There are no organic changes, but there may be tremor when somatic anxiety is a feature. There may be a single episode (lasting from weeks to years), an episodic course or continuous symptoms. More usually the course is chronic and in two thirds of patients it lasts for more than 5 years. The prognosis is worst in early onset cases and also when onset occurs during the involutionary period. Many patients may require hospital admission.

The differential diagnosis is considered to be difficult in many cases, and Karvarsarsky states that in some patients schizophrenia can only be confidently excluded after decades! The earlier the onset the more likely that this will prove to be the diagnosis.

Differential diagnosis
Zavilianskaya (1987) writes about the need to differentiate between the neuroses, in which there is real psychogenesis, and the neurosis-like disorders, in which the symptoms are similar, but with no psychogenesis. A typical case where this would be important would be that of a middle-aged man presenting with asthenia. There are implications for treatment in deciding whether it is due to neurosis or arteriosclerosis. Generally, if there are changes in memory and the speed of mental processes it is more likely to be a neurosis-like condition due to arteriosclerosis rather than a true neurosis.

The distinction is not always absolute, of course. There may be somatic pathology in neurosis, and at certain times there may a psychogenic process in patients with neurosis-like disorders. Vein has drawn up four groups:
1. Neuroses with no signs of a brain lesion.
2. Neuroses arising in the context of residual brain damage.
3. Neuroses combined with ongoing brain pathology.
4. Neurosis-like syndromes.

He claims that in this fourth group psychogenesis never applies. Zavilianskaya (1987), however, argues that this is too rigid a view and that one cannot exclude the possibility of psychogenesis in this group. Such patients might also have experienced a traumatic event which then complicates the picture.

Neurosis-like disorders are common. Zavilianskaya (1987) quotes the figures from the psychoneurological dispensary in Kiev. Over the period 1980-1983 there were 1783 patients and of these there were 813 with neurosis-like disorders. The conditions that presented in this way were:

Schizophrenia 46
Cyclothymia 277
Head injury 144
Cerebral arteriosclerosis 92
Somatic illnesses 254.

She writes that this accords with the literature, showing how commonly the neurosis-like conditions occur. She argues against simply applying symptomatic treatment measures, making a case for pathogenetic psychotherapy in cases where there are disordered otnoshenia (relations/attitudes).

Aetiology
The different Soviet concepts of neuroses inevitably mean that there are various different theories with regards to aetiology. The view that the neuroses are psychogenic disorders is gaining ground, mainly due to the influence of Karvasarsky (1980) and work carried out at the Bekhterev Institute in Leningrad. The views about aetiology discussed here are drawn mainly from this source. The term psychogenesis has a different connotation to its usage in the West. It does not imply that the neuroses have no organic basis and that they happen "in the mind", but is taken to mean that psychosocial factors are important in aetiology. It also carries the implication that the processes are not simply due to a pathological lesion in the brain, but that they reflect adaptive responses. Aetiology is still considered multifactorial, with an interaction between biological, social and psychological factors. A psychotraumatic event may be the main immediate cause of the neurosis, but its impact is modulated by a complex interaction of other factors, both genetically determined and acquired. Psychosocial factors determine symptoms, but the basic predisposition ("soil") often becomes more significant when the course of the neurosis is drawn out. Predisposing factors might include some accompanying somatic illness or organic cerebral insufficiency. However, Karvarsarsky (1980) also stresses that a prolonged course may be due to unresolved conflicts, features of personality, relationships or the "mental set". Occasionally, he warns, the course might be prolonged by inappropriate symptomatic treatment (ie drugs) instead of psychotherapeutically based treatment.

This is because symptomatic treatment might not allow the disrupted relationships, the original cause of the neurosis, to be reconstructed.

Karvarsarksy (1980) claims that diagnosis is more culture-bound in neuroses than in other disorders, commenting that the decrease in hysteria and the increase in neurasthenia probably reflects changes in society, particularly with regard to education and knowledge, and the decrease in superstition. There are fewer patients with hysterical manifestations such as blindness or paraplegia, and patients with these kinds of symptoms are more likely to come from remote rural areas.

Genetic aspects
Soviet and Western studies are mentioned with regard to the role of genetic factors, particularly in obsessive-compulsive disorders. Karvarsarsky (1980) makes the curious point that Freud had most of his success with hysterical patients, in whom there seems to be the smallest genetic component.

Structural changes
Karvasarsky (1980) reports on the work of Vein and Rovstein who attempt to explain all neurotic phenomena in terms of structural brain lesions. They report, for instance, that right sided brain lesions produce more emotional and vegetative disturbance. Vein claims to have shown that organic damage, including that due to minor infections, can lead to personality changes. Karvarsarsky criticizes the findings on the grounds that patients in specialist centres who have extensive investigations are an atypical group, by virtue of the referral system, and are more likely to have organic changes than other neurotic patients. He supports this by quoting an early pneumoencephalography study at the Bekhterev. Neurotic patients with long-standing, persistent headaches were likely to have changes - either atrophy or enlargement of ventricles, but those with simple neuroses did not. He also quotes other work indicating that the changes were commoner in hysteria, occurring in about two thirds of patients, whereas only about a third of other neurotic patients had some abnormalities. This early work is questionable because of the absence of adequate control data. It does, however, indicate that organic factors do play a role, especially in prolonging the course of a disorder.

Soviet studies reveal that somatic illnesses are closely associated with the neuroses. Half of all neurotic patients have chronic gut disorders and a fifth chronic cardiovascular disorders. It is thought that these influence the course of the neuroses.

Biochemical theories
Karvasarsky (1980) refers to 70 years of work in this area at the Bekhterev Institute in Leningrad, pointing out the limitations of the work due to methodological problems. The more reliable findings would suggest that catecholamine levels are high in neurotic patients with insomnia, in certain types of stress headaches and when there is a diencephalic lesion (see page 191). In contrast to Western work most of the studies on cortisol function suggests that levels are lower in neuroses, especially asthenics, compared to controls, and this is thought to be due to exhaustion of the hypothalamo-pituitary-adrenal axis. However, under conditions of stress there are increased cortisol levels in neurotics, and this is especially the

case when there is no organic component. Changes in thyroid function have also been found in patients with neurosis, particularly neurasthenia, and this is related to somatic anxiety symptoms.

Neurophysiology and psychophysiology
There is a large body of neurophysiological and psychophysiological work in neurosis. Karvasarsky (1980) writes that there is a shift away from simple analysis of reflexes to the examination of complex aspects such as personality and consciousness. He points out that clinical-experimental work on the biological correlates of stress proves the relevance of materialist psychophysiology for psychogensis. Thus EEG responses to verbal stimuli which are related to aetiologically significant experiences may reflect the psychotraumatic situation, especially in rapidly developing neuroses. EEG changes also correlate with mental states. Thus, asynchronized fast (beta) waves are associated with emotional excitability and lability. On the other hand with general weakness and fatigue there is less beta and more alpha activity. There is some work to suggest that each neurosis has its own pattern of EEG activity. Obtrusive neurosis is associated with more fast waves and neurasthenia with slow waves. As might be expected there are more EEG changes when there is an organic component so that in neurasthenia with diencephalic insufficiency there are marked bursts of frontal slow-waves bursts. The biological correlates of the syndrome of asthenia (which can occur in any of the three forms of neurosis) include EEG changes, decreased reaction time and decreased period of active attention. In addition there is lower amplitude and longer latency with Walter's E-waves (expectation waves). There is recent work on the relationship between cortex and sub-cortex, with use of EEG and other neurophysiological measures. There are also studies on the relationship between biochemical and EEG variables.

Pavlovian theory. Pavlov's concept of the experimental neurosis suggests that the neuroses are caused by over-strain of the higher nervous system from outside factors, either because they are too great or too prolonged. In early Soviet Psychiatry this was seen as the main factor in the clinical formation of neurosis (Davidenkov, 1963). The "soil" was essentially genetic, and Pavlov considered neuroses were a continuation of the normal repertoire of behaviour, with the form of neurosis determined by the nature of the weakness of the nervous system. The "artistic" type of person was seen as being more prone to hysteria, whereas the "intellectual" type was more prone to psychasthenia, which he considered to be a neurotic disorder. It would now be thought that these people are more prone to obtrusive disorder. Intermediate types are prone to neurasthenia.

Another important concept was that of the "dynamic stereotype". This is the individual's pattern of response to the environment. Experimental neuroses, and, presumably, real life neuroses occur with sudden changes in the dynamic stereotype. These can be seen as the equivalent to having a bad (essentially inconsistent) upbringing with lack of proper boundaries, confused messages and so on. It results in disruption of conditioned reflexes and disorganization of behaviour, dissonance between cortical and subcortical structures which produce somatic changes. Certain types of higher nervous system are considered more susceptible: the weak, which is less adaptable, the imbalanced and the excessively mobile. Disruption may be due to three main factors: over-strain because of excitation, inhibition or excess mobility. This, then, is the "soil" for the effects of psychological trauma. The development of neurosis is not innate or due to "simple, mechanistic processes" (as with behavioural models), but a combination of individual susceptibility and environmental factors.

In hysteria there is thought to be strong inhibitory tone in the cortex and hence a predominance of the subcortex. This results in mood swings, leading to suggestibility and emotionality. In psychasthenia the first signalling system is weak, so that there is weak information coming in through the organs of perception. Thus the experience of the environment is weak and distorted. Incoming signals (eg social cues) determine behaviour and if these are weak or distorted behaviour will be socially inept or inappropriate. If the second signalling system (language) predominates this will dominate and there will then be excess rumination and intellectual distortion of the outside world. This mechanism is thought to apply to obtrusive neurosis, accounting for the excessive intellectual activity, for instance the obsessional ruminations. Neurasthenia is characterized by "inertia" of the brain. The main element is over-strain caused by overload. Both inhibition and excitation fail. In the first phase there is weakening of cortical inhibition resulting in insomnia, irritability and excitement. In the second phases both inhibition and excitation are weakened, so the person tires easily, loses the ability to concentrate and has mood swings. In the third phase inhibition is predominant, mainly to protect the organism from over-strain, resulting in a lethargic, apathetic picture with more depression. The hypersthenic form of neurasthenia corresponds to the first phase and the hyposthenic to the third phase[2].

Personality
Clinical studies suggest that personality is normal in the simpler neuroses where there are only one or two symptoms. In hysteria, on the other hand, patients tend to have abnormal personality traits and in neurasthenia up to a half of the patients have asthenic personalities. Karvasarsky (1980), however, considers that there is little evidence to support the view that neurosis is simply decompensated psychopathy ie that hysteria is decompensated hysterical psychopathy and neurasthenia is decompensated asthenic psychopathy. He argues that it is better to think in terms of variations or accentuations of normal character. The importance of the distinction between psychopathy and an accentuation of character is that psychopathy is seen as pathological and maladaptive, so that social functioning is affected. This is not the case in the accentuations of character found in neurotics, who normally (that is in the absence of conflict-producing situations) function well. Thus, neurasthenics are seen as conscientious and responsible, working well, although tending to be sensitive to criticism. The obtrusive premorbid personality is low in self-confidence, activity and decisiveness, with more anxiety and suspicion, but again tending to be responsible and conscientious. This, incidentally,

---

2.   Pavlov's work has been continued by many workers, most notably Ivanov-Smolensky, who suggests that in hysteria the presence of increased suggestibility is related to a disturbance in the three vertical brain systems. Thus, disturbance in the cortico-pyramidal system, which is related to intellectual function, speech and actions, results in hysterical symptoms. The cortico-extrapyramidal system, related to emotional activity, results in changes in basic instincts and increased affectivity. Changes in the ascending reticular system alter the regulating tone of the brain.

is said to make them more susceptible to conflicts in the "moral-ethical" sphere. Hysterics do not come out of this so well, in that they are described as excessively self-confident and egocentric.

Early environment

Karvarsarsky (1980) writes that there is need for more empirical work in this area, quoting research which found a high incidence of loss of an important relative in childhood in neurotic patients. This occurred in about 40% of all patients, and in half the cases it was due to divorce. No mention is made of controls, but the figures for divorce are clearly not different from the normal population. The high death rate may be significantly different, but, in view of the fact that the research was carried out in Leningrad, on a population which would have included many who were born before or during the Second World War, this is not certain (Leningrad was under siege for three years during the Second World War and over a half of its population perished). He discusses work on broken families which suggested that absence of father might be significant in the aetiology of hysteria and neurasthenia and the absence of mother in obsessive-compulsive disorders. There were similar trends in controls with "mild" forms of the disorders. There were, however, some differences within the neurotic population, in that hysterics were more likely to have been in orphanages (13%) than the rest (3%). He writes that although there is much work on obvious disruptions in childhood more work is required to investigate conditions within intact families.

Life events

Karvarsarsky (1980) writes that 25% of neurotics have poor marriages, 12% have problems at work, and in 12% of cases the death of a close person is reported. In the majority of cases it is only prolonged difficulties that are significant in aetiology. He gives a long list of different types of problem, mainly related to the family, but also to work difficulties. Work issues tend to be more significant for men and home circumstances for women, perhaps surprising in a society where the vast majority of women work. The high incidence of neurosis in students in further education is commented on. Bojanova (1974) argues that the pressure of further education is a cause of neurosis, or at least a factor in the decompensating process. There is a large body of work on choice of job and job satisfaction. No major findings with regard to neurosis have emerged, although, as might be expected, a negative attitude to work or a badly organized work schedule are potentially damaging.

The type of conflict also tends to vary across the neuroses, so that work difficulties are found more commonly in neurasthenia, and family and sexual difficulties in hysteria and obtrusive neurosis. He quotes a small study of 40 patients in which they tried to quantify the unsatisfied needs producing the conflicts. The main areas were:

1. Needs related to adequate social attainment
2. Needs in the areas of love or sex. These were only present in 15% of cases, he writes, "in contrast to psychoanalytic thinking".
3. Needs related to friendship.
4. Difficulties with self-expression and self-assertion.

Karvasarsky (1980) also writes about iatrogenic causes of neurosis, produced either by the doctor, the hospital investigations or other patients. Although personality is again critical it is important to be aware that the doctor's behaviour and the quality of the interaction may be a factor in a proportion of patients. Although it is rarely a leading cause of neurosis, it may provoke a neurosis that could have remained latent.

Karvasarsky (1980) stresses the difficulty of research in the area, and again there is the issue of lack of controls. This does, of course, present serious difficulties, in that what is central to Miasishchev's theory of *otnoshenia* is the distinction between serious life events and pathogenetic ones. Miasishchev considered that the situation at work or in the home were not in themselves important in aetiology, because similar difficulties are found in healthy people; symptoms arise when these are combined with a pathological attitude. Thus, a particular experience may be pathogenic for one individual, and not for another, and even serious difficulties will not distress some people. The key point, then, is that the theory of *otnoshenia* sees the combination of the event and the attitude/relationship as being pathogenetic.

Zavilianskaya (1987) considers the role of frustration in producing neurosis. She writes that being able to withstand frustration does not depend only on the strength of the nervous system, but also on help and moral support from other people. This gives a sense of protectiveness, mutual support from within the "collective", and increases the hardiness of an individual to adverse experiences.

The role of life events in the aetiology of mental illness is still controversial in Western psychiatry. The Miasishchev theory of *otnoshenia* might help to account for why there have been conflicting results in life events work in physical, psychosomatic and psychiatric disorders. The theory suggests that life events provoke conflicts, but these will produce neurosis only if they have a central place in the person's system of *otnoshenia*. Thus, life events are important but are only aetiologically significant if they occur in the context of a particular *otnoshenia* [3].

Treatment

Some of the treatments, both biological and psychotherapeutic, are discussed in more detail in Chapter Six. The treatment of neurosis is generally thought to be difficult, requiring the use of complex measures, although psychotherapy is the mainstay of treatment according to Karvasarsky (1980). Much is made of the quality of the doctor/patient relationship, and the appropriate behaviour of the doctor. Social measures are aimed at resolving the conflict and the traumatic situation. These might involve trying to change the environment in order to get the patient away from the traumatic situation.

The goals of psychotherapy depend on the clinical picture and the stage of the disorder, also on the content of the traumatic situation. In the acute stage it is used to calm the patient and reduce tension. Patients need to be taught about their condition and about the approach to treatment. The primary mechanisms in the development of the neurosis are linked to the patient's life history and his intrapersonal conflicts. Secondary mechanisms, which prolong the symptoms, are

---

3. This approach is in keeping with the work of Brown and Harris (1978) on the contextual rating of life events and vulnerability.

linked to difficulties in interpersonal relationships and actual life situations and problems. Thus, individual psychotherapy is generally indicated for the primary mechanisms and group psychotherapy for the secondary. It might also be appropriate to include the different symptomatic group therapies such as rational therapy or autogenous training. The later stages of treatment are directed towards reconstruction of the disturbed relationships and the disruption in the social and microsocial environment, changing unrealistic expectations, resocialization and return to work.

Karvarsarsky discusses pharmacological treatment methods, stressing that drugs should not be used just because other methods fail and criticizing the notion that drugs only bring symptomatic relief or are a sign of the failure of psychotherapy. The timing is seen as important. Thus, drugs given late in treatment might hinder progress by interfering with psychotherapy. He sees the correct use of drugs as opening the door for psychotherapy. Drugs are especially useful in the early stages when there is often marked anxiety. Even a short course of symptomatic treatment will improve psychotherapeutic contact, giving the patients faith in the possibility of a cure. Moreover, because they tend to normalise mood the patients are able to work faster at resolving the psychotraumatic situation.

Tranquillisers are the mainstay of treatment, but use is also made of neuroleptics and antidepressants. Drugs are sometimes used intravenously. In more prolonged cases, where there has been neurotic development, most psychotropics lose their efficacy. Drugs should be changed around, also attempts made to target drugs at particular syndromes. Karvasarsky describes the relative efficacy of different drugs on each of the different neurotic syndromes. Herbal remedies, tonics and psychostimulants are also used, as are various measures such as rest, diet and exercise.

Obsessive and phobic syndromes are recognized as being notoriously difficult conditions to treat, often being resistant. They can be treated with behaviour therapy, but Karvasarsky considers that this is only effective in the long-term if it is combined with pathogenetic psychotherapy. Benzodiazepines, sometimes combined with amitriptyline and other antidepressants, are used, as, occasionally, are the neuroleptics. Various forms of physiotherapy may also be used.

Treatment of the asthenic syndrome depends on the stage of the disorder. In the hypersthenic stage sedatives may be necessary. During the hyposthenic stage stimulants, either naturally-derived products such as ginseng or drugs such as sidnocarb, are used. Another group of drugs used here are the tonics. These include vitamins, aloa and the nootrope, aminalon. Other treatments include massage, electrophoresis with calcium chloride and acupuncture.

Hysterical symptoms are mainly treated with psychotherapy, and this is one area where Karvasarsky sees more of a role for suggestion and hypnosis rather than insight-oriented pathogenetic psychotherapy. Physiotherapy might also be used. Hypochondria is considered difficult to treat and a wide range of drugs have been used. These include the tranquillisers, small doses of antidepressants, stimulants such as sidnocarb. Physiotherapy is thought to have an important role in many cases.

The Handbook (1983) is more concerned with biological and social approaches.

The use of rational therapy is suggested and there is no mention of pathogenetic psychotherapy. In hysteria it is suggested that the first step should be to eliminate possible traumatic psychological circumstances or to reduce their impact or influence. Psychotherapy is seen as having a central role, especially rational therapy. There should be regular, persistent goal-directed talks whose aim is to correct the patient's attitude to the cause of the illness. The obsessive-compulsive form is treated with rational therapy and various tonics in mild forms and possibly with tranquillizers and antidepressants in more severe forms. In neurasthenia a range of treatments are suggested including tonics, vitamins, valerian, bromides, tranquillisers and occasionally antidepressants. The role of physiotherapy and exercise is mentioned. Sanatoria are considered useful, but admission to hospital for more severe forms is suggested. There is emphasis on rest, sleep and work. Social measures include possible changes of employment and measures to reduce the source of emotional stress.

Treatment of the neurosis-like disorders
These conditions have a similar syndromal presentation to the neurotic disorders, for instance anxiety or asthenia, but they are not true neurotic disorders in that there is no psychogenesis. They occur in patients with endogenous psychoses, alcoholism, arteriosclerosis, trauma and various somatic illnesses. Zavilianskaya (1987) writes that psychotherapy is often appropriate, even though the disorder is not psychogenic. She lists a wide number of treatments, reflecting many of the features of the Soviet approach to treatment, including what would be considered fringe in the West. Various drugs are used, including nootropes, tranquillisers (including older ones like valerian and the bromides), vitamins and various tonics, many derived from herbal preparations. Exercise and physiotherapy are also considered important. An interesting additional treatment is the use of immunostimulants [4].

Outcome and prognosis
Karvasarsky distinguishes between symptomatic and genuine success in treatment. He writes that behaviour therapy might treat a symptom, but that the difficulties and conflicts remain. This is not too dissimilar to the position often taken by psychoanalysts. He does, however, condemn psychoanalysis for not being sufficiently concerned about symptoms, often ignoring these and seeing the only goal as the achievement of some kind of inner resolution.

Smulevitch (1983) writes that prognosis in neurosis is generally good, but tends to be worse if there are complicating factors such as the effects of involution and arteriosclerosis.

Comparative aspects
The neurosis category has been dropped from DSM-III and the neurotic disorders are distributed across various groups such as anxiety and depression. This is criticized on the grounds that it has implications about aetiology which are not justified. Smulevitch (1983) argues that the neuroses have enough features in

4. These preparations are listed in Medical Preparations (1985) as general biogenic preparations derived from animal and vegetable sources eg spleen extracts, yeast preparations.

common to justify retaining the use of the term and suggests that the concept of a single neurosis might make more sense [5].

Karvarsarsky (1980) criticizes both ICD-9 and DSM-III, mainly on the grounds that the syndromes of anxiety, hypochondria, depersonalization and depression are described as independent forms. He considers this unsatisfactory because the clinical picture may change over a short period of time ie from one syndrome to another. He also argues that they are not classified according to any convincing theoretical basis. Depersonalization is thought to occur in the neuroses only rarely and should not be included at all. The DSM-III notion of multiple personality is not recognized as a disorder, and there is scepticism about the concept. Any vaguely similar presentation would probably be seen as a form of malingering.

A criticism of DSM-III is the fact that panic disorder has been enshrined as a separate entity on rather doubtful grounds, mainly the so-called anti-panic effect of certain drugs, imipramine and the MAOIs [6]. On clinical and demographic grounds it is hard to distinguish between the different subgroups of anxiety disorders (Lancet, 1986a). Moreover, antidepressants, including imipramine, work in all anxiety states, not just panic attacks (Tyrer, 1986). On the other hand, DSM-III lumps the phobias and the obsessional-compulsive disorders together, suggesting that there may be a common mechanism underlying both disorders. Reflecting this, the Comprehensive Textbook of Psychiatry (1985) agrees that it is hard to distinguish obsessional states from phobias and argues that the difference is not to do with the clinical picture but the different underlying psychological processes. Thus, in phobias the anxiety, which is related to Oedipal conflicts, stems from fear of harm from external things and the mechanisms involved are displacement and projection. In obsessional states the anxiety, which is related to pre-Oedipal conflicts, is about what harm the patient might do and the mechanisms involved are isolation and undoing. Although many psychiatrists would find these concepts implausible it is clear that they have influenced the classificatory system.

A feature of the main Soviet classification is the absence of Anxiety State as an independent syndrome [7]. It seems odd to Western psychiatrists that something so common should not be recognized. The Soviet view, however, it that it is just because it is so common that it cannot be considered an independent syndrome ie it is too widely distributed across other disorders, psychoses as well as neuroses. Many of the patients diagnosed as anxiety state in the West would be classified under neurasthenia in the Soviet Union. The loss to Western psychiatry, particularly in the English-speaking world, of asthenia and neurasthenia, can be seen in terms of nosological empire building on behalf of the affective disorders [8]. The case described on page 172 illustrates this. Most Western psychiatrists would diagnose the young man as suffering from depression, and the fact that he didn't feel particularly depressed would lead to the use of the term masked depression. This diagnosis is, of course, no more correct than the Soviet one. It is simply that a

5. This view has also been put by Tyrer (1985) who used the term "general neurotic syndrome".

6. It has been argued that the promotion of panic was a marketing exercise for particular products with "anti-panic" activity (in particular alprazolam).

7. As already discussed, the term anxiety does not readily translate into Russian, although the word strakh (fear) describes what is essentially the same emotion or feeling. Thus, anxiety state (300.0) in ICD-9 is translated as Neurosis of Fear for the purpose of discussion rather than clinical usage.

8. There are several reasons for the expansion of the depression empire. One, possibly, is the promotion of research into the field by the manufacturers of anti-depressants.

Western psychiatrist given that list of symptoms has been taught to call it depression, whereas a Soviet psychiatrist has been taught to call it neurasthenia.

PSYCHOPATHY

Psychopathy has the same meaning in Soviet psychiatry as the term personality disorder has in English-speaking psychiatry. It refers to all the personality disorders, not just psychopathy or antisocial personality disorder. In the "Handbook" it is described as a pathological disorder characterized by disharmony of aspects of the personality (Smulevitch, 1983). The disharmony is mainly in the emotional and volitional aspects of the personality with the intellect generally remaining intact. Shmaunova (1985) in the Manual writes that psychopathy develops as the result of the interaction between environmental factors, mainly social, and a biological insufficiency of the nervous system which is innate or acquired early in life.

Gannushkin's early work remains influential [9], especially his attack upon the idea that the psychopathies were stationary and immutable. He described a gradual development of psychopathy throughout life, characterised by different reactions and phases, essentially a dynamic process. Gannushkin's basic criteria are:

1. The personality traits are innate and comparatively stable. However, psychopathic traits undergo changes throughout life and may develop in different directions.
2. They affect the whole personality.
3. They prevent the person from having a normal interaction with the environment and impair social adaptation.

Smulevitch (1983) writes that psychopathy should be distinguished from specific characterological divergences which are compensated for and which result in pathology only during periods of stress. These should be thought of as accentuations of character. It is also necessary to distinguish psychopathy from the psychopathic-like conditions which arise during the course of endogenous psychoses. The personality disorders are not absolute entities, but are on a continuum with personality accentuations and with normal personalities. Lichko (1986) mentions various terms that are used for the majority of patients in the intermediate groups where psychogenic factors seem to be more important. The terms include marginal psychopathy, pathocharacterological formation and psychopathic development.

Snezhnevsky (1983) writes that in the psychopathic disorders there is disturbance of mental function characterized by instability, weakness and disharmony of various mental processes and responses which are inappropriate to the stimuli that provoke them. There may be impatience, quarrelsomeness, marked lack of self-control and explosions of fury. There may also be poor social adaptation and various sexual deviations. In other cases the main feature is mental exhaustion, emotional lability, lack of spontaneity, reduced mental activity and easily provoked confusion. However, it is also stressed that although social adaptation is impaired, psychopathic patients may be highly intelligent and have

9. Gannushkin (1933) "Klinika psikhopatia" Sever, Moscow is widely quoted.

exceptional abilities in particular spheres.

The different types of psychopathy listed by different authors vary. The main ones described are:

Asthenic

Asthenic patients are anxious, irritable, weak, easily fatigued. They tend to be dissatisfied with themselves and lack self-esteem and self-confidence. They are shy, over-sensitive and impressionable.

Psychasthenic

Definitions of this vary, but it has some features in common with obsessional or anankastic personality disorder. Patients are irritable and easily fatigued. They have a critical attitude towards themselves and are prone to excessive self-doubt, self-analysis and self-control. They are rigid, finding that new situations provoke marked anxiety, and have obsessional traits with obsessional ruminations and rituals.

Schizoid

Patients are withdrawn, shy and autistic. Other traits are secretiveness, pedantry and meanness. There may be sudden, unexpected affective reactions, often provoked by attempts to break into their private, secret world.

The asthenic, psychasthenic and schizoid types are sometimes classed together under the "inhibited" group.

Affective

This is characterized by mood disorders. It is sometimes divided into *hyperthymic*, *depressive*, and *cycloid* types, reflecting the different directions the mood takes. *Hyperthymic* patients are high in energy, sociability and risk-taking. They tend to be hypersexual and aggressive, without necessarily having any cruel or vicious tendencies (which would be seen as more psychosocially determined). The Manual (1985) also quotes the *emotionally labile* type.

Paranoid

Patients are distrustful, suspicious and tend to get fixed on a narrow set of ideas and experiences. These are usually unpleasant or negative, and they take a one-sided and dogmatic view of these. Other traits are defensiveness, obstinacy, rigidity and an increased sense of their own importance. They may believe that they are singled out for special attention and tend to interpret events to fit in with their view of things. In situations of prolonged conflict, either at home or at work, their ideas may become delusional.

Hysterical

These patients are superficial, egocentric and attention-seeking. Behaviour may be showy and demonstrative. They find it difficult to tolerate stress and tend to deceive themselves and others. They are suggestible and often naive. There may be affective outbursts.

Excitable (explosive) or epileptoid
Patients are highly impulsive, irritable and prone to outbursts of anger and aggressive behaviour. They may also be cruel, tyrannical and unforgiving. Lichko (1986) writes that this group are prone to sexual deviations. The term epileptoid does not imply any proneness to fits.

Unstable
In this there is a poor threshold of attention and inability to concentrate. Patients generally resist long-term goals and are more interested in pleasure-seeking and entertainment.

Sexual deviations
Sexual deviations are generally included under the psychopathic disorders. They are not considered to be separate types of psychopathy but are said to occur more commonly in patients with psychopathy and across the range of psychopathies. They are thought to be acquired as a result of distorted patterns of relationships within the family or as a result of unfortunate conditioning during early sexual experiences.

Aetiology
According to Shmaunova (1985), psychopathy develops as the result of the interaction of environmental factors upon a biologically insufficient nervous system. This may be innate or acquired early in life. The early physical damage may be due to trauma, infections or toxins, which includes alcohol. Thus, the role of genetic factors is recognized, but these are not considered sufficient to produce psychopathy. Genes might produce an inert nervous system with a dominant second signalling system, but to develop psychasthenia from this one would need other, environmental, influences [10]. These might be physical, but the role of social factors is emphasized. This includes the effects of upbringing, faulty education, prolonged mental trauma, especially during the formative years of personality development, and current life events.

Kerbikov (1971) described acquired psychopathy arising in people with no predisposition, distinguishing this from "core" or constitutional psychopathy. The term is not in general usage, but the concept is incorporated into the notion of pathological development of personality in which the innate or constitutional element is considered to be much less significant than environmental factors.

Course and development
Because the environment continues to modify the development of personality (and, therefore, personality disorder) the clinical picture is never static. Personality traits

---

10. Some authors attempt to explain the psychopathies in terms of Pavlovian typology. In hysterical psychopathy it is thought that there is predominance of the first signalling system over the second signalling system, essentially of subcortical over cortical regions. In psychasthenia the opposite applies. Lakosina and Trunova (1983) show that the responses to verbal stimuli are stronger in psychasthenic psychopaths as compared to hysterical psychopaths. According to them the theory would also suggest that patients with psychopathy have an emotional deficit. They tested this by carrying out detailed psychophysiological testing on groups of patients with hysteria and psychasthenia and found less emotional intensity and fewer affective reactions in psychasthenia. The interaction between the cerebral cortex and subcortical structures is thought to be reflected by the orienting reflex which was also different between the two groups.

may intensify or ameliorate over time and psychopaths "decompensate" under certain environmental conditions. Hence the emphasis that patients should be in the right social environment, both work and family. Puberty is seen as a critical stage in the development of personality disorder.

There may be brief changes in functioning due to decompensation or a reaction of the personality to particular circumstances, followed by a return to the previous level of functioning. The clinical picture during the period of decompensation is varied and depends upon the type of psychopathy. There may also be prolonged pathological developments of the personality, generally the result of continuing baleful influences. On the other hand, a good environment might promote favourable development. Thus, in someone with an explosive personality disorder a favourable environment might lead to the development of secondary compensatory features of the character which would play a defensive role against the primary explosive characteristics.

In addition to these environmentally-determined stages it is thought that there are phases which do not have any obvious environmental influence. In all the types of psychopathy there may be brief dysthymic phases or prolonged, severe affective (depressive) phases, possibly lasting from six months to two years.

Pathological development of personality

Pathological development of personality is said to differ from constitutional psychopathy in that social factors are more critical in their formation (Manual, 1985). They develop as a result of prolonged exposure to unfavourable social factors, for instance unresolvable psychotraumatic situations, and, more commonly, poor upbringing in a family which distorts the development of the child. Sexual deviance is more likely to occur in these circumstances. It is recognized that this is a controversial area in that the relationship between this and psychopathy is far from clear. Smulevitch (1985) writes that in comparison to those with constitutional defects of personality patients with pathological development of personality have a richer emotional life and are less immature. The onset tends to be later and more gradual.

Diagnosis

Writing about disturbed adolescents Lichko (1986) stresses that it is important to distinguish between normal mischief, the normal period of opposition to authority and genuine psychopathology. He refers to Gannushkin and Kerbikov and writes that in psychopathy abnormal behaviour persists because of "manifest deviation in character formation". In psychopathy the abnormal traits are evident "...in all sorts of situations. Everywhere, a hyperthymic teenager will boil with energy, a hysteroid will be striving after special attention, and a schizoid will create a coccoon around himself." Psychopathy cannot be diagnosed unless there is this picture of *total involvement of the personality*. He considers that it is much harder to judge the stability and totality of the traits in adolescence and that time is required to make a proper diagnosis. Thus, a sensitive adolescent might want to be alone a lot between the ages of 16 and 18 and this might be confused with schizoid personality. Social maladjustment in a troubled adolescent without psychopathy may be continuous, but is more likely to be related to stressful events.

Karvasarsky (1980) discusses the differential diagnosis between these disorders and the neuroses. In psychopathy, both innate and acquired forms, there is a stable pathocharacterological state, although it has its own dynamic. The damage to personality is more fundamental whereas there is more influence of the environment in neurosis. Moreover, only a part of the personality is affected in the neuroses and there is better insight into the condition. The neurotic syndrome of asthenia is distinguished from asthenic psychopathy by the fact that in psychopathy the individual becomes asthenic whenever tired, not just episodically at times of crisis or in difficult situations. Other Soviet authors are less convinced by the clear distinction between the two sets of disorders, essentially seeing them as being on a continuum which reflects a balance between what is particular to the personality and to the environment.

Portnov et al (1987) argue that psychopathy is an over-used term and question the basis on which the diagnosis is made. They claim that true psychopathy is transitory and is related to delayed development of the pubertal stage. This tends to improve with time. Other patients, according to their follow-up studies, should really be classified into other groups. Many are due to oligophrenia, traumatic encephalopathy and slow-flow schizophrenia. These tend not to improve to the same extent over time.

The prevalence of psychopathy in the general population is generally put at around 5% (Smulevitch, 1987)[11].

Classification

There is little consistency about the classification of the personality disorders. There are various clinical classificatory systems based on the types described above. Lichko (1986) writes that in the 1960s Kerbikov attempted to classify them into two basic types, according to Pavlov's typology. These were the excitable and the inhibited types, but that this did not cover the hysterical, schizoid and paranoid types. He added a hysteroid group later.

One classification of the psychopathies is:

Excitable (explosive)
Paranoid
Hysterical
Inhibited (includes asthenic, psychasthenic
    and schizoid)

An adapted version of the ICD-9 is also given in the Manual (1985) and is used for administrative purposes, although the modified Soviet version does not include the category 301.7: Personality disorder with predominantly sociopathic or asocial manifestation [12].

Treatment

Social, environmental and educational approaches are considered to be the mainstay of treatment in psychopathy. Patients need to be in the right environment

---

11. Vaillant and Perry (1985) quote 5-15% for various Western studies. Because of the different diagnostic criteria the figures cannot be compared.

12. The 301.7 slot is given to Psychopathy of emotional blunting types or heboid psychopathy.

and away from baleful influences. There is emphasis on work therapy, vocational guidance and the correct working environment. Psychotherapy, generally of the rational, directive kind, is thought to be indicated with relatives in order to help to create a therapeutic family atmosphere.

Medical treatment is only appropriate during decompensations. The range of drugs used include neuroleptics, tranquillisers and antidepressants. The treatment depends on the nature of the reaction. Thus in an affective reaction or during an affective phase drug treatment would be as for affective reactions in other disorders. Lakosina and Trunova (1983) claim that treatment with small doses of chlorpromazine combined with the stimulant sidnocarb is effective in psychasthenia. Chlorpromazine suppresses overstimulation of the hypothalamus and sidnocarb activates the weak reticular influences of the brain stem, boosting the sub-cortical influence. This is said to fit in with the aetiological theory, that is the notion that the cortical first-signalling system is dominant compared to the sub-cortical second-signalling system.

Comparative aspects

An obvious difference between the Soviet and Western concepts of psychopathy is the different emphases placed on the notion of the stability of the traits and the effects of the environment. The idea that there are innate, immutable personality traits is rejected in Soviet psychology and psychiatry. The Soviet view is that personality is not a fixed entity but a set of behavioural patterns which are characteristic of the individual. These change as the person develops and as the environment around him changes. Nothing is fixed by the time of adolescence from within this conceptual framework. By contrast, most Western schools of psychology or psychoanalysis consider personality traits to be enduring and predictable and fixed by the time of adolescence. DSM-III defines personality traits as "enduring patterns of perceiving, relating to, and thinking about the environment and oneself..". It does, however, go on to say that the manifestations of personality disorders "..often become less obvious in middle or old age." [13].

There is some inconsistency in the Soviet position in that the very definition of psychopathy suggests that the traits are stable. The difference, then, becomes one of degree.

"Sociopathy"

One of the major differences in the classification of the personality disorders is the lack of any category for antisocial or sociopathic personality disorder in the Soviet system [14]. It is argued that one should not introduce sociocultural values into clinical definitions and descriptions. Thus, Karvasarsky (1980) criticizes the Western usage and writes that the carrying out of antisocial acts should not be regarded as a clinical sign [15]. It is argued that anyone can carry out antisocial acts and this definition raises the question as to what point someone, say with

---

13. ICD-9 defines personality disorders as "deeply ingrained, maladaptive, patterns of behaviour generally recognizable by the time of adolescence or earlier and continuing throughout most of adult life, although often becoming less obvious in middle or old age."

14. Schneider's classification also excluded antisocial behaviour from the criteria for defining abnormal personality. He considered that psychopathic personalities cause suffering to themselves or to others. This may include antisocial behaviour, but this is secondary to the personality disorder.

psychasthenia, is shifted over into the antisocial group. The fundamental objection, however, is that it does not allow for the effects of the environment. The same personality type might lead to quite different behaviours in different sociocultural environments. Thus, someone with a "sociopathic" personality who finds himself in the kind of social environment that promotes obvious antisocial behaviour and leads him into the hands of the law will end up with a diagnosis of sociopathy. Someone with a similar personality in a different social environment might end up with a successful career in politics or medicine. The diagnosis of sociopath is thus made on sociocultural grounds, on the grounds of class, background and education. This criticism is not altogether justified in that the definition of sociopath is in fact fairly specific about the duration and pattern of antisocial behaviour, and there is no suggestion that any kind of antisocial activity allows you into the category. Thus, Vaillant and Perry (1985) stress that antisocial personality disorder is not synonymous with criminality. It is also questionable as to whether the argument about the differentiation between clinical and social criteria applies only to sociopathy. It could be argued that some of the clinical criteria in other types of psychopathy or personality disorder are no more than descriptions of certain types of social behaviour.

ANOREXIA NERVOSA
Anorexia nervosa is another disorder which Soviet psychiatry sees as having been given an artificial status as a disease entity. The Handbook (1985) describes anorexia nervosa as a syndrome which may occur as a feature of neurosis, psychopathy or neurosis-like schizophrenia. It is also recognized as a separate disorder, although this is essentially considered to be a type of pathological development of the personality. The point is made in the handbook (1985) that there is very low hereditary factor, that only 1% of siblings have anorexia whereas 17% of siblings have some other serious psychiatric disorder. This is seen as evidence for its nosological heterogeneity.

Patients are described as having personality traits which include rigidity, pedantry, punctuality and accuracy and are said to be over-attached to their mothers in many cases, also having a marked dislike of separations. There may also be hysterical personality traits. Emotional conflict in the premorbid personality is seen as important and it is thought that mothers are often over-protective. Endocrine dysfunction is found, but it is recognized that this might be secondary to starvation. Rollin (1972) discusses the Soviet view that disorders in the diencephalon or endocrine system are of aetiological important, but also quotes a leading child psychiatrist as saying that unpleasant experiences during the critical phase of pubertal sexual development may be important.

The symptoms are described as the refusal to eat and over-valued ideas about size and body image which are considered as being close to dysmorphophobia. Patients develop a dislike for large people with big appetites and begin to take part in food preparation and feeding their siblings. Weight loss leads to amenorrhoea. There may be increased exercise. The differential diagnosis is mainly related to

15. The Soviet psychiatrist Ganushkin, whose work in the 1930s on psychopathy is often quoted, did, however, include an antisocial type in his classification.

189

differentiating between anorexia in the borderline disorders and schizophrenia with the anorexic syndrome. In schizophrenia it is thought that there will be more extreme, irrational dysmorphobia, for instance with bizarre convictions about the body and bizarre feeding patterns. "Vomitomania", odd vomiting behaviour which produces a kind of frenzy or ecstasy, may also be a feature of schizophrenia. This is seen as being distinct from the more controlled vomiting behaviour which occurs as a feature of anorexic personality development or in patients with what would be called bulaemia nervosa in the West. "Vomitomania" is considered a serious feature, part of a set of near-delusional behaviour patterns. This distinction between the different types of vomiting perhaps accounts for some of the confusion about its significance in the West. Vomiting was originally described by Russell as "an ominous variant of anorexia", but at the same time the behaviour occurs in mild bulaemia which is common in the population.

Other features such as depersonalization, senestopathia and obsessional symptoms may suggest schizophrenia. Other diagnostic issues are between true anorexia and the anorexia of depression with secondary food refusal.

The Handbook (1983) describes two phases of treatment. The non-specific stage consists of restoring reasonable body weight. This might last for two to four weeks and consists of refeeding, if necessary intravenously and without the consent of the patient. Small amounts of insulin might be used to stimulate appetite. Neuroleptics might be used for sedation or the prevention of vomiting during artificial feeding. Specific treatment includes the introduction of a normal feeding pattern. Drugs are used according to symptoms. Autogenic training might be used when there are vegetative symptoms. Psychotherapy is used, especially rational therapy, occasionally with hypnosis. The effects of weight loss on health are emphasized. It is considered important to work with the relatives, planning a reasonable approach to meals. In Leningrad there is greater emphasis on psychotherapy, especially work with the family, which might include a period of separation from the mother.

"MINOR" ORGANIC DISORDERS

These terms encephalitis, diencephalitis and arachnoiditis are used in a way which is largely unfamiliar in the West. Recently there has been less emphasis on them in Soviet psychiatry, perhaps partly because of Western influence and partly because the disorders are treated mainly by neuropathologists (neurologists). Thus, they are not mentioned in the Manual of Psychiatry (1985). The following account is taken mainly from Karvasarsky (1980), the Handbook (1983) and Umansky (1989).

Arachnoiditis.
Arachnoiditis is essentially a mild form of meningitis in that the pathology is not restricted to the arachnoid membrane alone. It refers to mild, localized forms of meningitis in which there are adhesions in limited areas, resulting in restriction to the normal flow of cerebrospinal fluid. The clinical picture will depend upon the location and extent of the disorder [16]. Karvasarsky (1980) writes that about one third of cases of arachnoiditis are of uncertain aetiology, one third are due to trauma and one third to some kind of infection.

Decompensation (generally with raised intracranial pressure) occurs in the context of other illnesses, often minor, which might affect the circulation. The main symptom is headache, which tends to be diffuse, dull and persistent, and is often brought on by mental or physical stress. It can occur once a week or less than once a month, and may last from hours to days. Patients may end up taking many pain-killers. It is sometimes migraine-like, pulsating, with or without vomiting. There may be changes in the field of vision, also vertigo and, possibly, motor or sensory disturbances. Occasionally there are fits.

Examination may reveal paleness or blurring of the optic discs. On examination there may be increased CSF protein, widening of lateral and third ventricles (due to secondary hydrocephalus). It is recognized that this condition is hard to diagnose, but a clear history of trauma or viral infection followed by persistent headache would be the most characteristic presentation.

Encephalitis.

The term chronic encephalitis would probably be better to describe what is meant by this condition which is thought to be due to viral infections. Headache is a prominent feature, but in addition there will often be mood changes and impaired memory and attention. The headache is more profound at the beginning of the illness, often diffuse and very severe, possibly described as bursting. There may be general sleepiness during the day. Odd sensations in various parts of the body are described, especially in the head. Descriptions such as "everything burns (or flows or squelches) inside my head" may be given. Depersonalization and derealisation may be present. There is generally an acute presentation followed by a chronic course, characterised by relapses and a slow, gradual worsening. There is general malaise and patients have a sticky, monotonous quality to their complaints, what has been described, perhaps unkindly, as "encephalitic tiresomeness".

Various physical symptoms and signs may be present. Vegetative signs include dizziness, hypersalivation and there may be eye signs, including diplopia or ptosis. Investigations might show increase in CSF protein, signs of hydrocephalus, cortical atrophy and a large subarachnoid gap. A history of an acute onset is present in about 70% of cases, and without this is hard to diagnose. Outcome is considered better than in the past.

Diencephalitis.

The diencephalon refers to subcortical structures, especially the thalamus, hypothalamus and mammillary bodies, and this disorder is said to be due to trauma, intoxication or, more commonly, a chronic, recurrent viral neuroinfection. There are various stages of the condition: an early stage with anxiety, depression and loss of drive; an intermediate stage with mixed features; a later stage with neurosis-like and hypochondriacal features, also asthenia. Unlike true neurotic syndromes there will be no psychogenesis. There may be disturbances in water, fat and carbohydrate metabolism, temperature regulation, vegetative symptomatology. These may include vegetative crises, especially with cardiovascular symptoms.

There are various features that aid diagnosis. There may be increased intra-

---

16. In the West arachnoiditis generally refers only to the spinal column and a complication of myelography.

cranial pressure with enlargement of the third ventricle or lateral ventricles. There are characteristic EEG changes: dysrhythmia and/or polymorphic, slow activity, with occasional bursts of high amplitude alpha, slow theta and delta waves, especially over the fronto-temporal area.

Sleep
Sleep is markedly disturbed in these disorders. In encephalitis the insomnia persists and is resistant to treatment. There is disruption of the day/night rhythm, with sleepiness during the day and wakefulness at night. There is a similar picture in diencephalitis, in which there is particularly stubborn insomnia. Arachnoiditis presents with more varied patterns, generally less severe insomnia. Treatment measures for the insomnia, whether psychological or pharmacological, are less effective than for the insomnia found in the neuroses.

Social factors and outcome
The importance of social factors is stressed by some authors. Koniukhova (1985) reports on a follow-up study of the three disorders (arachnoiditis, encephalitis and diencephalitis) and writes that the outcome does not depend upon extent of the neurological changes but on the degree of personality disturbance, the neurotic manifestations and environmental factors. The outcome was surprisingly poor: 15 patients were doing well, 27 were coping, but had inadequate social/work adaptation and were still in touch with the services, and in 12 there was bad social/work adaptation.

Treatment
Treatment generally consists of mild, non-specific measures, including diet, rest, acupuncture, various psychotherapeutic measures and some of the fringe approaches discussed in chapter 6. Antidepressants and benzodiazepines are sometimes used.

Comparative aspects
These disorders are considered to be common in the Soviet Union and the source of considerable morbidity. It is perhaps surprising that they are scarcely recognized in the West and most books on psychiatry or neurology do not describe them. It seems unlikely that this is because they are simply artefactual, especially as the syndromes describe some of the features found in affective disorders and the neuroses: disturbances of vital functions, especially sleep, appetite and libido, also the changes in temperature regulation, water intake, fat and carbohydrate metabolism. The discrepancy may simply be due to the different theoretical positions. There is some tendency for the Western dualist tradition to promote the view that something is either psychological or organic. A disorder is considered psychological if no obvious organic disorder can be demonstrated. This is likely to be the case if symptoms and signs are vague and there are no predictable serious sequelae to a syndromal presentation. The symptoms are seen as typical or atypical manifestations of neurotic or affective disorder. Once a psychological disorder has been diagnosed, and nothing obviously serious or life-threatening is apparent on the organic side, it is generally assumed that no further investigations are required

192

or relevant. This approach is fostered by the fact that Western neurology is still concerned mainly with the motor and sensory systems, so that this range of disorders rarely comes under neurological scrutiny.

There is perhaps a parallel with the controversial myalgic encephalomyelitis (ME) or post-viral fatigue syndrome. This is said to be the consequence of a viral infection and some of the symptoms are similar to those found in depression, although in ME there is anhedonia rather than depressed mood. Other features of ME include fatigue, weakness after exercise, unsteadiness, memory loss and inability to concentrate. There seem to be features in common with the disorders described above.

The vegetative disorders

The vegetative disorders cover a number of syndromes due to changes in the activity of the autonomic nervous system. They may present with continuous symptoms or as dramatic, episodic *vegetative crises*. There may be over-activity of the sympathetic or parasympathetic nervous system or both. Sympathetic over-activity is common in all neuroses, and results in increased pulse and blood pressure, sweating and dry mouth. Parasympathetic over-activity, in which there may be a decrease in pulse and blood pressure, hypersalivation (especially nocturnal), increased gut motility is less common. The *vegetative crisis* refers to an acute episode in which there are symptoms suggestive of autonomic nervous system over-activity eg sweating and tachycardia. They generally last for 10-30 minutes and occur once or twice a month.

Some authors, including Karvarsarksy (1980), argue for a psychogenic aetiology. Vein and Rodshtat (1974) consider that the vegetative disorders are due to local lesions in the brain. They argue that mediobasal lesions of the temporal lobe produce paroxysmal parasympathetic vegetative disorders, often with a monosymptomatic picture, for instance gut or cardiovascular symptoms. Hypothalamic pathology produces sympathetic or mixed pictures, either continuous or as vegetative crises. There is also an age-related disorder of cerebral vegetative dysfunction, thought to be due to pathology of the brain-stem, generally caused by arteriosclerosis.

Treatment is directed to dealing with the acute episodes and also correcting vegetative dysfunction between. During an episode treatment is essentially symptomatic. In sympathetic crises this might involve the use of lytics such as chlorpromazine or piroxan. In parasympathetic crises small doses of anticholinergics might be used. Antihistamines and benzodiazepines are also used. For increased sympathetic tone between episodes a combination of sympatholytics (stimulants such as nicotinic acid, dihydroergotamine) and cholinomimetics may be used. For increased parasympathetic tone, cholinolytics (either central or peripheral, depending on the level of the lesion) are suggested. Relative insufficiency of the sympathetic system is treated with various vitamins or calcium. Remedies which act on both systems are recommended when there is insufficiency of both sympathetic and parasympathetic tone.

Panic attacks or vegetative crises?

In the West the vegetative states are incorporated into the various neurotic syndromes, generally being considered as the somatic manifestations of anxiety. Perhaps the most specific syndrome in this respect is DSM-III Panic Disorder which would be classified as a vegetative crisis by most Soviet psychiatrists. Although there is no mention of the subjective feeling of fear/anxiety during the vegetative crisis (it essentially describes what happens to the body) it would seem likely that these feelings are present during the episodes. "Panic attacks" and "vegetative crises", therefore, can perhaps be considered to be more or less synonymous [17].

---

16. Several Western studies suggest that the concept of the vegetative crisis might be as useful as that of panic. Nesse et al (1984) demonstrated disorders of adrenergic function in patients with panic anxiety. Matuzas (1987) reported that 50% of patients with panic attacks had evidence of mitral valve prolapse, and there is evidence that mitral valve prolapse might be due to over-activity of the sympathetic nervous system. This would seem to be linked to the concept of hyperadrenergic states (Lancet, 1987a).

Chapter Eleven

ALCOHOLISM AND DRUG ADDICTION

ALCOHOLISM

Shumsky (1985), in the "Manual of Psychiatry", writes that alcoholism in the social sense refers to the excessive use of alcoholic beverages leading to disturbances which affect the individual and society. In a medical sense it is considered a form of toxicomania in which the substance abused is alcohol. He describes various stages of alcoholism, along with the different syndromes, psychotic and otherwise, that develop. These include the personality changes found in alcoholism.

On aetiology he writes that alcohol is used because of its effects on mental and physical state and that it has relaxing, sedative and euphoriant effects. He considers that the need for this effect is greater in people with neurotic or psychopathic traits, although social and psychological factors are also important. These include tradition, education, the micro-social environment (family life), physical and mental strain, psychotraumatic events. A genetic component is also recognized, although the aetiological role of physiological factors is not established.

Bekhtel (1984) describes the importance of personality and of defence mechanisms in perpetuating alcoholism. These are mainly denial, repression and rationalization. He writes that "... one of the main elements in such an explanatory system is the alibi. The alibi system is essentially an attempt to construct an individual psychological concept justifying drunkenness. So as not to acquire the reputation of a drunkard, every instance of imbibing alcoholic beverages and of alcoholic excess must be explained and justified from the stand-point of social norms and rules. Weighty arguments are presented as to why excessive drinking was necessary in each particular situation. The person will remain quite sincere in all this. With time, the range of situations accompanied by the imbibing of alcohol gradually expands, and the alibis pile up, creating a permanent state of being in an unusual situation. The illusion is created of a confluence of circumstances in which it is simply impossible not to drink. When no alibi is any longer sufficient to explain regular drunkenness, an explanatory system of a universal type emerges, postulating drunkenness as a style of life ("a hopeless life"). ..... Even partial acknowledgement of the extreme nature of the patient's drinking produces a sense of guilt, which in turn gives rise to expiatory behaviour. Society and other people relate to the person in a condemnatory, even hostile, manner. The person feels guilty and endeavours to mitigate his guilt by conscientiously doing what is required of him. When sober, such people are very meticulously dressed, are always exaggeratedly polite, sugary, accommodating, and immediately ready to fulfil any desire one may have. The development of this expiatory behaviour is the basis of the myth that all alcoholics are nice people. They are simply forced to be nice because of their problem. The person acts in a way that will restore his esteem in the eyes of others and allay his guilt. This quality makes these people essential in some enterprises, in which they perform the most undesirable tasks and work overtime in exchange for being pardoned for their absenteeism."

According to Lichko (1986) the pattern of alcohol abuse depends upon personality traits. Thus, hyperthymic personalities may indulge in wild binges, taking these to excess as they are prone to do in all aspects of life, for instance with various adventures, sexual or otherwise. Hysterics put on a show of drinking bravado to gain attention. Schizoid individuals may also abuse alcohol, but this is likely to be in small, regular amounts, mainly in an attempt to relieve tension.

There has been a considerable amount of work into the biological aspects of alcoholism, much of it at the Serbsky Institute. There have been various theories with regard to changes in catecholamine metabolism having a role in the formation of psychological and physical dependence. According to Anokhina (1985), alcohol releases noradrenalin but in the withdrawal phase there is a gradual depletion, possibly explaining some of the behavioural effects of alcohol. In chronic alcoholics there is a compensatory mechanism with a gradual increase in catecholamine turnover. Prolonged intake also inhibits activity of dopamine beta hydroxylase so that dopamine accumulates in the brain, a possible mechanism to explain vegetative and motor dysfunction, tremor and some of the psychopathology.

Because of the emphasis on premorbid personality there is no distinction between primary and secondary alcoholism, although "symptomatic" alcoholism, occurring in psychiatric disorders such as schizophrenia is recognized.

10% of alcoholics in the Soviet Union are women. Babayan (1985) writes that they have a more severe course of the disorder, with marked deterioration in personality and, often, severe mood swings. Because of the lack of insight and negative attitude to treatment they are harder to treat and need a more intense approach with more education and psychotherapy.

There are different figures on prevalence and incidence. As shown in Table 8, the number of people registered with the narcological dispensary in 1989 was 1.5% of the population [1]. There are differences between the republics with Russia, Moldavia, Latvia and the Ukraine coming out badly and the Central Asian republics well. Perhaps unexpectedly, Georgia and Armenia had the lowest figures.

---

1. Kornilov et al (1987), giving the results of a survey of 550 workers at a chemical plant, report that 4.7% suffered from chronic alcoholism.

Table 8: *Patients (per 100,000 population) with alcoholism on dispensary lists and patients presenting for the first time (National Economy, 1989).*

	1980	1985	1986	1987	1988	1989
Patients on the dispensary list	1235	1613	1618	1628	1598	1494
Patients presenting for first time	206	217	196	181	154	149

Treatment

Babayan (1985) describes the narcological service run by specialist psychiatrist-narcologists who treat drug addicts and alcoholics. There are narcological treatment rooms within dispensaries, and there is also a narcological service in its own right which was established by the Ministry of Health in 1975. This has a same range of in-patient, partial hospitalization and out-patient facilities, along with workshop and industrial facilities. There are plans to site the narcological dispensaries nearer to the general population, for instance in the medical departments of industrial and agricultural enterprises, general polyclinics, and even in "sobering-up stations".

Partial hospitalization facilities are considered particularly valuable. The day hospital provides a full range of therapy, but avoids isolation from the family. The night "prophylactoriums" allow a person to continue with his daily work. At hospitals and day units attached to the work place the course of treatment generally lasts for six months. 40% of pay goes to the narcological service and the rest to the family. It is said to be twice as effective as out-patient treatment or the usual narcological departments linked to psychiatric hospital. There are also courses of evening treatment for patients continuing working who want their treatment to remain confidential [2].

According the Shumsky (1985) the first stage of treatment is concerned with acute symptoms and the physical state due to intoxication or withdrawal. The aim of the second stage is to suppress the pathological urge to drink and the third stage aims to reduce the likelihood of relapse. Treatment is generally out-patient based. In the acute stages a wide range of physical treatments, including vitamins, drugs and sulphazin injections may be used [3]. At all stages the drug treatment is targeted at whatever syndrome presents. In the phase of active treatment he recommends conditioned reflex and sensitization treatments. These are forms of aversion therapy, using substances such as apomorphine. Psychotherapy in various forms is considered to be crucial at each stage of treatment, both as an adjunct and to motivate the patient to make use of the other forms of treatment. Supportive therapy is indicated for at least five years, and the mainstay of this is

2. A high success rate is claimed from a centre for the confidential treatment of alcoholism in Tadzhikistan, according to the newspaper Trud (7.9.1984).
3. Sulphazin is no longer in use.

psychotherapy. Rational psychotherapy and hypnotherapy are used, often in groups. Family therapy may be necessary to alter pathogenetic conditions at home. Drugs and aversive therapy may also be used. In some centres a combination of psychotherapy, conditioning and a sensitizing approach is used. Admission to hospital is still considered important for many patients. Babayan (1985) argues that this should be long enough to allow thorough investigation and detoxification. After discharge the patient should move on to the dispensary for observation and continuing supporting treatment.

I visited a large narcological dispensary in Leningrad with in-patient facilities for 300 patients. Patients came from a wide range of sources - the psychiatric service, the general medical polyclinics, various trades unions or from the work-place. Some patients were remanded for treatment by the courts. The usual regime was 10 days detoxification with drugs and vitamins followed by 35 days treatment with apomorphine, antabuse or a similar slow release preparation, Espiral. Other treatments included drugs, for instance lithium, and, more rarely, small doses of insulin. Hypnosis, group and individual psychotherapy were also used, and there was a psychologist at the dispensary who had the main responsibility for psychotherapy. Staffing levels were high. There was a patients' abstinence club. It was claimed that 30% of patients were abstinent for one year and that the other 70% drank less. The rate of alcoholic psychosis was markedly reduced.

There has been much in the popular and medical press about the treatment of alcoholism since the start of the anti-alcohol campaign. Many are different forms of rational therapy, suggestion and hypnosis, but with most emphasis on various types of behaviour therapy, for instance "affective counterattribution" - associating unpleasant experiences and sensations with the smell or taste of alcohol.

Social issues

The role of alcohol in Russian culture has achieved a kind of mythical status both within the Soviet Union and in the rest of the world. Despite all the campaigning there remains a somewhat ambivalent attitude to the "tradition" of alcohol use. Babayan (1985) makes the point that people move from being consumers of alcohol to abusers to chronic alcoholics. He stresses the historical tradition of alcohol consumption in Russia, writing that alcohol is drunk "both in sorrow and in joy". He also emphasizes the difference between alcoholism and drug addiction, arguing that they should not be lumped together. He attempts to justify this on the rather dubious grounds that the human body has its own endogenous alcohol, that alcohol is a more natural substance which is also categorized with foodstuffs and is used in flavouring. He argues that alcohol should be restricted on health grounds, but not forbidden altogether as with the narcotics. Babayan was writing before the 1985 campaign and his rather fuzzy attitude has been criticized.

In May 1985 the Central Committee of the Communist Party passed a decree "On Measures to combat drunkenness and alcoholism" leading to a series of different measures [4]. These included a reduction in the production of vodka and strong wines and restrictions of opening hours for shops, also a publicity campaign. A campaigning organization sponsored by Komsomol, the Soviet TUC and the Ministry of Health was also established. These set up anti-alcohol clubs in parts of

4. There have been earlier anti-alcohol campaigns, for instance one in the 1970s (Hyde, 1973).

the country and began a new magazine "Sobriety and Culture" [5]. There were also to be stronger punitive measures taken against people who were drunk at work. Various polls suggested that the public were behind the measures [6]. An article in Pravda (1987a) suggested that the campaign had met with some success. There had been fewer working hours lost due to alcohol, the number of alcohol-related crimes had fallen by 26% and there was a reduction in the number of people brought to sobering-up stations. The article, however, condemned the slackening pace of the reforms and the increase in home distiling of spirits [7]. It proposed stricter measures and more stringent punishment for offenders.

Table 8 seems to suggest that the changes are beginning to have an effect on the prevalence figures for alcoholism [8]. The measures have had an effect on official intake of alcohol as shown in Table 9 [9], but there is anecdotal evidence that there has been an increase in the consumption of various substances such as perfumes and cleaning fluids.

Table 9: Litres of absolute alcohol consumed per head of population
(National Economy, 1987)

1960	3.9
1970	6.8
1980	8.7
1984	8.4
1985	7.2
1986	4.3
1987	3.3

Comparative aspects

The stereotyped view that alcoholism is a peculiarly Russian or Soviet problem is not borne out by the epidemiological evidence, either in terms of the prevalence figures for alcoholism or in terms of alcohol consumed. The National Economy (1987) quotes the 1986 figures for litres of absolute alcohol consumed per head of population in various countries: Bulgaria 9.2, GDR 10.3, FRG 9.0, Italy 11.0, France 13.9, USA 8.1, Britain 8.4. This compares with a figure of 4.3 litres in the Soviet Union. There is little doubt that this does not reflect the whole picture. These are All-Union figures and the lower intake in certain parts of the country, for instance the Central Asian Republics, gives a higher figure for areas such as the

5. The medical press reports various enterprises along these lines, for instance a sobriety club called "Inspiration" set up by the chief doctor of the psychoneurological dispensary in the Tulskoi oblast, a few hundred kilometres south of Moscow (MG 21.8.1987). It aims to rehabilitate and provide prophylaxis and there are close links with industry and schools. There are also articles which criticize the small number of doctors who have joined the All-Union voluntary organization for sobriety. A number of cities such as Yaroslav and Gorky were identified as particularly unenthusiastic (2.10.1987 and 9.10.1987).

6. Again, this is not particularly new. Hyde (1973) writes that a poll of Izvestia readers showed that 40% favoured prohibition at that time.

7. One consequence of the increase in the production of samogon or home-distiled spirit was the disappearance of sugar from the shops and the introduction of sugar rationing.

8. Nemtsov et al (1989) give figures to show that the prevalence of alcoholic psychosis correlates with the purchase of alcoholic beverages. They write that regression analysis indicates that if the purchase of beverages was reduced to 28% of the 1984 level there would be no alcoholic psychosis!

9. Wortis (1950) quotes an average consumption of 2 gallons of vodka per person for 1913 which dropped to 1 gallon per person by the 1930s. Prohibition was introduced in Russia in 1914 and lasted until 1925. One result was a massive increase in moonshining.

Russian Republic and the Ukraine. There is still considerable home-distiling in the Soviet Union, and alcohol is also obtained through a wide number of different sources. Despite these factors, however, there is little evidence to suggest that alcohol presents a significantly greater problem in the Soviet Union than it does in many other parts of the world.

There is evidence to support the Ledermann hypothesis that alcoholism and alcohol-related problems, including morbidity, mortality and crime, are linked to the overall per capita consumption of alcohol (British Medical Journal, 1985). This would tend to suggest that the rate of alcoholism is determined by the availability and price of alcohol. A number of European countries, notably in Scandinavia, have acted on this to ensure that alcohol is priced relatively highly and that availability is restricted. In many Western countries, however, alcohol has gradually become cheaper relative to other items such as food and clothing. In Britain the consumption of alcohol has doubled over 25 years as the real price of drink has halved (Lancet, 1988a) [10]. Indeed, Britain now has a higher per capita consumption of alcohol than the Soviet Union and up to 1.3 million people have a severe alcohol problem.

An Editorial in the British Medical Journal, "The Politics of alcohol" (1985) discusses social and fiscal policies with regard to alcoholism. It suggests that the position of the British government has been that this is a medical problem and that it is not the job of the government to intervene. Various reasons are suggested, including the parliamentary drink lobby and the fact that in 1983-1984 tax and excise on alcohol brought in £5,825 million per year (Steele, 1985) [11]. With 7.3% of disposable income being spent on alcohol this represents massive income for the drinks industry (Lancet, 1988a). An additional factor may be that governments both in Britain and the USA have been influenced by the political ideology of the libertarian right, the move away from state control to the notion that individuals should take responsibility for their own actions and health.

The disease model of alcoholism is used as an argument against social measures aimed at cutting down the overall consumption of alcohol. It implies that most people can drink as much as they like and that alcohol is only a problem for the minority population of alcoholics. The increasingly popular Minnesota method of treatment is committed to the disease model and takes a vaguely revivalist approach based on total abstinence (This is the world of "Hi, I'm Tom. I'm an alcoholic."). In Britain the treatment is used mainly in the private sector, often run by doctors with limited psychiatric experience.

DRUG ADDICTION (NARCOMANIA)

Smulevitch (1985), in the Manual, defines toxicomania (narcomania) as a condition of temporary or chronic intoxication due to the use of various natural or synthetic

10. From 1950 to 1976 the consumption has increased from the equivalent of 5.2 to 9.7 litres of pure ethanol. Over the same period conviction for drunkenness went up by 100%, deaths from cirrhosis by 60% and hospital admissions for alcoholism by 2500% (Lancet, 1984).

11. To this can be added the other gains to the exchequer in terms of income tax from employees in the drink industry. The argument seems to be weighted in favour of the drinks industry, despite the fact that the costs of alcohol in terms of the demands on the health service and other agencies and losses to industry is £1600 million (British Medical Journal, 1985).

toxic substances. The characteristic features are an insuperable desire for the substance, a tendency to increase the amount used and psychological, sometimes physical, dependence on the substance. Smoking marijuana is recognized as a form of toxicomania although without marked psychological or physical changes. The main danger is seen as the increased likelihood of using more dangerous substances such as morphine. Rarely there are associated psychotic states. Addiction to tranquillisers and also smoking tobacco are included as types of toxicomania.

Until recently, narcomania was not considered to be a major problem in the Soviet Union. Babayan (1985) wrote that there had been a dramatic increase in drug addiction in the West over the previous few decades, but said that it "seems incredible" that there were so few cases of narcomania in the Soviet Union. Since then, however, there has been recognition of the issue in the Soviet Union, although it would seem to be on a small scale by comparison to the West. Table 10 gives the number of drug addicts registered with dispensaries as well as those patients presenting for the first time [12].

Table 10: *Patients (per million population) with narcomania on dispensary lists and patients presenting for the first time (National Economy, 1989).*

	1980	1985	1986	1987	1988	1989
Patients on the dispensary list	136	149	171	215	243	255
Patients presenting for first time	13	35	58	86	60	54

The Afghan war was implicated as a possible factor in introducing young conscripts to drug use, mainly marijuana. This is also readily available from the many wild species of the hemp plant grown in the Central Asian Republics [13].

Treatment

According to Smulevitch (1985), in-patient treatment is necessary in opiate addiction. In the acute stage the emphasis is on various drug regimes, and, in the acute stage of withdrawal, diet and vitamins, physiotherapy and work therapy. The regime of in-patient treatment may last for two months, after which several years of follow-up in out-patients is recommended. On discharge it is considered important to maintain contact through psychotherapy and to organize work and activity. Tranquillisers might be indicated.

12. Levin, in the newspaper Ogoniok (4.6.1988), writes that although 50,000 patients are registered with dispensaries the real number of drug addicts is in the region of 120,000.
13. There has been an active campaign to destroy these and in Tadzhikistan more that 25 million wild shrubs were destroyed. One problem was that many plants were grown on state and collective farms (Pravda, 1987b).

The broad interest in drug abuse is reflected in press articles about new developments, for instance new units in Tadjikhistan and Volgograd (MG 19.8.87 and 21.10.87). An article with an optimistic tone describes the Byelorussian republic's psychiatric hospital in Minsk where young drug addicts are treated with a combination of more traditional approaches, including medication, but also curative baths, physiculture and various forms of exercise (MG 26.2.88). There is emphasis on giving the young people new interests. Another article describes a cooperative workshop attached to a narcological dispensary in Uzbekhistan (MG 30.12.1987). This was set up on the initiative of the director and is now self-financing after an initial loan from the state bank, Gozbank. There are 130 workers, all from the narcological dispensary. Again there is a note of optimism. On the other hand there is a rather disgruntled article from a sector psychiatrist-narcologist in Moscow complaining about the doctors getting in on the "drugs bandwagon" (MG 13.5.1988). He writes that they might or might not be influenced by longer holidays and 25% higher pay. He maintains that this work should not fall to any old surgeon or army doctor but that adequate training is required, including knowledge of drug treatment and psychotherapy.

Comparative aspects

The Soviet view of drug addiction in the West is rather similar to the Western view of alcoholism in the Soviet Union. According to Pravda (1987b), there are thirty million drug addicts in the USA and this is considered to be engendered by socio-economic conditions. The same article reports that there are only 46,000 people with a medical diagnosis of drug addiction in the Soviet Union. This figure is seen as high and is the result of imitative behaviour, pushers and "lack of spiritual values". The article emphasizes the need for stricter policing methods as well as more emphasis on the medical treatment of the addicts.

The ethos of treatment in the Soviet Union is directed towards getting people off drugs, using long admissions where necessary to break the habit. Therapeutic optimism is strongly encouraged. In such a context the idea of methadone maintenance treatment is an alien one. By contrast, methadone is widely used in many Western countries. New York (which has half a million drug addicts of whom about 200,000 inject opiates intravenously) has a total of 35,000 of its inhabitants maintained on methadone [14].

---

14. There was opposition to the "Rockerfeller" methadone programme from radical black groups in the early 1970s. They saw it as a way of sedating blacks and Hispanics and keeping them from being politically active. The AIDS epidemic has given a different perspective to this issue.

Chapter Twelve

MENTAL HEALTH LEGISLATION
AND FORENSIC PSYCHIATRY

Mental health legislation is largely concerned with the detention and treatment of patients against their will. Rates of compulsory detention vary considerably from country to country. The Soviet Union has one of the lowest rates of compulsory detention amongst the countries with developed psychiatric services with about 3% of all psychiatric admissions being compulsory. In the USA, by comparison, the proportion is 25%, although this rises to 50% in the public sector (Roth, 1989). In Britain about 10% of all admissions are compulsory [1]. Despite these figures, there has been considerable controversy, both within the Soviet Union and in the rest of the world, about the nature of the Soviet legislation and its application.

Forensic psychiatry can be seen as having two different, but related, roles: the treatment of mentally ill offenders and the provision of a system for society to deal with certain groups of mentally disordered antisocial and/or dangerous people. The fact that these two roles may on occasions be in conflict underpins much of the controversy about the role of forensic psychiatry both in the Soviet Union and in the West.

There is some material in English, although it varies in quality and much of it is now dated. There is a Soviet book on forensic psychiatry which has been translated into English (Morozov and Kalashnik, 1970). Medvedev and Medvedev (1971) and Bloch and Reddaway (1977 and 1984) discuss aspects of the legal system and forensic psychiatry in the Soviet Union. Lader (1977) gives a brief comparative account of Soviet and Western forensic psychiatry. More recent information is available in the "Report of the U.S. delegation to assess recent changes in Soviet Psychiatry" dated July 12 1989 with its preliminary Soviet Response. Schizophrenia Bulletin (1989; volume 15, number 4) discusses aspects of dangerousness and involuntary commitment in the USA and USSR.

MENTAL HEALTH LEGISLATION

Zharikov (1983) compares mental health legislation in a number of different Western countries, giving a favourable impression of the position in Britain. He goes on to describe the Soviet procedures for the compulsory admission of patients, which he says are regulated by instructions from the Ministry of Health. According

---

1. This figure seems to be rising. Recent statistics suggest that in London as many as 40% of admissions may be compulsory.

to Zharikov (1983) and Babayan (1985), the basic criterion is that patients must be a danger to themselves or to others because of mental illness. There is a list of the kinds of mental illness that are considered grounds for detention, and these are similar to those in the new legislation (see below). Affective and neurotic reactions, antisocial behaviour and psychopathic personality traits are not indications, but chronic alcoholics and drug addicts may be admitted and treated against their will. Patients must be seen by a commission of three psychiatrists within 24 hours of the involuntary admission and all three must be in agreement that the admission is appropriate [2]. Subsequently a similar commission has to meet at least once a month.

Although the numbers of compulsory admissions in the Soviet Union are relatively low [3] there have been criticisms related to individual cases of unnecessary admission. There has also been criticism within the Soviet Union about the restrictive nature of the mental health legislation and the lack of adequate protection for patients' rights. In late 1987 the Presidium of the Supreme Soviet ratified new legislation covering various aspects of psychiatry and these came into force in March 1988. The measures included legislation on compulsory detention and measures to safeguard the rights and welfare of patients. An important change was the introduction of the right of patients, relatives or their legal representatives to challenge in court the decision of the chief psychiatrist or commission of psychiatrists with regard to compulsory detention (*MG* 6.1.88). It makes it an offence for a psychiatrist to wrongfully admit someone to a psychiatric hospital.

This legislation is described in an announcement in the Korsakoff Journal of Neuropathology and Psychiatry (1988; 11, 149-158). Patients may be admitted to hospital against their will or against the will of their relatives if they are a danger to themselves or others because of mental illness. The nature of the mental illness is defined and it is stipulated that the danger to self or others must be due to hypomania, depression or systematized delusions or due to abnormal behaviour arising as a result of psychomotor excitement, delusions, hallucinations, passivity phenomena, impaired consciousness, pathological impulsivity or mood changes. Abnormal behaviour because of intoxication and antisocial acts in someone with a personality disorder or neurosis is not grounds for admission. The Chief Psychiatrist in each republic and province has responsibility for monitoring procedures and also acts as arbiter. The patient has the right of appeal to the court against the decision of the chief psychiatrist or the psychiatric commission.

There is evidence that the number of admissions overall fell after the introduction of this legislation. This may partly be due to what some Soviet psychiatrists see as a general climate of "anti-psychiatry". There has been much internal criticism of psychiatry in newspapers including Pravda, Komsomolskaya Pravda, Izvestia and the Medical Gazette. Some psychiatrists claim that there is excessive and ill-informed criticism by journalists who do not understand the issues and argue that the new legislation will act against the interests of patients [4].

The new legislation has not changed the criteria for compulsory detention in

2. Patients or relatives have the right to name a psychiatrist of their choice to sit on the commission, although this rarely happens. Medvedev and Medvedev (1971) describe the process and discuss some of the issues.

3. The figures are more striking taken in the context of a smaller total number of admissions per capita population. This can be calculated on the basis of the smaller number of beds and longer periods of admission (see chapter 3).

4. Similar concerns were expressed by some British psychiatrists after the introduction of the 1983 Mental Health Act.

any fundamental way. However, ready access to the courts means that it will be easier for patients and their relatives to challenge these. The concern of some Soviet psychiatrists is that it will lead to a rigid interpretation of the notion of danger to self or others. In discussion with a psychiatrist and psychologist in Leningrad I was given an example of a patient who they thought was a problem because of the new legislation. The patient was a doctor, the head of a large polyclinic, who had become over-active and was arriving at work in the early hours of the morning, several hours before she normally did, telephoning people at all hours, re-organizing everything and everyone, being critical and argumentative. The psychiatrist considered her to be hypomanic in that she had pressure of speech and flight of ideas as well as over-activity and sleep disturbance. However, because she was not a danger to herself or to others in any obvious sense they were wary of compulsory admission. She herself was well aware of the issues and had told a psychiatrist that she would take him to court if he tried to admit her.

There is a cautionary note in the journal about the new instructions on involuntary hospitalization with regards to disturbed behaviour in patients with hypomania (Polischuk, 1989). The point is made that in some cases there is only slight affective disturbance which would not necessarily account for the behaviour. This would not, therefore be grounds for hospitalization even in patients known to be manic-depressive. The author warns that non-psychiatrists in particular may be confused about this point.

New legislation
Following on from the edict of the Presidium of the Supreme Soviet described above, there has been a more comprehensive review of the mental health legislation. A draft form of the new legislation has been prepared for wider consultation and is given in full in Medical Gazette (*MG* 27.7.1990). The legislation concerns broad issues such as the duties and responsibilities of psychiatrists, the provision of care in hospital and the community. It details patients' rights with regard to access to information, access to adequate community care and civil rights in general. There is particular emphasis on the rights of patients in hospital with regards to appeals, complaints, the right to see a lawyer or priest alone.

Article 22 allows urgent hospitalisation for 24 hours on the grounds of mental illness and danger to self or others on the decision of one doctor or psychiatrist. Within the 24-hour period the state procurator must be informed and the patient must be examined by a commission within 48 hours.

Article 23 allows non-urgent admission on the grounds of mental illness and danger to the patients health or safety and can only be implemented with the sanction of the procurator.

Patients brought into hospital on *either* article 22 or article 23 must be seen within 48 hours (excluding public holidays) by a commission of psychiatrists which has the right to discharge the patient. The patients must be seen by a commission every month for six months (after which time there is a six-monthly review). Patients, relatives and legal representatives have the right to be at the commission hearing.

There have been various comments on the legislation in the columns of Medical

Gazette, including an article from the Independent Psychiatric Association which suggests, among other things, that there should be more legal assistance for patients.

Patients' rights

According to Babayan (1985), patients with severe psychiatric disorders who are found to be legally incompetent by a special medical board (a forensic psychiatry commission) may lose certain civil rights. He writes that there are strict criteria for this and that it is not based simply upon a particular diagnosis or admission to hospital. There may be other consequences such as exemption from military service. Most civil rights, for instance the right to education, welfare and so on, are retained. A commission may be called to determine the validity of marriages and other civil transactions made when someone was mentally ill. These may be judged as having no legal standing and may be annulled. However, if mental illness developed after the transaction or marriage then these do not lose their legal standing. Marriages can be annulled on the grounds of mental illness by application of the spouse. The capability of bringing up children will also be determined by the commission, but parental rights are never lost on the grounds of mental illness.

According to Zharikov (1983) the rights and interests of the patient are paramount. Mental illness in itself does not mean there is an automatic change in the patient's legal standing, and decisions about removal of rights should be made on the basis of the patient's capabilities and the degree of disturbance. This should be kept under review. Snezhnevsky (1983) writes that in patients with schizophrenia legal capability depends upon the mental state at the time of the legal transaction. Patients who are actively psychotic or have severe defect states are not legally competent, but he stresses that even in severe illnesses there is a need to make careful individual assessment of capability.

Guardianship

In severe and chronic disorders, if a patient continues to be legally incompetent for a prolonged period of time, arrangement may be made for guardianship *(opieka)* with a view to safeguarding the interests of the patient. The following outline of guardianship arrangements are derived from Zharikov (1983) and Babayan (1985). Guardianship must be obtained through a court of law which has to declare someone legally incompetent. Patients must be unable to understand the significance of their legal acts and unable to carry out their social responsibilities. Guardianship is under the supervision of the executive committee of the local Soviet (the district Soviet of peoples' deputies) and is the responsibility of the health department. The implementation of guardianship is done by a special commission, usually consisting of the chief psychiatrist of the dispensary, the patient's sector psychiatrist and the "social-work" nurse. The commission assesses the patient's mental state, selects a guardian and attempts to look after the interests of the patient. This might involve ensuring that his property is secure, cancelling debts if necessary, resolving issues to do with children. The commission produces a statement on whether the examinee is mentally ill, whether or not he should be pronounced legally incompetent and placed under a guardianship. The conclusion may be challenged within a month by anyone involved and it is possible to call for a new commission and a new medical examination.

The guardian is usually a relative, and may use the dispensary service for advice. He is responsible for carrying out the patient's legal transactions and must give a yearly account of the patient's financial position and expenditure. As well as looking after the social interests of the patient the guardian should attempt to ensure a healthy environment for the patient and encourage him to make regular visits to the dispensary and comply with treatment. The guardian is directly responsible to the commission and thus to the executive committee of the district Soviet and any irregularities are punishable by law. A guardianship order cannot exceed two years.

Consent to treatment

Patients who are compulsorily admitted may be treated against their will and in practice legislation for compulsory treatment is encompassed within this. According to Babayan (1985), compulsory treatment may be given in hospitals but also in out-patients within guide-lines laid down by the Ministry. Duration depends upon the individual case. He writes that, in contrast to "the problems in the West," the law protects patients by ensuring close scrutiny of drug treatment. Some treatment methods, including psychosurgery, are banned. There are instructions from the Ministry of Health with regards to the application of ECT which he refers to as a "traumatic method" of treatment. There are strict limitations on the number of applications and restricted indication for its use. ECT is very rarely given against a patient's will.

Mental health legislation in the West

Most countries in the world have some provision for involuntary admission on the grounds of mental disorder. The details of the different mental health acts vary according to the criteria used to justify compulsory detention, the personnel involved, the length of detention and the appeal procedures. All criteria for compulsory detention stipulate that patients should be mentally disordered, although there is much variation in how this is defined. Along with the mental disorder criterion it is usual for there to be an additional requirement. This may be relatively stringent, for instance requiring that a patient be a danger to himself or to others. Somewhat "looser" criteria include disability, danger to health, not being able to cope or care for oneself.

The USA

Each state has its own mental health legislation and there have been recent changes in the legislation in many states. States such as New York and California are considered to be more "liberal" in making it harder to arrange for involuntary admissions. All require evidence of mental illness, although in most states this simply means that the criteria for one of the DSM-III disorders has to be fulfilled [5]. There are greater variations with regard to the other criteria. The trend is towards dangerousness to self or others but other criteria such as severe disability,

---

5. These are notoriously loose and allow a wide range of conditions to be considered as criteria for compulsory detention. They include the personality disorders, adjustment disorders and "oppositional disorder" (see page 249). Several studies show that about one in five of the young adult population meet DSM-III criteria for mental disorder (eg Regier et al, 1988).

inability to cope or to care for oneself are still in use in many states. There is generally some restriction on patients' discharging themselves after voluntary admissions. This may involve a period of up to a week of holding power whilst the psychiatrist applies to the court to prevent a voluntary discharge.

In New York, article 9.39 of the Mental Hygiene Law covers emergency admissions. One physician of any specialty can sign the order and the criteria are that the person must be mentally ill, which means fulfilling DSM-III criteria, and must be either suicidal or threatening harm to others. It also allows the police to bring someone to a designated emergency centre (usually city hospitals but also some private hospitals) for assessment for a "9.39" admission. The order applies for 15 days after which it can be changed to a "2PC". The "2PC" is the two physician certificate which is intended to enforce admission when other treatment would be insufficient. A family member petitions for the certificate, although in the absence of a family member this can be a guardian or hospital administrator. The "2PC" is still used in cases of mental illness where the patient is in need of care rather than being a danger to self or others. However, a number of court cases, for instance that of the celebrated Billie Boggs, are pushing the "2PC" in the direction of the "9.39" in requiring evidence of danger to self or others. The looser criteria are opposed by various civil liberties groups.

Britain

The current legislation is based on the Mental Health Act of 1983. Section 4 allows detention for up to 72 hours. It stipulates that a patient is suffering from mental disorder and requires the signature of one doctor and a social worker [6] or nearest relative. Section 136 allows a police officer to remove someone who appears to have a mental disorder from a public place to a "place of safety" which may be a psychiatric hospital. The person may be detained for up to 72 hours. Section 2 allows detention for up to 28 days and requires the signature of two doctors and a social worker or nearest relative. Section 3 allows detention for six months for treatment. The patient must be suffering from a mental illness or from some form of mental impairment or psychopathic disorder. It also requires the signature of two doctors and the social worker or nearest relative. This section may be extended for six months and then on an annual basis. The British legislation defines mental disorder as mental illness, arrested or incomplete development of mind, psychopathic disorder and any other disorder or disability of mind. There is no further definition of mental illness. The further grounds for admission are protection of others or the interests of the patient's own safety or health.

Other countries

There are major variations in mental health legislation throughout the world. Some of the important differences concern the use of criteria in addition to danger to self and others. Switzerland, for instance, allows detention on the grounds of not being able to care for oneself and is thus similar to Britain which allows detention on the grounds of danger to health. In Switzerland the legislation is implemented by a court-appointed police doctor who may be called in by a relative or some other doctor. Japan has some of the loosest mental health legislation in the world and,

6. Employed by local government.

according to Cohen (1988), compulsory detention is allowed on the opinion of one doctor on the basis of vaguely defined mental illness with no other criteria. Some Middle Eastern and third world countries appear to have virtually no legislation designed to protect the interests of patients subject to compulsory detention.

Appeals

The appeal procedures are also subject to considerable variation. In the USA a patient can appeal at any stage of his detention. There is generally a delay before the court hearing which involves the judge coming to the hospital. In Britain there is no right of appeal from the three day sections. With sections 2 and 3 there is a right of appeal to a tribunal which consists of a psychiatrist, a lawyer and a lay person. This usually meets several weeks after the patient's appeal. In Switzerland a tribunal of two psychiatrists and a lawyer should meet within two weeks. From this it is also possible to appeal to the civil court.

Consent to treatment

The legislation with regard to compulsory treatment varies in the different American states. In some it is covered by the admissions legislation. In some states it is necessary to obtain court approval for the treatment of involuntary patients. Emergency treatment may be allowed but this is usually taken to mean control of disruptive behaviour rather than treatment of psychotic symptoms. There are sometimes delays of several weeks before hearings take place. In New York treatment can only be given if there is immediate threat to life. Paradoxically, patients in the Emergency Room may be treated for up to a week without any further legislation being invoked.

According to Appelbaum (1988) the rights of the individual vary from state to state. In most states patients have the right to refuse treatment, even when compulsorily detained. In the overwhelming majority of cases, however, when this comes to court the patient's right is overridden. Patients have the right to refuse specific procedures such as ECT in some states, for instance California and Massachusetts. In Britain drug treatment is covered by the sections for compulsory admission under the Mental Health Act of 1983. A second medical opinion is required from a doctor appointed by the Mental Health Act Commission if a patient refuses ECT or refuses treatment with drugs after he has been on them for over three months [7]. A controversial issue is compulsory treatment in the community. As yet there is no such legislation in Britain. A number of American states have statutes which allow for compulsory out-patient treatment. The criteria are usually dangerousness or the probability of dangerousness and a court appearance is necessary to implement this. There are a number of other approaches. For instance, a patient may be bound by the court to appear at out-patients for follow-up and if he fails to do so will be admitted automatically. Treatment may be a condition of probation for certain offenders, especially those with personality disorders and perversions. In Massachusetts a judge can find a patient incompetent to consent to treatment and therefore order treatment until such time as he is competent again. One problem of the legal intervention is that treatment plans endorsed by the courts may be for specific drugs and dosages, leading to rigid and inflexible treatment regimes.

7. There are few cases where the psychiatrist's opinion about the need for ECT has been overturned (Cohen, 1988).

Patients' rights

Most Western countries have few legal restrictions on the rights and activities of psychiatric patients, although it is almost universal to have legislation for implementing some form of guardianship on the grounds of mental illness. Some of the restrictions appear to be semi-official, for instance the entry restrictions to some countries (including the USA) on the grounds of mental illness. Employment prospects are clearly affected by a history of mental illness and in some countries including the USA there are a number of jobs in which checks on mental health records are made and some diagnoses, for instance schizophrenia, bar entry. Japan again appears to come off badly in this area. According to Cohen (1988) there is a wide range of restrictions on the activities of ex-patients, for instance not being allowed to go into public baths, have a driving licences or hold certain jobs such as being a cook.

Comparative aspects of legislation

Mental health legislation may be loose either because of the vague definition of mental illness or because of the accompanying criteria. In Britain patients must be a danger to self or others or to their health. This is open to wide interpretation. Roth (1989) quotes studies showing that clinicians have poor inter-rater reliability for assessing whether or not patients can care for themselves. In practice it means that most patients with serious psychiatric disorders can be detained against their will. This may be seen as a loop-hole in the legislation or applauded as a wise provision which is in the interests of patients. The second loose area is with regard to the definition of mental disorder. This is left open to the judgement of the individual psychiatrist in Britain. The apparently tough legislation in some American states which requires a person to be a danger to self or others allows for this in the context of any DSM-III disorder. This includes personality disorder, adjustment disorder and oppositional disorder. These criteria are broad and vague and some are essentially based on social rather than clinical criteria.

The impact of the legislation is shown up in cross-national comparisons of the demographic profiles of patients detained compulsorily. There is selective admission of younger males in the USA and older females in the UK (Segal, 1989). Segal (1989) argues that this is because involuntary commitment in most states in the USA is based on dangerousness whereas in Britain and some other European countries it is based on the need for treatment criterion. It can be argued that mental health legislation in the USA is geared less to the needs of the mentally ill than to the necessity of dealing with socially dangerous behaviour in the large segment of the population who at any one time meet some of the DSM-III criteria for "psychiatric disorder".

Cohen (1988) is critical about the laxity of much of the legislation. He maintains that in Britain there is a tendency to use known colleagues to implement the 1983 Act and this makes it easy to detain and treat patients against their will. In Israel a single psychiatrist can detain someone in hospital for seven days. He reports that this can happen without the patient even being seen, for instance on the word of a general practitioner over the telephone. He is severely critical of the

8. See footnote 1 on page 203.
9. In the Soviet Union the Trade Unions act in a kind of social work capacity.

situation in Japan where the criteria are so loose as to be almost meaningless. More serious is the fact that most compulsory admissions are for long periods of time to private psychiatric hospitals. Patients can be detained indefinitely by a single doctor who might be the owner of the psychiatric hospital. There have been other criticisms (eg Lancet, 1986b and 1987). There is no legal protection for patients in a country in which 75% of the admissions are involuntary. In 1981 there were 250,000 involuntary patients in Japanese mental hospitals, which at a rate of 2.5 per 1000 population makes it ten times higher than anywhere else in the world.

In comparison to many countries the Soviet Union has relatively stringent legislation with regard to compulsory detention. It defines the types of disorder that may be grounds for compulsory admission. One problem in this area is that there are no established international criteria with regard to involuntary detention in hospital. There are moves towards greater involvement of the judiciary and also for making dangerousness the main criterion for detention, although, as discussed above, these developments may not necessarily be in the best interests of those suffering from psychiatric disorders. An additional problem is that dangerousness is hard to predict (Steaman, 1983).

Numbers of patients compulsorily detained
The proportion of compulsory admissions to voluntary admissions in the Soviet Union is low, with most sources reporting that about 3% of all admissions are involuntary, a figure comparable to the 3-4% reported a quarter of a century ago by Bazelon (1967). The figure compares with 10% in Britain [8], 25% in the USA (50% in the public sector) and 75% in Japan.

Several explanations are proffered for the national differences. Soviet psychiatrists argue that their system of care is better so that patients' relapses are detected and admission can often be avoided. They also maintain that patients trust their doctors because of the long period of time they have known them, especially in the dispensary. Critics would maintain that the reasons are more to do with the greater degree of conformity in society and the authoritarian, bureaucratic nature of the various organizations involved. It is argued that relatives and trade union organizations put pressure on patients to go along with psychiatrists' decisions [9]. Patients might well trust their doctors in many cases, but they also know that if they don't do what the doctor advises they can be admitted anyway. This is true, although the same argument applies in any society. Bazelon (1967), who mentions this as a possible factor in the low rates of compulsory detention in the USSR, writes that it "differs little in practice from the time-honoured American tradition of inducing a patient to undergo voluntary commitment by threatening the commencement of involuntary commitment proceedings ...". Few psychiatrists (or social workers) can be unfamiliar with this practice.

FORENSIC PSYCHIATRY
Zharikov (1983) writes that forensic psychiatry is a branch of psychiatry which is concerned with the rights of the mentally ill and the question of whether or not he should be held responsible for punishable offences. According to Babayan (1985), Soviet legislation is designed to protect the interests of the mentally ill and to safeguard society against socially dangerous acts by the mentally ill.

Historical

Zharikov (1983) writes that there was a progressive pre-Revolutionary tradition of forensic psychiatry, associated with psychiatrists such as Balinsky, Korsakoff and Kandinsky who were familiar with the concepts of partial insanity and diminished responsibility, but that the system at that time prevented its implementation. The revolution allowed forensic psychiatry to develop, mandating a forensic psychiatric examination whenever there was doubt about the mental state of the accused. In 1919 the Moscow City health department first sent psychiatrists to prisons in order to detect mental illness, and one of the first psychiatrists involved in this was Krasnushkin who helped to found the Serbsky Institute of Forensic Psychiatry in 1921 (Babayan, 1985). However, Babayan (1985) considers that the early post-revolutionary guide-lines allowed too wide a range of conditions to qualify for non-responsibility and that in 1925 a conference redressed this. It was accepted that crime was a social phenomenon requiring jurisprudence not psychiatry. The 1919 guide-lines which allowed non-responsibility on the grounds of mental illness at the time of sentencing was changed to require evidence of mental illness at the time of the offence [10].

The current position

According to Babayan (1985), a forensic psychiatric examination can be requested by any investigative or judicial body or by the defence at any stage of the proceedings: before or during trial or before sentencing. It is also possible to request a mental state examination on a plaintiff or witness in civil court proceedings. There are departments of forensic psychiatry attached to some dispensaries and psychiatric hospitals. In major cases or difficult cases there may be a forensic psychiatry commission with a second commission being appointed if there is disagreement.

Non-responsibility or non-imputability is defined by Article 11 of "The Fundamentals of Criminal Law of the USSR". Someone is not criminally responsible if, at the time that they committed the offence, they were in a state of non-imputability, that is that they were unable to realize the nature of their acts or to control them as a consequence of chronic mental illness, temporary derangement of mental activity, mental handicap or some other morbid condition. According to article 12 a person is not relieved of criminal responsibility if he was merely drunk at the time of the offence. However, if there is evidence of a psychotic state related to alcohol this may be grounds for non-imputability. Articles 58-61 cover the compulsory measures that the person may be subject to.

The legal criteria for non-imputability are that there must be some medical disorder and that the intellectual ability to realize the nature of one's actions or the volitional ability to control them must be lost. A medical diagnosis alone is not sufficient to define non-imputability. Thus, epilepsy or chronic mental illness without profound personality changes may not be grounds for non-imputability. Moreover non-imputability does not rest on the nature of the diagnosis. If one

---

10. According to Lader (1977), many minor disorders were still grounds for non-responsibility in the 1930s and "the question of legal sanity was decided by psychiatrists in terms of the optimum treatment for that particular offender in his context in society". He writes that a reaction then set in and psychiatrists were criticized for designating almost anyone with any kind of emotional instability as legally non-responsible. It is probable that Babayan (1985) is correct and that this change in policy actually took place in the 1920s.

expert diagnoses manic-depression and another circular schizophrenia the grounds for non-imputability may be just the same. If a person was imputable at the time of the offence but then develops some mental disorder so as not to be able to realize the nature of his acts or control them he may be subject to compulsory medical treatment and then subject to punishment for the offences on recovery.

There is no plea of diminished responsibility. According to Morozov (1985) the concept of diminished responsibility departs from the principles of thorough forensic psychiatric evaluation. He maintains that people are either responsible or not, a surprisingly absolute view in the context of the Soviet concept of mental illness [11]. On pragmatic grounds he maintains that accepting the principle of diminished responsibility would mean that special institutions would be required. He argues that most people with diminished responsibility are psychopaths and experience has shown that concentrating such people in one institution has a deleterious effect upon them. Moreover there is no benefit to them to have their conduct considered non-responsible. He rather succinctly states that the only way of treating the *imputable* psychopath is by participation in a regime of collective work with a view to reconstruction of the personality and that "the Soviet correctional labour camp (prison) serves precisely this goal." As discussed below there are cases where psychopaths are considered to be non-imputable and it is important to stress that this particularly applies to paranoid development of personality.

There is also a theoretical objection to the concept of diminished responsibility in that it suggests the notion of partial imputability. This is taken to imply that there is a healthy part of the mind for some decisions and a morbid part for other decisions, a view which is considered illogical as all mental activity is interrelated. Zharikov (1983) writes that the notion is derived from the views of Esquirol about monomania, that outside a paranoid system a patient is normal and claims that there is no scientific basis for this idea [12]. He claims that the notion of diminished responsibility opens up the possibility of too much arbitrary interference with patients' lives by the law and allowing for "indefinite, unwarranted isolation".

With regards to the humanitarian aspect of the diminished responsibility plea and the use of mitigating factors, Soviet psychiatrists generally maintain that it is not necessary for them to assume this responsibility. They claim that Soviet courts are well aware of mitigating factors and always take account of social and family circumstances in sentencing and so do not require psychiatrists for this.

The consequences of being found not responsible are varied, and do not involve admission in all cases. According to Zharikov (1983) a person may remain under the observation of the sector psychiatrist or be placed under the care of relatives. The period of observation is not fixed, but is reviewed at least six-monthly. A commission to terminate the observation or treatment is called when the patient recovers or is no longer a danger. Patients may also be admitted to general psychiatric hospitals or one of the nine special psychiatric hospitals. These were under the aegis of the Minister of the Interior but have recently moved over to the Ministry of Health.

---

11. The materialist basis, along with the concept of a continuum and intermediate forms, might suggest that there should be degrees of responsibility.
12. The Soviet concept of delusion is stringent in that one of the criteria are that for an idea to be delusional it must affect all aspects of the mental functioning. See page 23.

Schizophrenia

Snezhnevsky (1983) writes that in schizophrenia psychotic features or personality change would be grounds for legal non-responsibility if patients were not aware of their actions or in full control of them. This would not apply to patients with episodic schizophrenia in whom there had been, say, a single episode with full remission and no personality change. The most difficult cases are patients with slow-flow schizophrenia or those who have developed post-process psychopathic-like states. In these patients it is necessary to take into account individual aspects of the case: the extent of the defect state, the degree of personality change, the circumstances at the time of the crime with regard to how aware the patient was of his actions and how able to control them. He makes the point that care is required as there may be concealed schizophrenic processes as revealed by fragmentary delusions or affective changes in the post-process psychopathic-like states.

Psychopathy (personality disorder)

Smulevitch (1983) writes that in the majority of cases psychopaths should be considered fully responsible for their actions. Exceptions would be cases of severe psychopathy with loss of insight and the inability to modify behaviour. Patients might also be considered not responsible if they carried out a crime during a phase of decompensation or during a reaction, for instance an affective reaction. Patients with paranoid development of character may be considered not responsible if they have delusional ideas or over-valued ideas with loss of insight.

Korolev (1983), from the Department of Psychiatry at the Second Medical Institute in Moscow, emphasizes the distinction between psychopathy and antisocial behaviour. He writes that psychopaths may be "engaged in normal, legal activity even in the presence of marked clinical disorders. Indeed they are often engaged in hypersocial acts (expressing altruism, philanthropy etc). Such people may themselves be engaged in a struggle against antisocial activity." He also stresses that the antisocial or illegal behaviour of psychopaths is not necessarily linked to their psychopathology. He is critical of the simplistic view that all behavioural abnormalities in people with psychiatric illnesses or psychopathy should be ascribed to their mental illness. He argues that this issue needs further investigation, especially with regard to establishing the appropriate medical and non-medical measures for dealing with antisocial activity.

Comparative aspects

Early tests for insanity in England were concerned with behaviour and aspects of cognitive function. The most significant development in forensic psychiatry was the introduction of the M'Naghten Rules [13] with its verdict of "not guilty by reason of insanity" which applied if it could be shown that a person was not able to form guilty intent (that he was not "mens rea"). The rules state that a defendant is not guilty if, at the time of the commission of the act, he suffered from a defect of reason arising from disease of the mind such that he did not understand the nature of the act or did not know that it was contrary to law. The diminished responsibility

13. In 1843 Daniel M'Naghten shot Edward Drummond, the private secretary to the Tory Prime Minister, Robert Peel, having intended to shoot Peel himself. It was demonstrated in court that M'Naghten believed that he was being persecuted by the Tories.

plea came into the Homicide Act of 1957 by way of the common law of Scotland. This reduced a murder charge to manslaughter if it could be shown that the person had an "abnormality of mind" which "substantially impaired his mental responsibility for his acts..."

In the USA the M'Naghten rules are still the sole test of criminal responsibility in several states. However, the difficulty of determining guilty intent has led to the Guilty But Mentally Ill (GBMI) verdict which was introduced in 1975 in the State of Michigan and has since been adopted by several other states. It still requires a definition of a mentally ill person. In the state of South Carolina this is defined as "a person afflicted with mental disease to such extent that for his own welfare or the welfare of others he requires care, treatment or hospitalization" which is essentially a broad social definition. On the whole the GBMI verdict allows a broader scope for applying psychiatry to the judicial process. However, the verdict can also keep people within the criminal justice system, and some states, Indiana for instance, allow the death sentence with a GBMI verdict.

The Durham rule was introduced as a result of a ruling by Judge Bazelon in 1954. This held that a defendant was not guilty if the act was the product of mental disease or mental defect. The rule was abandoned because of the vagaries of defining mental disease but the basic principle of the approach remains, for instance in the American Law Institute test. This states that a person is not responsible for criminal conduct if, at the time of such conduct, he lacks substantial capacity either to appreciate the criminality (wrongfulness) of his conduct or *to conform to the requirement of the law* as a result of mental disease or defect. Mental disease or defect does not include abnormality manifested only by repeated criminal or antisocial conduct. The joint statement of the American Bar Association and the American Psychiatric Association in 1982 suggested a return to the notion of non-responsibility defined on the basis of whether a defendant has a mental disease or not, but to limit this to its effect on cognition and leave out the question of self-control or impulsivity.

The concept of diminished responsibility is in use in some states, but not others. Fitness to plead requires someone to be aware of court procedures, to be able to instruct his lawyers and understand the significance of a plea of guilty or not guilty. The "unfit to plead" plea is similar in the UK and USA and is generally applied only to defendants who are mentally handicapped or are psychotic with lack of insight.

The basic criteria for non-responsibility are similar in the Soviet Union and the English-speaking world. The Soviet criteria incorporate the main features of the M'Naghten rules in allowing non-responsibility if the defendant is not aware of his actions. However, they are broader in that they also allow non-responsibility on the grounds that a person is not to control his actions as a result of mental illness[14].

The over-use and under-use of forensic psychiatry
The discipline of forensic psychiatry has to define a position in relation to two contrasting opinions: the view that all crime can be understood as some form of

---

14. Some American states have incorporated this criterion, for instance as the "irresistible impulse" criterion, in the past. In Britain, and some American states, control does not come into the issue of non-responsibility but is the key element of the diminished responsibility plea.

"psychiatric" disorder [15] and the view that there is no place for psychiatry in dealing with people who break the laws of society. Szasz, perhaps the chief proponent of the latter view, talks about the evils of "confining law-breakers in mental hospitals as insane, without the benefit of a real trial" (Szasz, 1989) and maintains that forensic psychiatry is a weapon used by the state against the freedom of the individual. These contrasting views help to explain the quite different criticisms made of forensic psychiatry, that is its under-use and over-use. Either of these could be in the interests of the individual or of society as a whole.

The main charge against the Soviet Union is that it over-uses forensic psychiatry in the interests of society (or "the state"). Critics like Bloch and Reddaway (1977 and 1984) maintain that a number of psychiatrists collude with the agencies of internal security and put psychiatric labels on people who are unfairly charged with various crimes solely because of their political views. This is the main charge in the abuse issue and is discussed in more detail in the next chapter. Other authors, for instance Stone (1984), emphasize that it is necessary to distinguish between the question of legality and the question of whether or not one agrees with particular laws. Thus, the people named in the alleged abuse cases were in fact legally charged and detained.

A more general criticism of Soviet psychiatry is with regard to the over-use of forensic psychiatry in criminal behaviour, essentially the medicalization of crime. Despite the reservations of some Soviet psychiatrists it may be that patients with personality disorders are more readily referred for psychiatric disposal in the Soviet Union than in the West, certainly in Britain [16]. In the USA much depends upon the nature of the crime, the wishes and status of the defendant and the defence lawyer. Another factor is that some patients with personality disorder in the West would be diagnosed in the Soviet Union as having a psychopathic-like state in the context of an endogenous psychosis. They would, therefore, be considered as being more obviously within the province of psychiatry [17].

The wider criteria for non-responsibility, especially for patients who, from the Western perspective, have personality disorders, does produce greater potential for abuse and for allegations of abuse. This is partly mainly because there is little evidence that psychiatry can achieve much for this group. The debate might be conducted in quite different terms if treatment was clearly and demonstrably effective.

The USA can also be charged with the over-use of forensic psychiatry in acting against the interests of the individual. This is based on the fact that psychiatric intervention often results in longer periods of detention than ordinary criminal disposal. Lader (1977) writes that in the USA over half of those found unfit to plead spent the rest of their lives in hospital. Although this situation has probably

---

15. Guze in the USA has argued that up to 90% of felons have psychiatric disorders, with only half of these being accounted for by personality disorders.

16. It is hard to find empirical data on this. Criticisms made within the Soviet Union give some indication that, as in the West, many mentally ill offenders end up in the prison system (eg Gluzman, 1989). The discussions of the Supreme Soviet on the provisions for the mentally ill included further recommendations about treating mentally ill offenders in hospital rather than in the prison system (Medical Gazette, 6.1.88).

17. The point has already been made that the Western cross-sectional approach to diagnosis turns schizophrenics into personality disorders. In this context the study of Coid (1987) is of interest. He reviewed 131 psychopaths in Broadmoor and Rampton. 55% had been admitted in the past, generally with some category of mental illness. The majority had been treated with psychotropic drugs and 29% had been treated with ECT in the past.

changed there is no doubt that in certain categories of offence, especially more serious crimes such as rape and murder, a committal to a psychiatric hospital will be much longer than a routine sentence. In 1983, in Jones vs USA, the Supreme Court ruled that someone could be held indefinitely in a mental hospital even if the original offence warranted a lesser sentence. In 1975 Michael Jones had tried to steal a jacket from a shop. After his arrest he was seen by a psychiatrist and diagnosed as a paranoid schizophrenic. After plea bargaining he was sent to St. Elizabeth's hospital and had been there for seven years when he appealed.

A more familiar charge against the practice of forensic psychiatry in the West, especially the USA, is that it is over-used in the interests of certain individuals, namely those with enough money to buy their services. This only applies, of course, where the results of psychiatric intervention result in evading punishment, receiving shorter periods of detention or escaping the death penalty. Soviet psychiatrists have also been accused of giving false diagnoses to enable people to evade custodial sentences or military service (Medical Gazette of 31.7.87, 2.3.88 and 11.11.88). However, as these are considered to be criminal offences in the Soviet Union, they should probably not be considered in the same light as the charges made against Western psychiatrists.

The main criticism in the West is of the under-use of psychiatry in people with clear-cut mental illnesses. Many studies indicate that a high proportion of the prison population are mentally ill and that treatment in prison is far from adequate (see page 241). It is argued that the closure of the mental hospitals has meant that many mentally ill offenders end up in prison and are treated in an inhumane manner. There are, however, several reasons for the high proportion of mentally ill in our prisons and it is perhaps too simplistic to explain it away solely on the policy of deinstitutionalization. The current situation has arisen over the course of many decades and is closely linked with the theory and practice of psychiatry. Concepts of mental illness, the approach to diagnosis and the system of out-patient care (or lack of it) all affect the issue. A common situation arises in the forensic examination of someone with a chronic disorder who is seen at a time when there are no obvious psychotic features. In the West, certainly in Britain, the cross-sectional approach to diagnosis often means that someone like this is considered as eccentric or personality disordered. The patient-offenders therefore end up with the judicial system rather than the psychiatric system. Whether this is better or worse from the point of view of the offender is debatable, although it might be more appropriate to subject the question to some fairly basic research. The issues become more clear-cut when the death penalty is involved. Here, most people, with the exception of Szasz [18], would see that forensic psychiatry might have something definite to offer the patient. In the USA, however, there is evidence that this does not happen in the case of certain disadvantaged groups. Lewis et al (1986) report that of 15 prisoners who were awaiting the death penalty 6 had schizophreniform psychoses and 2 had manic-depressive disorder. All had a history of head injury and in five cases there were major neurological signs. In a later paper they report that there were 37 male "juveniles" awaiting the death penalty (Lewis et al, 1988). These were people who had been sentenced to death before

18. He argues that there is a "fate worse than death". He suggests that M'Naghten might have been done a disservice in having been saved from the gallows and having to spend 21 years of his life in the Bethlem and then Broadmoor.

the age of 18. The authors managed to see 14 of them, half of whom were black. They report that 9 were psychotic and 7 had been psychotic before the offence. Most had long histories of psychiatric disorder, neurological damage, severe physical or sexual abuse as children. Despite this only five had received psychiatric evaluation.

The services of the forensic psychiatrist may be used too little or too much. The balance of evidence suggests that the former criticism applies mainly to the USA where the availability of proper forensic psychiatry, acting in the interest of the individual, depends on socio-economic factors, mainly on being able to afford good defence lawyers and psychiatrists. The latter criticism may be made against Soviet psychiatry, although the evidence about this is largely anecdotal. The fundamental theoretical questions apply equally in the Soviet Union and the West. Perhaps the main one, touched upon by Korolev (1983), remains the question of imputability in a person who has some degree of mental illness but where the offence is not obviously related to the mental illness.

Chapter Thirteen

POLITICAL ISSUES IN PSYCHIATRY

One of the main underlying issues, never far from the surface of any psychiatric controversy, concerns the balance between the rights of the individual and the needs of society. Much of what is discussed below is related to this question. In general the West makes specific accusations about named individuals who are said to have suffered at the hands of a collectivist society. The traditional Soviet counter-argument has been to identify disadvantaged groups who suffer under the Capitalist system. The charges can perhaps be divided up into sins of omission and sins of commission. The finger pointing from West to East usually points at a sin of commission whereas the East to West finger points at sins of omission.

The chapter will give a brief outline of the charges made against Soviet and Western psychiatry before going on to discuss some general issues raised by these accusations.

CHARGES AGAINST SOVIET PSYCHIATRY
Criticisms of Soviet psychiatry come from within the Soviet Union as well as from outside. The main charge from external sources concerns allegations of systematic abuse of psychiatry for political purposes. Internal criticisms are generally about individual cases of corruption and abuse as well as conditions within the psychiatric service.

Allegations of abuse of psychiatry for political purposes
The issues discussed here have become the source of major controversy in psychiatry and have caused ill-feeling amongst psychiatrists throughout the world, with accusations of dishonesty, treachery and betrayal. The result is that there are large discrepancies between what is said by the different factions and it is difficult to make an objective appraisal of the evidence. My approach, therefore, will be to summarize the accusations and then present the Soviet response.

There is some irony in the fact that until the present criticisms Soviet psychiatry was held up as an example of an enlightened system for the care of the mentally ill. Many early writers commented favourably on the system of community care, day facilities, rehabilitation and the restricted use of beds [1]. Another irony is that one

---

1. These include Ziferstein (1966), Auster (1967), Hein, (968), Sirotkin (1968), Visotsky (1968), Fuller Torrey (1971), Rollin, 1972), Allen (1973), Holland (1975).

of the early criticisms of Soviet psychiatry was that mental illness was *under-diagnosed* in order to get people back to work (Szasz, 1961).

The main accusation according to Bloch and Reddaway (1977 and 1984) was that sane people were admitted to psychiatric hospitals and treated against their will because of their politically unacceptable views. They claim that there were a number of core psychiatrists who were pivotal participants in the alleged abuse, among them Morozov, Lunts and Landau at the Serbsky Institute and Snezhnevsky and Vartanian at the Institute of Psychiatry, and that other psychiatrists "reluctantly collude with the politicisation of their discipline out of a blend of indoctrination, passive conformism and sheer fear." They maintain that political and religious dissenters were arrested by the security services who would then get a psychiatrist to examine them and certify them as not responsible for the offences they were alleged to have committed. They were therefore subject to psychiatric disposal rather than entering the prison system. The people involved were usually charged under Article 70 of the criminal code for anti-state activities or Article 190-1 for slandering the Soviet system. Another common criticism has been that people are admitted directly from official departments where they go with complaints. Koryagin, speaking at the Royal College of Psychiatrists in October 1987, claimed that people were being hospitalized directly from the waiting-room of the Central Soviet Presidium [2].

There is a related criticism that conditions in the Soviet Union, especially for dissidents, are such as to produce mental illness and that dissidents are "driven mad" by psychiatrists, for instance through the use of psychotropic drugs. In a similar vein, other critics have examined the medical and psychiatric status of certain dissident groups. Robinson and Berger (1988) suggest that there is a high incidence of psychosomatic and psychiatric disorder amongst "refuseniks" which they attribute to the altered status associated with applying to leave the Soviet Union.

The main sources for most of the allegations are the books by Bloch and Reddaway (1977 and 1984) and Wynn (1989). There are other sources, including the personal accounts of Tarsis (1967), Medvedev and Medvedev (1971), Bukovsky (1978) and Podrabinek (1980). There are letters and articles in newspapers and medical journals, some of which are quoted in this text or in the above sources. These come from journalists, victims of alleged abuse, Western psychiatrists and Soviet psychiatrists who have left the Soviet Union. The main primary source is the Samizdat publication "A chronicle of current events", produced in the West by Reddaway. Amnesty International relies upon secondary sources, mainly the Samizdat publications [3].

According to Bloch and Reddaway (1984) sane people with dissident views were incarcerated in pre-Revolutionary Russia and the practice continued throughout the early years of the revolution. However, it was only from the 1960s

---

2. This, incidentally, is not denied by Soviet psychiatrists who say that people with paranoid delusions often present themselves to various official bodies with petitions and complaints. There are parallels with the West. For instance, Shore et al (1985) describe the so-called "White House Cases", referring to people who approach the White House or other government offices and are interviewed by a Secret Service agent. If the person is considered potentially dangerous to himself or to others because of an apparent mental illness he is taken directly to a psychiatric hospital in Washington. The authors describe the demographic details of 328 patients who were admitted in this way over a three year period. The commonest diagnosis was paranoid schizophrenia.

3. The main Amnesty International publication was their booklet "Prisoners of Conscience in the USSR" (1975).

onwards, with the growth of civil rights movements within the Soviet Union, that there was awareness of the issue in the West. Two events in 1965 were the real beginning of the campaign [4]. One concerned the admission to hospital of an interpreter known to a group of British students, an issue that was taken up by the media and Amnesty International. The other event was the publication of the novel "Ward 7" by Valery Tarsis, an autobiographical novel describing his experiences of being in a psychiatric hospital in Moscow [5]. In the novel, Tarsis describes his experiences in a psychiatric hospital in Moscow and suggests that a group of sane dissidents are detained in hospital by party functionaries such as a Professor Stein who "believed that all mental disorders were caused by a mysterious malfunctioning of the body and refused to have any truck with the soul.." Ironically, (in that Professor Andrei Snezhnevsky has been a target for later critics) one of his characters is a Professor Andrei Nezhevsky, described as a tall man in his seventies with a world reputation as a psychiatrist and a "follower of Ghandi", who is sympathetic to dissidents.

In 1968 the Action Group for the Defence of Human Rights was formed in Moscow and had an outlet with the emergence of the Samizdat publication the "Chronicle of Current Events" which reported cases of alleged abuse. In June 1970 there was widespread publicity, both within the Soviet Union and in the West, about the admission of the geneticist Zhores Medvedev to Kaluga psychiatric hospital, a provincial town about a hundred miles South of Moscow [6]. In July 1970 an interview with Vladimir Bukovsky, in which he made allegations about the abuse of psychiatry, was broadcast by CBS television in the USA. A year later Bukovsky sent material to the West via a French emigre organization with psychiatric reports on six dissenters. Bukovsky has remained one of the key figures in the campaign and in his book "To Build a Castle: My life as a dissenter", Bukovsky (1978) describes his experiences of Soviet psychiatry as well as the prison system [7]. He was first arrested in 1963 and was sent for assessment to the Serbsky Institute after which he was admitted to the Leningrad Special Hospital. He remained for about a year without any form of treatment and describes one doctor, Kalinin, who, in the Leningrad tradition, looked for evidence of malaria, alcoholism or psychopathy, but who eventually considered him to be a malingerer

4. There were earlier charges laid against Soviet psychology. Hutton (1960) claimed that the Notting Hill race riots were provoked by "red psychologists" from Moscow who had managed to infiltrate gangs of teddy-boys in order to provoke disturbances with a view to bringing about world revolution.

5. The title is derived from Checkov's short story "Ward 6" which is about a doctor admitted to his own hospital. Tarsis makes his political stance clear. He sees communism as a conspiracy of the lesser beings, referred to as apes, to be fought by superman. Certain philosophers, Nietzche above all, are described as aristocrats of the spirit whose thinking is on a different plane to that of the "Philistine Marx" who is followed only by "blockheaded talmudists".

6. Zhores Medevev, along with his historian brother, Roy Medvedev, discuss this episode in their book "A Question of Madness" (1971). Zhores Medvedev was admitted to the psychiatric hospital on the recommendation of a local psychiatrist. Concern about his mental state seems to have arisen after his appointment with the chairman of his local Soviet to discuss his son. Medvedev was eventually admitted compulsorily to Kaluga Hospital. Because of the adverse publicity received by the case (there was pressure from leading Soviet writers, film-makers and scientists, with the chief psychiatrist of the hospital, Alexander Lifshits, receiving numerous visits, letters and telephone calls) there was a commission from Moscow which made a diagnosis of "psychopathic personality with paranoid tendencies" and recommended discharge. Despite this he remained in hospital for a total of three weeks, apparently without receiving any form of treatment. The book gives a good account of legal issues and the procedures of civil commitment and commissions. There is discussion of the nature of diagnosis and the political issues.

7. He describes many features of the regime and conditions at the time. There is a section on those he says were criminals who were pretending to be schizophrenic in order to evade justice. "During the day the sane patients gathered in the dining room, while the loonies were chased into the corridor. There was a television set, and we also played cards and drank there. Practically no attention at all was paid to the loonies, except when some comical madman wandered in and some fun was to be had from teasing him."

trying to evade justice. The commission disagreed and diagnosed him as suffering from "psychopathy of paranoid type in stage of compensation" and discharged him. However, in 1965 he was compulsorily admitted to a Moscow psychiatric hospital and later transferred to a hospital outside Moscow. He writes that he was considered to be sane by doctors at both of these hospitals and then transferred to the Serbsky Institute where the psychiatrists had a similar view. A commission held in Spring of 1966 was undecided and he was discharged again at the end of the summer of that year. He was in the Serbsky again in 1971 where a commission reported that he was sane but that it was possible that he had suffered from a schizophrenic-like psychosis in 1963. In 1976 he was released to the West in exchange for the Chilean Communist, Corvolan.

Semyon Gluzman was the first of a small number of Soviet psychiatrists who have been involved in the campaign. In 1971 he carried out an unofficial assessment of General Grigorenko, perhaps the most celebrated of the Bukovsky cases. In 1972 he was sentenced to prison for anti-state activities. Along with Bukovsky he wrote the widely-quoted "Manual on Psychiatry for Dissenters" which was published in Samizdat in 1974 and by Reddaway in the Chronicle of Human Rights in the USSR in 1975 [8].

The first international condemnation came in January 1971 when the Canadian Psychiatric Association endorsed a report from one of its sections condemning "alleged wrongful detention in mental hospitals in the USSR of seemingly healthy individuals whose views and attitudes are in conflict with those of the regime." In 1971 Reddaway set up the working group on the internment of dissenters in mental hospitals. This included Bloch, a psychotherapist, with whom he subsequently wrote two books on the subject. One of the key areas for the campaign was the Soviet membership of the World Psychiatric Association (WPA). The working group attempted to raise the issue at the WPA by circulating the six case histories sent out by Bukovsky. However, according to Bloch and Reddaway (1977), they were blocked. They maintain that the WPA did not debate the issue "thanks to strong-arm support from WPA Secretary-General Denis Leigh".

The campaign was intensified throughout the 1970s and there was frequent correspondence in the press, especially the Times. In 1973, during a WPA conference on schizophrenia held in Moscow, a group of 13 Western psychiatrists visited the Serbsky Institute. Several different versions of the events emerged, but the main result was that there were further allegations about the abuse of psychiatry. After this a WPA working party on ethical issues was set up by Leigh. Several national bodies pressed to have the issue raised at the Sixth World Congress of the WPA in 1977. Early in 1977 Bloch and Reddaway's book "Russia's political hospitals" was published [9]. At the WPA congress in Honolulu there was an active lobby from Bloch and various emigre Soviet psychiatrists. There was a plenary session on ethics which turned into an attack on Soviet psychiatry with various speakers from the floor and a number of resolutions condemning Soviet practice. A review committee to monitor psychiatric abuse was set up chaired by Professor Costas Stefanis from Greece with representatives from

8. Gluzman now works as a psychiatrist in Kiev, in the Ukraine, and is adviser on psychiatry to the Minister of Health

9. The title, presumably bland for American taste, was changed to "Psychiatric Terror" in the American edition.

the USA, Japan, Iran, West Germany and Brazil as well as the USSR. In 1977 the WPA elected a new Secretary-General, Peter Berner. The campaign continued within the WPA with various individual cases being presented to its committee on the abuse of psychiatry.

In Moscow in 1977 a "Working Commission to Investigate the Use of Psychiatry for Political Purposes" was established and sent out 24 bulletins over the next three years. The founder members included Alexander Podrabinek, a feldtscher in the Moscow ambulance service [10]. Two psychiatrists, Koryagin and Voloshanovitch, were involved. Voloshanovitch emigrated to Britain in 1980, but Koryagin was arrested and imprisoned in 1981 [11].

In the West various national organizations began to take up the issue actively. In 1978 the Royal College of Psychiatrists set up the Special Committee on the abuse of psychiatry. This body accused Snezhnevsky of involvement in the abuse and argued that his honorary membership of the Royal College should be rescinded. In 1980 Snezhnevsky was asked by the Council of the Royal College to appear before the Court of Electors which he declined to do, resigning his honorary membership, an action considered by Bloch and Reddaway (1977) to be "an admission of unprofessional conduct". The campaign continued as visits were made to the Soviet Union to examine dissenters. The "International Association on the Political Use of Psychiatry" was established in 1980 in Paris by Bukovsky. In Britain there was a campaign to have the Soviet Union expelled from the WPA, with Bukovsky and other members of the "working group on the internment of dissenters in mental hospitals" (set up by Reddaway in 1971), playing an active role. The Royal College of Psychiatrists, under a new President, Kenneth Rawnsley, pressed for expulsion. In June 1982 the American Psychiatric Association also called for expulsion and other national bodies, including the Danish and the Swiss, joined in the demand. The Canadians, although they had been involved in the campaign early on, were now against suspension or expulsion. There were now several resolutions to be put at the Seventh World Congress of the WPA to be held in Vienna in July 1983. However, in January 1983 the All-Union Society of psychiatrists, the Soviet psychiatric association, resigned its membership of the WPA.

The campaign now turned to other international bodies as more individual cases were publicized and there were demands for the removal of certain people in important positions in Soviet psychiatry. Within the Soviet Union Koryagin remained in prison and in 1985 an appeal was made in the Bulletin of the Royal College of Psychiatrists for Western intervention on his behalf. Koryagin was released in February 1987 and returned to his home town of Kharkov before coming to the West later that year. He spoke to the Royal College of Psychiatrists in October 1987, claiming that the persecution of dissidents was inherent in the Soviet system of psychiatry and that any form of political protest could be

---

10. In his book "Punitive Medicine" (1980) Podrabinek claims that "thousands" of healthy people were in hospital for their political beliefs and that most Soviet psychiatrists acquiesce in this. He publishes a "white list" of the victims and a "black list" of psychiatrists. He condemns the various treatments used, including sulphazine and high doses of haloperidol and chlorpromazine (the doses that he quotes are lower than those in routine usage in the West). He maintains that nothing will improve until the communists are out of power.

11. In 1981 Koryagin's paper on "Unwilling Patients" appeared in the Lancet (Koryagin, 1981). He stated that the people he saw on behalf of Working Group were psychologically healthy. They had been considered paranoid by psychiatrists who had diagnosed schizophrenia in 30% and psychopathy in 70%.

considered diagnostic of schizophrenia. He singled out Tarsis as an early victim and made particular reference to the involvement of certain forensic psychiatrists, including Lunts and Landau. At the Annual General Meeting of the Royal College in 1988 a motion was put by Bloch that the Soviet Union should not be re-admitted into the WPA unless they met certain conditions, one of which was that they should confess their previous mistakes.

In 1988 the Soviet Union had reapplied for membership of the WPA and according to Rich (1989) the WPA European Regional Executive met in April 1989 and provisionally accepted re-entry of the Soviet Association. This was sponsored by the President, Dr Costas Stefanis of Greece, who had been the chairman of the committee of abuse.

Soviet officials were in correspondence with various American bodies and eventually arrangements were made for a team to visit Moscow with representative from the APA and NIMH, under auspices of State Department. In March 1989 there was a two-week tour of American psychiatrists along with psychologists, lawyers and a state department official, along with Reddaway. The 26-man visit was led by Robert Farrand, Deputy Assistant Secretary for Humanitarian Affairs at the State Department and by Dr Loren Roth of Pittsburgh University. They visited four hospitals and four special hospitals, having free access to the hospitals, patients and records. They used their own translators and interviewed 15 in-patients and 12 discharged patients. Their report [12] acknowledged that they were given "unprecedented opportunity to interview and assess systematically a group of involuntarily committed forensic psychiatric patients of its own choosing...". According to the report there was "no evidence of any past or current mental disorder" in nine of the twelve discharged patients. According to the report the practice of "hyperdiagnosis" persisted, especially in the "psychopathy" and "schizophrenia in remission" diagnoses. Once again the symptom of "delusions of reform" is referred to [13]. The report also comments that patients retained their diagnosis of "schizophrenia" or "psychopathy" despite changes in clinical status. It condemns the fact that patients are denied certain rights and that medication, especially sulphazine and atropine, is sometimes used in a punitive way. It states that the conditions in most Special Psychiatric Hospitals were unduly harsh and restrictive.

The report made a large number of recommendations about diagnostic practice, treatment, conditions and procedures. It also recommended continued professional contacts between the USA and the USSR, follow-up visits to the Soviet Union and reciprocal visits by Soviet psychiatrists, and the establishment of an international commission to review psychiatric abuses in any nation.

A preliminary Soviet response [14] made a number of points. The authors referred to a lack of "clinical analysis" and called for joint reviews on the cases as they were unable to "understand the logic of the clinical thinking of the members of the American delegation". They refer to the "one-sided attitude on the part of the

12. "Report of the US delegation to assess recent changes in Soviet Psychiatry" to the Assistant Secretary of State for Human Rights and Humanitarian Affairs, US Department of State (July 12 1989).

13. It is stated that "demonstrating for reform, or being outspoken in opposition to the authorities" was defined in some patients as being a symptom ("delusion of reformism") or a diagnosis ("sluggish schizophrenia"). It is difficult to see how this view could be reconciled with the high level of such political activity in the Soviet Union at the time.

14. "Preliminary Soviet Response" to the report (S.V.Borodin and S.V. Polubinskaya June 28 1989).

U.S. psychiatrists....who did not take distinct psychotic states in the case histories of the patients into account, and even clearly overrated the facts of subjective memories" (this relates to the issue of longitudinal as opposed to cross-sectional diagnosis discussed in chapter 2). However, according to the document "...a number of patients who did not pose a physical threat to those around them had unjustifiably been under forced treatment for a long time". It also accepts the criticism of treatment with sulphazine and atropine coma and reports that the Ministry of Health is developing guidelines to ban their use. There is much discussion of the legal issues and the fact that an Independent Commission for Psychiatry is to be established is mentioned [15].

At the WPA congress in Athens in October 1989 the All-Union Society was readmitted to the WPA by a vote of 219 to 45 with 19 abstentions on condition that there should be a visit to the Soviet Union by the WPA review committee within one year. There was a lengthy debate, much concerned with the question as to whether or not the Soviet delegation would say that abuse had taken place in the past. A statement was read which said that "previous political conditions created an environment in which psychiatric abuse occurred for non-medical, including political, reasons" [16].

Internal criticism

An independent psychiatric association has been established in Moscow by Podrabinek and a small group of Soviet dissidents, ex-patients and some doctors. They aim to expose alleged abuses and they maintain that there are still psychiatric political prisoners [17].

Three main positions are reflected in the columns of the Medical Gazette: the official establishment view, the official opposition and the unofficial opposition. Two psychiatrists from the Bekhterev Institute in Leningrad, Lichko and Popov, in an article "Psychiatry at the Cross-roads", are critical of the All-Union Society of psychiatrists for a number of reasons, including its withdrawal from the World Psychiatric Association in 1983, but they also condemn the Independent Psychiatric Association, mainly for its pre-occupation with Snezhnevsky's classification (MG 19.11.1989). There is a response from Zharikov and Lukacher, defending the past actions and current working of the All-Union society (MG 20.12.1989). In the same edition there is also a response from Savenko, President of the Independent Psychiatric Association, most of which is a condemnation of the nosological concepts of Snezhnevsky and Ivanova-Smolensky. The Independent Psychiatric Association reflects the strong "anti-psychiatry" lobby growing within the Soviet Union and now finding a voice in the press. Despite its relatively small

15. Some of the unofficial responses have been more critical. The competence of the translators and interviewers has been questioned. It is claimed that when interviewing the patients there was an uncritical readiness to accept the patients' account of events. The superficial level of the clinical interview also raised doubts about the ability of the psychiatrists and translators to evaluate psychopathology. The cross-sectional "check-list" approach was condemned and also that little allowance was made for the fact that they were talking to patients or ex-patients who were detained against their will, who had strong political views and who were well aware of the purpose of the interview.

16. The WPA review committee visited the Soviet Union in June 1991 and voiced concern about various issues including conditions, treatment, the dispensary system, diagnostic criteria, the mental health legislation in practice, the structure and leadership of Soviet psychiatry and the pace of reform, but "found no evidence of new cases of political abuse of psychiatry" (Report by the WPA team of the visit to the Soviet Union, Birley et al, July 1991).

17. According to Amnesty International and Podrabinek about 30 dissenter-patients remained in hospital (Cornwell, 1989a).

size, it appears that there are already a number of opposing factions within this body, reflecting shades of opinion from reform of psychiatry through to a more extreme "anti-psychiatry" position (MG 20.12.1989).

Other internal criticisms are concerned with conditions within the psychiatric services, for instance over-crowding and shortage of staff, drugs and equipment (MG 31.7.87). There have also been criticisms of the training of staff and reports about corruption in mental hospitals (MG 21.7.87). There were reports on the visit of American psychiatrists to inspect hospitals and examine the charges that sane dissidents are locked up against their will (MG 1.1.89).

A number of different newspapers, including Pravda, the party newspaper, and Izvestia, the state newspaper have taken up issues to do with psychiatry. In the Summer 1987 Komsomolskaya Pravda, the newspaper of the communist youth organization, discussed Western allegations of abuse and interviewed Soviet psychiatrists about this. Subsequently, the same paper carried an article about the apparently wrongful detention of a twenty year-old woman who was always reading "Marxist-leninist literature" and was too out-spoken about her radical views. It also raises the issue of bribery, reporting on psychiatrists receiving bribes to give people diagnoses to avoid prison or army service.

In July 1987 Izvestia claimed that two women, one of them an Intourist Guide, had been wrongfully detained in a psychiatric hospital, reporting that the psychiatrist involved was subsequently dismissed. The February 1989 issue of the theoretical journal "Kommunist" wrote that "psychiatric abuses are far from eradicated" and that "the ministry circular of March 1988 would be fine if it wasn't so general, and full of mere declarations whose sense becomes less and less clear as time goes by. It contains no concrete rules guaranteeing patients the practical use of their rights."

A major article in Medical Gazette (MG 2.3.88) entitled "Psychiatry: to a new frontier" discusses various controversial issues about the different concepts of schizophrenia and the implications for mental health legislation. The articles stresses that psychiatrists with a sense of duty towards their patients have always been cautious about the social consequences of diagnostic labels and have to balance the interests of the patient and those of society. The problems of stigma are discussed and they describe a common example of someone who becomes ill during his military service. The fact that this is recorded on his army ticket means that his chances of finding particular types of work are prejudiced even if he has had a long remission. The paper questions why the diagnosis needs to be recorded in the first place, especially when it may have been made on the basis of a single medical opinion. It argues that in many cases there are mistakes in diagnosis, especially in young men having difficulties in adapting to new conditions. It suggests that the trade unions should be taking up these issues.

The Medical Gazette also reports an interesting case of bribery and embezzlement in a psychiatric hospital in the Sverdlovsk oblast (MG 11.11.1988). It began when a new chief psychiatrist, a Doctor Yarus from the Ukraine, was appointed in 1971 at the age of 33. He wanted to rebuild the old, crowded hospital and is described as having been full of energy and enthusiasm. The project began in the late 1970s and the article makes the point that readers will be aware that to get anything like that off the ground was a heroic undertaking. Problems soon began with builders who needed "commission". Yarus and the chief nurse began to sell absolute alcohol, in all 463 kgms for 15,000 roubles, as well as claiming wages for false staff on the pay-roll (shades of Gogol). He also received "lavish gifts" from the parents of those whom he had saved from serving in the army in his capacity as president of the dispensary forensic psychiatric expert commission. He continued to work actively for the hospital, keeping constant pressure on builders, and the result was a highly successful building. It is described as having plenty of space, good facilities for patients and excellent workshop facilities with a special factory attached. At this point his crimes came to light and the chief psychiatrist and one colleague were sent to prison, with four others getting a conditional discharge and being allowed to return to work. The chief psychiatrist, interviewed from his prison cell, claimed that he'd only ever wanted to help patients, that his diagnoses had never been wrong just because they were also "good deeds". He hoped that he would be able to return to his hospital and work there as a junior doctor in one of the workshops.

At the 8th All-Union Congress of Neuropathologists, psychiatrists and Narcologists in October 1988 there were complaints about lack of proper equipment, especially scanning equipment such as CT, MRI and PET. There was also condemnation of the conditions of buildings and facilities. There was criticism of the standard of psychiatrists themselves, the fact that they are often poorly qualified and adopt a hackneyed approach to treatment, ignoring psychological and social factors in their patients.

The dissident psychiatrist Semyon Gluzman (1989), writing in Medical Gazette, discusses the process of diagnosis, claiming that diagnostic criteria are vague and shift over time [18]. He criticizes conditions and the lack of sufficient beds and also condemns certain treatment methods, especially the use of sulphazine in pyrotherapy. He condemns the low cultural level of the population, including doctors, maintaining that doctors in this context, with the daily grind of living, are unlikely to be of good quality. He accepts that there are better establishments, the institutes, where facilities and drugs are better, but argues that doctors are still cogs in a totalitarian system. He also maintains psychiatrists are hampered because they cannot change the poor conditions that patients find themselves in (he quotes noisy workplaces and alcoholic husbands). He stresses that what is important to a patient is not the actual label, but the fact of being called mentally ill and the consequences that this has. He accepts that many dissidents are mentally ill and gives one of his own clinical examples to make the point that delusions of reform are delusions first and foremost. However, he maintains that a doctor has a duty to the patient and must *doubt* on behalf of the patient. He writes that people with mental illness may be socially adapted and may understand perfectly well when they are breaking the law. If he breaks the law and is charged, for instance, with slandering socialism, then to claim that this is exclusively due to mental illness is an abuse of psychiatry. He accepts that it is not possible to stop individual doctors from abusing psychiatry

18. He writes, for instance, that where one psychiatrist sees a schizophrenic, another sees a mild neurotic. He quotes German psychiatrist talking about the "feel" of schizophrenia. He criticizes the Soviet concept of psychopathy, arguing that the broad description can be widely too applied. His main criticism is for Snezhnevsky for "creating" a new form of schizophrenia, adopting a rather sneering tone when discussing slow-flow schizophrenia. He writes that the boundaries have again changed and that Smulevitch now regards it is as a borderline form. He also quotes varying opinions amongst psychiatrists at the Serbsky Institute, making the point that even leading experts disagree about criteria.

in their official capacity but the state must ensure that the possibilities for this are minimal and the law has to protect the patient's interest. He refers to the problem of the mentally ill in prison, quoting some authors as saying that 50% of the prison population are psychopathic or have alcohol-related problems. He blames various Soviet authorities, the late Daniel Lunts and also current forensic psychiatrists, who have denied the concept of diminished responsibility. The result is that young psychopaths go to prison, where, he maintains, they fare badly, for instance coming out with a damaged personality, drug addiction or homosexuality. He argues that the Soviet Union should look to "institutes of lowered responsibility" in the GDR, Bulgaria, Hungary and Czechoslovakia which provide intermediate facilities with treatment as well as detention.

Zagalsky (1989) in the literary journal, *Literaturnaya Gazeta*, makes a virulent attack on Soviet psychiatry and especially the "biological" schools associated with Pavlov and Snezhnevsky. He claims that Snezhnevsky's system of classification allows anyone to be sent to hospital. He regards Western psychiatry, with its Freudian leaning, as "humane". On a more practical note he berates the lack of resources going into psychiatry, referring to a hospital with no sanitation, and quotes the views of Semyon Gluzman. He refers to a number of recent cases of people he considers wrongfully detained and dwells on familiar themes with regard to delusions of reform, although without attempting to distinguish between the form and content of a symptom. He quotes the case of a girl he claims was "driven" to take an over-dose by a teacher and considers it a scandal that the girl is now in hospital whereas the teacher is still teaching. Tselmz (1989), in the same journal, gives another case uncovered from 1969 and calls on the Minister to investigate this and others.

There are several reports in the Soviet press about psychiatrists taking bribes to provide false diagnoses. Three Moscow psychiatrists were imprisoned for giving fake diagnoses of schizophrenia to criminals wanting to avoid responsibility for their crimes. The going rate was 5000 roubles. There were also charges with regard to falsifying medical reports in order to allow people to evade military call-up.

The August 1990 issue of "Kommunist", journal of the central committee of the Communist party, gives the number of people in psychiatric hospitals in Moscow as 71,000 (which is higher than the national average) and reports that "forced confinement to psychiatric hospitals has been practised on a massive scale" (this refers to the compulsory detention of the mentally ill). It calls for a radical shake-up in Soviet psychiatry and makes the rather perplexing suggestion that the psychiatric services should be withdrawn from the control of the Ministry of Health and made separately accountable.

Soviet psychiatrists' responses to the charges
This section is a compilation of the views of various Soviet psychiatrists that I have interviewed. Some spoke in their official capacity, but many were speaking unofficially. It will be followed by a brief report of the views of a number of Soviet psychiatrists in the West.

It is widely accepted that there have been abuses of psychiatry and that there may be other cases in the future. These are not considered to be inherent in the Soviet system of psychiatry but the result of incompetence [19] and, in rare cases, corruption. It is also accepted that there was excess caution in the past with regard to discharging certain groups of patients. These would include patients perceived as being a socially dangerous and thus would have included some people considered to be dissidents in the West. It was put to me that psychiatrists are more cautious about certain patients, for instance those with morbid jealousy, and this would extend to those in whom it might seem that their mental illness could lead to anti-social activity. The accusation that sane people are admitted to psychiatric hospitals because of their political views is considered to be without foundation.

A number of psychiatrists argue that the issue is less to do with psychiatry than with politics. The campaign is seen as politically motivated. The campaign about compulsory detention could only begin after deinstitutionalization had taken place in the USA and UK. Previously, when there were ten times more psychiatric beds per head of population in the West than there were in the Soviet Union, the case for systematic abuse would have looked thin [20]. Currently, there are roughly the same number of beds in the Soviet Union as compared to England (see page 64), although there are twice as many people per head of population in hospital in Scotland than in the Soviet Union. Depending upon what are counted as beds in the USA, the figure is again probably double the number of beds over the USSR (see page 62). Thus, there are fewer psychiatric admissions per head of population in the Soviet Union [21]. This, along with the fact that there is no obvious problem of the homeless mentally ill in the Soviet Union (implying that they are receiving hospital treatment when necessary), is cited as evidence that any kind of systematic policy to hospitalize dissidents would be impossible. Any such policy would mean that they would not be able to treat those with genuine mental illnesses because the system would be swamped with dissidents.

Another view is that the criticisms of Soviet Psychiatry are not dissimilar to those of Western Psychiatry made by various anti-psychiatry groups. It is argued that the attacks on Soviet psychiatry by Western psychiatrists are a way of scapegoating in order to deflect criticisms of their own practice. Western psychiatrists respond to the demands of the anti-psychiatry movement in the Soviet Union but ignore the accusations made by similar groups in the West.

The individuals concerned

In an article about charismatic religious sects Galanter (1982) writes: "When conversion is characterized by transcendental experiences and the acceptance of a highly deviant belief system, the phenomenology may even meet the DSM-III criteria of brief reactive psychosis ...". In the article he suggests that most of the members of contemporary charismatic religious cults and sects came from troubled families, mainly middle and upper-middle class backgrounds and that in over half there is evidence of long-term psychiatric disturbance [22]. There is little doubt that

---

19. One academic psychiatrist said that in his view some incompetent psychiatrists might not be able to distinguish between deviant thought and delusions. This could lead to a mistake but should be rectified by the commission.

20. In fact some critics do allege that abuse occurred in the late 1950s and others that it began under Stalin, implying the late 1940s or early 1950s.

21. Calculated on the basis that there are slightly fewer beds per head of population and that admissions are longer. See chapter 3.

22. Spencer (1975) reports a high rate of mental illness, especially of paranoid schizophrenia, amongst Jehovah's Witnesses.

if this article had appeared in a Soviet Journal, rather than the American Journal of Psychiatry, it would have been taken as further evidence of the abuse of psychiatry. It is quoted here to raise the issue of the overlap between mental illness and "dissent", political or religious.

One thing that has emerged from this controversy is that people continue to create false dichotomies. The extreme form of this is to hold the view that someone is either a dissident or a psychiatric patient and that there is no overlap between these categories as depicted in figure 4 [23].

Figure 4

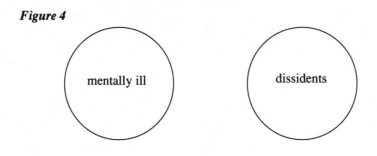

There is perhaps a tendency to fall into this trap if a person happens to be saying something that you agree with. This tendency to dichotomize has its roots in primitive concepts of mental illness, the idea that someone is either "sane" or "insane" and that in the separate world of insanity opinions and beliefs are somehow invalid. It can be argued that Jasper's view about the un-understandability of delusions has reinforced this view. More naturalistic concepts of delusions are perhaps less likely to lead to this kind of split.

Despite the opinions of some Western commentators there is nothing to suggest that Soviet psychiatrists hold the view that dissent indicates mental illness (as shown in figure 5).

Figure 5

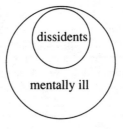

23. The dichotomy is most apparent in the field of forensic psychiatry, but is no more valid for that. West (1989) refers to Moran's suggestion that the attempt on Peel's life by Daniel M'Naghten might have been politically motivated in that M'Naghten was active in the Chartist Movement. At the same time West makes it quite clear that M'Naghten had paranoid delusions about Peel and the Tories.

I have read nothing in the psychiatric literature nor heard anything from Soviet psychiatrists that would indicate that there is a belief that dissidents must be mentally ill or that wanting to reform society is an indication of mental illness. The Soviet view is that the controversial dissenter-patients fall into the shaded area in the Venn diagram in figure 6. Thus, they are dissidents who also happened to have some form of mental illness.

Figure 6

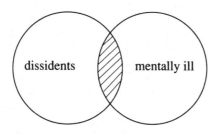

Some psychiatrists accept that there have been cases in which the issue was not clear-cut, giving the example of General Grigorenko. Thus, it is accepted that there is controversy about whether or not arteriosclerotic changes or a paranoid development of personality (see page 186) should be considered mental illness or grounds for non-responsibility. The difficulties in diagnosis are emphasized, also the changes over time and there is anger that Western psychiatrists judge someone to be "sane" or "insane" on the basis of an interview, often through an interpreter, perhaps some years after an episode of illness [24].

Those with experience of mental health tribunals in Britain will recognize that it may be difficult or impossible to elicit psychopathology from an actively paranoid patient when he is aware that his answers might be grounds for continued detention.

A second line of argument on this issue is that it makes no sense to use psychiatry for this purpose when the judicial system is well able to deal with people engaged in anti-Soviet activities. Soviet psychiatrists say that their critics must explain why a tiny proportion of the dissident population of nationalists, religious activists and refuseniks are singled out for psychiatric disposal. Available figures, even those given by the most severe critics, do suggest that only a tiny proportion of the various dissident groups are dealt with in this way. Thus, Bloch and Reddaway (1984) claim that there were 500-600 dissenter-patients over the period 1962-1984. They break these down into the following groups:

Civil rights actions 55%
Nationalist dissent 7%
Refuseniks 20%
Religious activity 13%

24. There have been several visits by Western psychiatrists (and others) bent on establishing the sanity of particular individuals. Wynn (1989), a retired Australian cardiologist who spoke no Russian, met a number of dissidents and wrote that he could "endorse the view that they are all sane."

These figures suggest that over the twenty year period there should have been 80 religious activists and 120 refuseniks amongst the dissenter-patients. The Soviet claim is that these figures represent the religious activists and refuseniks who were mentally ill, giving statistical evidence to indicate that this proportion is much lower than what one would expect from prevalence figures for mental illness in the general population.

It is not easy to get estimates of the numbers in the different dissident groups. In the 1960s and 1970s, according to Bloch and Reddaway (1984), there was a massive increase in various kinds of dissent, mainly nationalist and religious. This is given as the reason for psychiatry being used to contain the situation. However, it can also be argued that as the group of dissenters gets bigger the more people with some form of mental illness there will be within that group. Figures for active religious believers and nationalists vary from the tens of thousands to millions. It is somewhat easier to make an estimate of refusenik population through the number of emigration visas applied for and sent. There would be a measure of agreement for a figure of about 400,000 refuseniks past and present. Taking 1% as a conservative estimate of the point prevalence of serious psychiatric illness in a population would give a figure of 4,000 refuseniks with severe mental illness [25]. The Soviet argument is that Bloch and Reddaway's 120 dissenter-patient refuseniks are from this group of 4,000 mentally ill dissidents. The critical question is why should the 120 dissenter-patients be taken from the 396,000 healthy refuseniks rather than the 4000 that one would expect to be mentally ill. Even if this 4000 were accounted for separately, the question is why should just 120 people be dealt with in this controversial way and the other 396,000 ignored[26].

This argument, of course, rests on the assumption that various dissident groups are no different in terms of mental health from the rest of the population. There is certainly no evidence to suggest that dissident groups in any society have a lower prevalence of mental illness than other members of society and indeed it may be higher [27].

The critics
Soviet psychiatrists claim that their critics have made no attempt to understand Soviet psychiatry or to compare the different approaches in a rational way, based upon proper information. They maintain that the critics have taken a simplistic view that the Soviet political system is flawed and that Soviet psychiatry must also be flawed. The books by Bloch and Reddaway (1977 and 1984) are especially condemned as being no more than anti-Soviet propaganda. It is claimed that the main sources for the allegations come from anti-psychiatry dissident groups within

25. If 15% of the population meet the criteria for one or other of the DSM-III mental disorders this would yield a figure of 60,000!

26. One response to this argument is that it is the particularly troublesome individuals who are dealt with in this way. However, the evidence suggests that troublesome individuals are more likely to go through the prison system or be given exit visas.

27. Cohen (1989) quotes the dissident physicist Andrei Sakharov as saying that in his experience many dissidents were mentally unstable: "...the vast majority of people of this kind I have encountered were not mentally healthy. That's my personal experience which is unlikely to be representative of the global picture if only because mentally ill people are abnormally persistent, maniacal, so to say. An abnormally large number of such individuals sought contact with me and consequently there was a considerable proportion of mentally unhinged people round me."

the Soviet Union, also from right-wing emigre groups and "professional, careerist cold-war Sovietologists". They believe that a few extremists have duped some rather naive psychiatrists, and that others have taken up the cause for careerist motives or from anti-Soviet sentiments, based on strong religious or political beliefs. Those who refused to go along with the witch-hunt were discredited [28]. By contrast, there is no discussion of the political or religious motives of those active in the campaign against Soviet psychiatry.

Theoretical issues

One of the most widely quoted symptoms in reference to alleged abuse has been "delusions of reform". A widespread view is that the term can be applied to anyone who thinks that there is something wrong with Soviet society and has ideas or plans about improving matters. This relates to the question of form and content (discussed on page 35) and confusion between descriptive material and the criteria upon which diagnoses are made. It is not really justifiable to present incidental clinical material recorded in case records as if it were the criteria for making a diagnosis. Thus, Bloch and Reddaway (1977) show photographs of the alleged victims with captions such as: "...interned for handing our leaflets...interned for playing the guitar and singing his own songs....interned for applying to emigrate to Israel...". The argument can be illustrated with an extract from the American "Comprehensive Textbook of Psychiatry" (1985): "At their best, paranoid characters can assume a distant leadership role in movements for social reform....are often interested in mechanical devices, communication, electronics, and automation." Few psychiatrists would take these extracts to suggest that one might diagnose people who are "interested in mechanical devices" or those who "fight for justice" or "assume leadership roles in movements for social reform" as being paranoid.

There is still uncertainty about the distinction between diagnostic criteria and descriptive clinical features. This is sometimes due to ignorance, sometimes a deliberate attempt to obfuscate. Delusions of reform are delusions first and foremost, a point made by Gluzman (1989), and must therefore meet the criteria for delusional thinking which are strictly defined [29]. However, despite attempts to define strict criteria, problems are likely to remain for some time, both in the Soviet

28. There is some justification to this criticism. Bloch and Reddaway (1977) rather gratuitously describe Crome, someone who doubted the allegations, as a "British Communist". There is an attack on Sir Dennis Leigh, Secretary-general of WPA, for not joining in their campaign. He is described as "slippery, evasive, and condescending" and as an "empire builder". The setting up of the ethics committee by Dennis Leigh is described as "clearly a diversionary proposal." Bloch and Reddaway (1977 and 1984) talk about the betrayal of people like Bukovsky by the WPA. There are particular hate figures, for instance the unfortunate Daniel Lunts who is described as "small, morose and Jewish with an unhappy personal life." Babayan is referred to as "the wily Russian" (although, as his name suggests, he is Armenian). Vartanian is another key target and Wynn (1989) manages to bring in his wife, writing: "I imagine his wife has a collection of fur coats even a film star might envy." Vartanian's wife, Orlovskaya, is a distinguished neuropathologist and not noted for any sartorial elegance. Wynn (1989) also makes slightly odd insinuations about Sir Andrew Huxley, President of Royal Society. Bernard Lown, the Boston cardiologist who developed the defibrillator and went on to found International Physicians against Nuclear Weapons, is considered to be a communist stooge and is condemned for not replying to Wynn's letters.

29. Snezhnevsky (1983) emphasizes that mistaken beliefs are common in healthy people who are convinced of their authenticity. Although such mistaken conclusions are often held with stubborn conviction they cannot be considered as delusions. With a delusion it is not enough that the idea or belief does not correspond to reality, but there must be a pathological basis for the way it arose. The morbidity of a delusions comes from the general distortion of the relationships with people around them. Delusional opinions always refer to the patient and develop from ideas related to them. Delusions isolate people and are personal unshakeable convictions. By contrast over-valued ideas arise as the result of real circumstances which have achieved extreme significance for an individual and become emotionally loaded. For further discussion see pages 23 and 35.

Union and the West, about the boundary between delusional thinking, over-valued ideas and creative thinking. The fact that the content is often about political or religious issues suggests that there will be many controversies ahead.

Another clinical term at the centre of the controversy is "sluggish" or slow-flow schizophrenia. The controversy is partly fuelled by two common misapprehensions about this. The first is that it was a concept devised by Snezhnevsky and the Moscow school [30] and the second that patients with the disorder would be considered "normal" in the West. This is discussed in chapter 8. Kazanetz (1979 and 1989), who has been a consistent critic of the concept of slow-flow schizophrenia [31], makes no suggestion that the term is used for normal people. He writes (in the British Journal of Psychiatry): "There is no reason to subdivide verified cases of schizophrenia into rapidly developing and sluggish forms. According to the follow-up data, most cases of schizophrenia originally classified by the physicians as sluggish later proved to be manifestly typical cases of schizophrenia with prominent deterioration."

Official responses

In an interview in the Medical Gazette, Churkin, who was then the Chief Psychiatrist to the Ministry of Health, claimed that patients were being used as pawns in a political game and that they suffered as a result of this (MG 2.3.88). He gave examples where dissident patients had left the country and were soon in psychiatric treatment in the West. He claimed that he is regularly sent new lists of patients by the West which he investigated but that he had so far failed to find a single healthy person in hospital. He accepts that there have been cases where they found that out-patient treatment could have sufficed instead of hospitalization. Yegorov, a Ministry of Health official interviewed for British television by Cohen (1989b), admitted that there had been excess caution, with unnecessary admissions, in the past. On the same programme, Morozov, of the Serbsky Institute, said that most of the patients in the Serbsky had committed obvious crimes but admitted that there were still some "political" cases, although fewer than before. These were people with mental illness who incidentally held various dissident views. He maintained that a healthy person had never been admitted.

Kozirev, who was made chief psychiatrist at the Kashenko Hospital in 1987, is reported as saying that there is a "wall of misunderstanding" between journalists and psychiatrists" (Cornwell, 1989b). He accepts that there were mistakes and abuses in the past, but claims that these were never systematic. He asks why the authorities should pick out a tiny minority of dissidents for psychiatric disposal.

In April 1989 in Moscow there was a symposium on law and mental health, a joint meeting between the International Academy of Law and Mental Health and doctors from the Serbsky Institute (Lancet, 1989b). The purpose was mainly to review the 1988 changes in the law. Morozov, then director of the Serbsky, admitted that there had been unsatisfactory procedures for compulsory admission in the past and that some aspects of treatment were still unsatisfactory. The general

---

30. Bloch and Reddaway (1977) refer to the "sinister new illness of Soviet Psychiatry".

31. Kazanetz is referred to by Bloch and Reddaway (1984) as having incurred the wrath of the Soviet psychiatric establishment by challenging the Snezhnevsky concept of schizophrenia and publishing his controversial findings in an American journal (ie the 1979 article in Archives of General Psychiatry).

view was that the law had improved things, but that there was now excessive pressure on psychiatrists. Tikhonenko, the chief psychiatrist of Moscow, said that the number of admissions had fallen from 80,000 to 70,000 per year in Moscow.

According to Rich (1991a), Dmitrieva, the new head of the Serbsky Institute, criticized many aspects of Soviet psychiatry, in particular conditions and availability of drugs. She said that a narrow circle of psychiatrists, working with the KGB, had been involved in the treatment of dissidents. Rich (1991b) also reports that a Soviet Commission of psychiatrists have declared General Grigorenko to have been of sound mind.

Western responses

Aside from the frank critics of Soviet psychiatry there has been a wide range of Western opinion, from the more moderate [32] through to full support for what is perceived as the Soviet position [33]. There are also more exotic views, for instance those of Thomas Szasz who maintains that abuse is universal and an inevitable consequence of all psychiatry. Szasz, along with the Church of Scientology, who regularly quote him, regard the whole of the psychiatric establishment as part of a conspiracy aimed at social control and the curtailment of freedom of the individual with a view to promoting various aims such as taxation, collectivism, communism and world government. Western psychiatrists are condemned for being concerned only about the detention and treatment of patients in the Soviet Union, who, according to him, represent a tiny proportion of the victims of abuse in the Soviet Union and the West. Szasz (1988) responds to an article by Koryagin (1988) in the Lancet, condemning him for his "naive but unctuous professional chauvinism" in pleading for an end to psychiatric abuse for political reasons. He claims that one cannot distinguish between the so-called political abuse of psychiatry and any abuse. "Inasmuch as coercive psychiatric interventions necessarily rest on the (officially legitimate) use of state power, all such practices fall, by definition, into the domain of politics...". He reiterates his view that no involuntary intervention can be justified, saying that Koryagin "..adds his voice to the 300-year-old chorus complaining about the "wrong" people being locked up as insane - thus implicitly validating the legitimacy of psychiatric power and its inexorable consequences."

Wing (1974) refers to the different concepts of schizophrenia and differences in the systems of care. He argues that much of the debate is more about general social issues rather than psychiatry specifically. He suggests that there were about 20 people who might be detained on political grounds, with some having been in hospital before there was any question of dissent and others who held "complex theories" about various matters.

Wortis (1979), who had access to case records and interviewed several patients and psychiatrists, describes a patient who "had the delusion that the Soviet Union had fallen under the control of Jews who were persecuting him" and had "fantastic ideas of his own powers of leadership, described himself as head of an army...".

32. In a leader in the British Medical Journal, Wilkinson (1986) discusses the some of the issues and makes the point that the controversy about the issue is heightened because of the limited knowledge about Soviet psychiatry and calls for continuing international inquiry and collaborative research.

33. In a letter to the Times, Crome (1973) wrote that he had seen the Bukovsky case histories and that the material that was considered as evidence for abuse did not prove anything. Youssef (1973) wrote in similar vein to the Lancet. He also pointed out that there were political issues in the West with regard to issues such as unemployment and racism. Two eminent American psychiatrists, Wortis (1979) and Masserman (1986) raised serious doubts about the allegations.

Wortis reports that this patient was one of those listed by Bloch and Reddaway (1977) and had been mentioned as a case of psychiatric abuse in four different issues of the "Chronicle of Current Events". Wortis describes the Chronicle, the English version of which is edited and published by Reddaway, as a "clandestine, anonymous journal" and argues that this particular case casts doubt on the authenticity of the journal (which is the main source of information for most of the Bloch and Reddaway cases). He writes that he does not deny that there are cases of prejudice, cruelty, miscarriage of justice, misguided psychiatry and harsh conditions, pure error, but says that there must be more proof to support the idea that there is large-scale and systematic incarceration of dissidents.

Stone (1984), a forensic psychiatrist, gives a thoughtful account of the issues involved, particularly with regard to paranoia. He describes his psychiatric examination of General Grigorenko in 1978 when he was President-elect of the American Psychiatric Association. The Soviet view was that Grigorenko had cerebral arteriosclerosis and a paranoid development of personality. Stone reported that there was evidence for a cerebral atherosclerotic process (it was confirmed that he had had a stroke) but no evidence of paranoid ideation. He reproduces Snezhnevsky's letter in response to his findings - which stress the paranoid development of personality, the changing picture because of arteriosclerosis and, above all, of the difficulty of diagnosing paranoid symptoms, especially through interpreters.

Stone discusses the issues and draws a parallel between the case of Grigorenko, who considered himself to be a "pure Leninist", and that of an American General, Edwin Walker, whose extreme right-wing views and bizarre actions led the Kennedy administration to question his sanity and fitness to stand trial. Walker was eventually found competent to stand trial but the case was dismissed. Stone writes that paranoid ideation is particularly difficult to assess, and is often as much to do with acting on ideas as having them and as such touches closely upon religious and political ideas. He makes the point that Soviet psychiatrists were in disagreement about Grigorenko's mental state. He makes some suggestions as to the criteria for judging morbid paranoid ideation, suggesting that for legal purposes only "idiosyncratic paranoia with bizarre content" should count as mental illness.

Masserman (1986), a past president of the American Psychiatric Association, writes: "Conflicts arose when some professionals, particularly in Britain, repeatedly and publicly accused their Soviet colleagues of misusing psychiatry for the purpose of misdiagnosing, incarcerating and mistreating Soviet advocates of human rights and world peace as 'political dissidents'. Such condemnations in 1983 led to the indignant resignation of the Soviet All-Union Association of Neuropatholgists and Psychiatrists from the World Psychiatric Association. Although I too had been well aware that our speciality was occasionally misused for various purposes in many countries, including our own, it seemed unjust to condemn 30,000 Soviet psychiatrists for the alleged misconduct of a few". He continues: "While psychiatric theories and practices are no more uniform in the Soviet Union than they are in the US it has been my observation and that of others (including Ziferstein, Carson, Wortis, Kolb, Ponomaroff and others) that Soviet psychiatrists are as scientifically progressive, ethical, and humanitarian as we try to be in our country".

I interviewed several American psychiatrists who had visited or worked in the Soviet Union. One argued that the main factor was the difference between the two societies, especially as the collectivist system meant that Soviet psychiatrists were cautious about discharging patients because of fear of making mistakes, for instance with suicidal patients. Her own observations of a year working in Moscow had been that colleagues were professionally sound, if cautious, and that there was no evidence of abuse.

Emigre Soviet psychiatrists

I have interviewed nine Soviet psychiatrists who left the Soviet Union for various reasons [34]. Three believed that there had been systematic abuse, with two out of the three maintaining that the system and the diagnostic criteria allowed scope for abuse and that this had been regular practice in the past but had perhaps diminished recently. The third psychiatrist held firmly to the view that Soviet psychiatric hospitals are full of dissidents labelled as sluggish schizophrenia on the basis of having delusions of reform. This psychiatrist was unsure what the diagnostic criteria for delusions of reform were, but thought that they could be applied to anyone who disagreed with the system.

The other six psychiatrists that I spoke to considered that the political issues had been exaggerated. Two were scathing about the way in which some of their colleagues had taken up the issue. One maintained that he had not managed to get a job in Britain because he had not "co-operated" in the campaign. One described his own experience of "abuse". He said that one of his patients was a Soviet poet who was worried that the KGB were onto him because of his dissident views. He wanted to remain in hospital for a few months because he thought he was safe there and could also get a pension. Another psychiatrist, who held strong religious views and had left the Soviet Union because he felt it offended his human dignity, said that he personally had not come across any political abuse of psychiatry. He thought that the pressure on the Soviet Union was unjust in comparison to minimal response to the revelation of abuse in countries such as Japan. He argued that Japan should also have been dismissed from the WPA along with a number of Arab countries. A view expressed by two of the six was that the diagnostic criteria were reasonable, and applied fairly, but that once someone had received a diagnosis of schizophrenia then they were liable to have their dissident views or actions dealt with psychiatrically rather than through the judicial system. The common view was that there was excess caution with regard to admission and discharge, as compared to the West, and that this particularly applied at certain times, for instance certain public holidays or special occasions (eg the 1980 Olympics), when there was a desire to keep the mentally ill away from public places.

CHARGES AGAINST WESTERN PSYCHIATRY
This section is compiled from both Soviet and Western sources, the Western criticisms coming from within the established body of psychiatry and also from bodies that have an interest in psychiatry.

---

34. Several thousand Soviet doctors have left the country over the past few decades, amongst them hundreds of psychiatrists. Few of these have been involved in the campaign against alleged psychiatric abuse.

The main charges can be grouped in the following way:
1. Specific allegations of abuse.
2. The provision and availability of psychiatric care.
3. The influence of society.
4. Treatment.

Specific allegations of abuse

Beardshaw (1981) describes cases of abuse and neglect in British psychiatric hospitals. The charges included stealing from patients, poor standards of physical care, poor treatment, excess use of drugs and seclusion, assault, and patients' deaths caused by abuse [35]. Healy (1983) makes allegations about brutality and neglect in 16 different British hospitals. There are charges of physical and sexual assault, the use of high dosages of psychotropic drugs. The Bethlem Royal Hospital in London is criticized for its "barbaric" treatments including "tying children to chairs, locking them in padded cells...". The article alleged that staff who complained were isolated or moved on. There are allegations that violent beating of patients by staff is commonplace at Broadmoor and refers to the death a of 22 year-old patient after "a good kicking" (Hospital Doctor, 8.11.1984).

Some patients' groups in Britain complain of psychiatrists who do not listen to them, forcible treatment, abuse with drugs and ECT. There are broader criticisms that psychiatry is a powerful tool of society which is used to suppress dissent on occasions and that it is not just a question of there being bad psychiatrists, but that the whole practice of psychiatry needs reform (Multiple Image, Channel 4, 1986).

As previously mentioned, perhaps the most consistent source of criticism is from the most extreme of the anti-psychiatry groups, the Church of Scientology [36]. They hold numerous sworn affidavits from ex-patients with allegations of psychiatric abuse in the West and have published many books and pamphlets on the subject. Dalton (1973) lists reports of brutality, the use of drugs as punishment, the withholding of mail, unreasonable restrictions on visiting, bad food and conditions, for instance extreme cold or damp, false confinement, denial of religious practices, inadequate treatment and poor physical care. Garrison (1974) refers to psychiatrists as odd-ball, power-mad perverts. The Citizens Commission on Human Rights, a mental health reform group sponsored by the Church of Scientology, has had some success in placing articles in various medical and lay

---

35. The issue of physical abuse of patients is generally linked with institutional psychiatry. However, there is nothing to suggest that it is more prevalent in such settings than in private homes, group homes or hostels in the community.

36. In 1950 Ron Hubbard, a writer of science fiction, introduced a new school of psychotherapy with the publication of his book "Dianetics: the Modern Science of Mental Health". Like many new schools of psychotherapy there was little original apart from the terminology. Thus, the engram, the hidden conflict, has to be sorted out by a process of auditing, essentially a form of cathartic psychotherapy. In 1953 Hubbard founded the "Church of Scientology" and the movement adopted some religious views including a belief in reincarnation and, common to many such groups, Manichaean concepts of good and evil. The main enemies were psychiatry and communism, which were seen to be working hand in hand to destroy individualism. The movement maintains that there is no such thing as mental illness and has consistently attacked all forms of psychiatric care, including admission to hospital and physical treatment, most particularly psychosurgery and ECT. The movement claimed that because of their assault on psychiatry they were being persecuted by the American establishment, especially the medical and legal arms. The movement was banned in various countries including Britain, Australia and South Africa. In 1968 Ron Hubbard was declared an undesirable alien in Britain and denied entry by the British Government. Other scientologists were also prevented from entering the country. In 1969 scientologists were forced out of the National Association of Mental Health, the forerunner of MIND, because of a feared "take-over" (Dalton, 1973). In Britain the ban on Scientology was not lifted until 1980.

journals [37]. Scientology has a wider brief than detailing individual cases of abuse. Employing the slogan "Psychiatry Kills" it challenges the view that psychiatry is beneficial to people, claiming that millions have been harmed by its practice. It is also seen as part of a global conspiracy whose purpose is social control and world government.

There are scattered reports in the literature of the psychiatric disposal of awkward people. Baxter (1983) refers to allegations that in the USA student protesters were detained in psychiatric hospitals for their rebellious attitudes. Erlichman (1988) reports on the work of the American psychologist, Don Soeken, on whistleblowers, American civil servants who uncovered fraud. He writes that out of 233 whistleblowers 90% lost their jobs and 26% faced psychiatric and medical referral. Many of these were allegedly admitted to psychiatric assessment units by senior officials who had something to hide. There are also the so-called "White House Cases", described by Shore et al (1985) [38].

"Mind control"

It is ironic that one of the most alarming allegations directed against Western psychiatry concerns the first president of the World Psychiatric Association, Dr Ewen Cameron, also a past president of the Canadian and American Psychiatric Associations. According to the British Medical Journal (1988) it is well established that CIA, through a front organization, the Centre for the Investigation of Human Ecology, funded his research into "re-patterning" because of their interest in behaviour modification and "brain-washing" [39]. The idea of "re-patterning" was to delete maladaptive memories and replace them with helpful new memories. This was done by a programme of prolonged narcosis followed by massive courses of ECT (New Scientist 2.2.84; British Medical Journal, 1988).

The provision and availability of psychiatric care

Perhaps the most familiar charge made against American psychiatry is that it is geared towards those who can pay and denies adequate psychiatric care to certain sections of the population, essentially to those with serious, chronic mental illnesses [40]. The result is a high proportion of mentally ill amongst the homeless and the prison population.

In most industrialized Western countries some form of psychiatric care, essentially asylum placement, has been available free of charge for well over a

---

37. An example is an article with the memorable title: "ECT - why the sparks are flying". There seems to be a thin but distinct thread of humour running through much of the Scientology literature, although it is not clear whether this is deliberately intended.

38. These are discussed in footnote 2 on page 220.

39. According to the Lancet (1988b) the CIA were concerned about American servicemen taken prisoner in Korea who were persuaded to denounce their own country. The CIA set up the foundation to provide cover for research into "brain-washing". Ewen Cameron, an American citizen working in Canada was "an obvious port of call." For 6 years he reported to the CIA on the effects of multiple electroshock, drugs (including LSD) and continuous exposure to tape-recorded voices - "psychic driving". Cameron is described as a "chilly, sinister figure who studied the effects of cruel regimens in a basement out-of-bounds to colleagues, with the aid of two non-medical henchmen paid for indirectly by the CIA...experiments conducted in Canada because they would have been illegal in USA." The article clearly does not attempt to be objective as the language suggests ("chilly and sinister" is "shy and reserved" to his friends). Cameron's colleagues dismiss the allegations, and maintain that Cameron was not aware of the source of his funding. They maintain that the research was clinically oriented, as evidenced by the fact that it was all published.

40. Dorway and Schlesinger (1988) report on the increase in private "for-profit", that is non-charitable, hospitals over the past few decades. The proportion of private sector beds has increased from 10% in 1970 to 35% in 1986. More significantly the corporate "for-profit" sector has increased from 1% in 1970 to 15% in 1986.

century. It is still the case that even in the American system, dominated as it is by the private sector, there is a back-up system of state and county hospitals to provide for the socially disruptive mentally ill. In general, however, this provides a minimal level of treatment, essentially shelter and drug treatment during acute episodes of illness or long-term asylum for those unable to care for themselves.

The American system of financing medical care is through insurance and there are two programmes to cover those who cannot afford this. Medicare covers everyone aged over 65 and those registered as disabled. Medicaid is for the unemployed and those on very low incomes [41]. Medicare and Medicaid offer only limited cover, as do the cheaper insurance policies. They do not cover long-term psychiatric care. With Medicare, various "co-payments and deductibles" mean that only 45% of the health care needs of older people are met and those without private means are unable to afford any long-term psychiatric care (Roemer, 1987). Medicaid provides a limited range of care. Many psychiatrists and hospitals will not deal with Medicaid patients because of low payment levels. There are particular problems for those in low-paid employment who are not entitled to the state insurance programmes and are unable to afford insurance (or can only manage to pay the premiums on cheap and inadequate policies, covering, for instance, a few basic disorders such as appendicitis and trauma, certainly not psychiatric care). The result is that 15% of the population, 37 million people, have no insurance of any kind and are not on Medicare or Medicaid (Roemer, 1987) [42]. For many people in this section of the population the only psychiatry available to them would be the State Hospital.

There are also problems with the next rung up the ladder. Roemer (1987) makes the point that even with insurance there are problems for any kind of long-term care, especially on an out-patient basis. Many firms offer insurance cover as part of the terms of employment and the employee pays only a small proportion of the premium. However, there is a limit on the amount of psychiatric care provided, for instance 20 out-patient visits and 90 days in hospital. After that patients have to move on to the State facilities. It is not uncommon for patients to be in private hospitals until the insurance runs out and then transfer to a City or State hospital. This does, of course, have implications for the doctor-patient relationship which is generally held up as one of the successes of the American system. The reality, as one psychiatrist succinctly put it, is that the doctor-patient relationships lasts "just until the bucks run out". There are reports in the literature of patients being unwilling to go for treatment because of costs. A chronic mental illness such as dementia in one partner not infrequently means that the other partner has to sell the family home in order to pay for institutional care, leaving them homeless (New

41. There are 20 million people on Medicaid. The level at which Medicaid applies is well below the poverty linec (Lancet 1988c).

42. Silver (1989) writes that a similar number have only partial insurance or are insured for only part of the year. According to the New England Journal of Medicine (1988) there are about 65 million Americans, 30% of the population under 65, who have inadequate protection for serious illnesses or illnesses that would result in prolonged treatment. According to the Annals of Internal Medicine (1988) two thirds of people who are aged over 65 and living alone would become impoverished after 3 months in nursing home. "Medigap" policies which should fill in gaps for Medicare do not cover chronic illnesses and most private policies have cover limits of one year or $100,000.

43. The police are reluctant to deal with psychiatric cases, especially since a number of well-publicized cases in which there were unfortunate results due to police intervention. The most notorious case was that of Eleonor Bumpers. In New York in 1988 the police were called to deal with a psychotic woman, Eleonor Bumpers, who was resisting eviction and behaving in an apparently dangerous way. She was shot and killed by the police after she made to attack one of them.

A specific Soviet criticism of the Western system is the lack of a proper ambulance service, resulting in excess police involvement in the admissions of psychotic patients. This is perhaps more applicable to the USA [43] than most European countries.

The lack of an adequate forensic psychiatry service for sections of the population in the USA has been discussed in the previous chapter. The charge is that psychiatry ignores the genuinely needy, but comes to the aid of offenders who can afford good defence lawyers and psychiatrists [44]. This discrepancy is probably less marked in Europe.

A broader issue concerns the lack of facilities and the consequences for the chronic mentally ill. At the International Forum on Mental Health Law Reform organized jointly by the Japanese Society for Psychiatry and Neurology and the International Academy of Psychiatry and Law (in Kyoto in January 1987) there were severe criticisms by two American psychiatrists of what they called the "myth turned into nightmare", the dogma of community mental health care. They argued that deinstitutionalization had led to a big fall in the number of hospital inpatients in USA since 1955 and other countries with a big saving of public funds. The result was that the chronic mentally ill had gone into doss-houses and prisons or become homeless and vagrant. In Britain since 1954, 75,000 patients have been discharged from the psychiatric hospitals, but the local authorities, despite their statutory obligation, have only accommodated 4000 of these (Weller, 1988). In many places there has been no provision of any kind.

The result has been that many ex-patients have found their way into the prison system. Weller (1988) demonstrates an inverse relationship between the population in psychiatric hospitals and that the prison population, and argues that the increase in prison population is partly accounted for by more psychiatric patients are being sentenced, mainly because there is nowhere else for them to go [45]. This issue is particularly acute in Britain, which has one of the highest prison populations per capita in the world. It is estimated that 30% of prison population have some form of psychiatric illness and for female prisoners the proportion may be as high as 50%. Coid (1988) reports that most prisoners on remand with obvious psychiatric illnesses are rejected for treatment by the National Health Service. Those with chronic psychoses, organic brain damage or mental handicap are most likely to be turned away [46].

This issue might be less serious if there was evidence that prison could provide a reasonable standard of care for this group of offenders. However, conditions are often appalling with no treatment on offer apart from large doses of neuroleptic drugs, and in many prisons the regime includes isolation for 23 hours per day. There are allegations that prisoners are heavily sedated with neuroleptics in order

---

44. A cynical view might be that this is similar to the charges of corruption against certain Moscow psychiatrists who accepted bribes from criminals to produce false diagnoses.
45. Weller (1988) points out that in Britain 38 psychiatric hospitals are being closed and 26 new prisons opened, the first on the site of a closing psychiatric hospital.
46. This is partly related to diagnostic practice, in that schizophrenic defect states are often diagnosed as personality disorder. More critically, the shift to "community care" has meant that premises and staff to deal with this group are no longer available. In Britain spending on the prison service has increased, and, relatively, that on the health service decreased. To make any real impact on the policies of admitting mentally ill offenders there would have to be a considerable shift of resources.

to maintain order (Lancet 1988d, 1988e).

David (1988) discusses homelessness in the USA which is most serious in big cities like New York and Los Angeles. There are estimates of homelessness in USA varying from 300,000 to 3 million, the latter figure coming from the welfare organisations. 20-80% of homeless have some form of psychiatric disorder, mainly schizophrenia [47]. Bassuk (1984) examined a sample of the homeless who were living in the large urban "shelters" and reported that 91% had some form of psychological difficulty and 40% a major mental illness, mostly schizophrenia. He claims that the shelters are now "open asylums" where no treatment is provided. A study of the homeless in Britain found that one third were actively psychotic and a higher proportion had been treated for a psychotic illness in the past. A quarter had a severe physical illness, for instance tuberculosis, but the majority had no contact with the medical services [48]. The report states that in 1981 there were 14,000 direct access hostel beds in London but that in 1987 this had dropped to 3650.

Housing for the mentally ill is one of the areas where marked differences emerge between the two systems, although this has to seen in the context of the general housing situation. There is some irony in the fact that mental illness may actually improve housing prospects in the Soviet Union. Kosenko (1989) reports on the housing conditions of 10,000 patients in the Krasnodar region, comparing these before and after the illness. There was no overall change for patients with schizophrenia (64.4% had their own house, 32.9% a state flat, 2.6% a hostel, with 2.4% having a reduction in living space and 0.7% being homeless at the time of survey). In the other nosological groups, including epilepsy, trauma and manic-depression, housing conditions had improved as a result of the illness.

The influence of society
There is reasonable evidence to suggest that the conditions under which people live and work have an impact upon mental health. Thus, one might expect that the nature of society would influence the incidence and prevalence of psychiatric disorders. Mental illness, however, is common in all societies and the prevalence of major psychiatric disorders appears to be similar across different cultures and in different countries. Although some Soviet psychiatrists maintain that the neurotic disorders are more common in the capitalist West, there is no good epidemiological evidence to support this view. The similar rates of mental illness might suggest that the macrosocial environments share more similarities than differences, certainly with regards to their impact upon individuals. However, it may also be that it takes several generations before a change in the macrosocial environment has a fundamental impact upon the microsocial environment.

Unemployment
Several Soviet authors claim that the mental health problems in the West are in part due to the effects of unemployment. This has been debated extensively in the West, with, as yet, no clear-cut answers. There is an association between

---

47. According to the Annals of Internal Medicine (1986), there are 3 million homeless Americans, and of these 20% are "skid row alcoholics" with a high proportion of the rest being unemployed young people with psychiatric disorders.
48. Turner (1988) describes patients attending a community care (depot) clinic who were in a state of near starvation.

unemployment and psychological morbidity, strongest in middle-aged men with long duration since job loss (Jackson and Warr, 1984). However, this can not be considered as a simple causal relationship, although Melville et al (1985) showed that the rates of depression were significantly higher in men who became unemployed after involuntary redundancy, which, they argue, is less influenced by pre-exisiting morbidity. Platt and Kreitman (1985) demonstrate a strong positive association between unemployment and parasuicide, with the greatest risk being in the long-term unemployment. Smith (1985) reviews the issue in a series of articles, also discussing the relationship between suicide, parasuicide and unemployment. His general conclusion is that the mentally ill are most vulnerable to the effects of unemployment, but that this in turn becomes an aggravating factor and therefore of aetiological significance.

Individualism
The Soviet criticism of capitalist society (as distinct from the market economy) is that the emphasis on the rights of the individual is at the expense of the weaker members of society who are often over-looked and ignored. It is argued that the collective nature of Soviet Society ensures that people are not over-looked. Davidow (1976) contrasts the fate of troubled children in the Soviet Union with that in the USA. He quotes Gorman of the Executive Committee Against Mental Illness (at that time) as saying that many such children "are quite literally lost, bounced around from training school to reformatories, to jails, and whipped through all kinds of understaffed agencies until they vanish" [49].

The Soviet view is that this is partly due to a poor system of public welfare, but also due to the cult of individualism. The emphasis on individuals' rights means that the state is not empowered to intervene early enough. It is claimed that this does not happen in a collectivist society like the Soviet Union which implements its concern for its individual members through the public systems of welfare and health. More recently it has been acknowledged that there are severe social problems in the Soviet Union, but it is claimed that they are not on the scale of those in the USA and that the risk of children suffering at the hands of society is considerably less.

The issue of social control
Another traditional Soviet criticism of Western psychiatry has been that psychiatry is used to deal with disorders which are essentially due to social and economic conditions. Babayan (1985) writes that "..in a number of countries stubborn attempts are being made to blend psychiatry with politics, to use it as a means of pressuring people, of modifying their personalities". The relationship between psychiatric morbidity and social class, poverty and unemployment is cited in this context, and psychiatry is accused of papering over the cracks by treating the casualties of the system rather than tackling the basic social ills. Such arguments are less used now, partly because of the higher profile given to social problems within the Soviet Union.

---

49. An editorial in the New York Times (8.10.1982) reported that 150,000 children go missing every year in the USA and of these 50,000 vanish altogether. It is presumed that many end up being exploited. There are 10,000 child prostitutes in New York alone.

Criticisms of psychiatry as a means of dealing with social ills continue to be heard in the West. Cohen (1988) criticizes Assertive Case Management in which teams of mental health workers go out in search of the mentally ill. This developed out of Mayor Koch's 1987 clean-up campaign, an arm of which was the compulsory admission of the homeless mentally ill on the streets of New York (Thornicroft, 1988). The New York Civil Liberties Union fought the case of Billie Boggs, the name used by middle-aged black woman, Joyce Brown, a "bag-lady" who had been living on the streets for about a year. She was one of first people to be admitted to hospital in the campaign. The Civil Liberties Union successfully campaigned for her released, having apparently proved that she was not mentally ill. Subsequently, however, she was once again on the streets, begging and shouting at passers-by, and, according to psychiatrists, clearly hallucinating (USA today of 10.3.1988).

Several American psychiatrists have been critical of the way in which the Emergency Room (ER) is used, maintaining that it is often used inappropriately because there are no other facilities. They complain that the police use the ER to bring in disruptive people on the 9.39 section without adequate psychiatric grounds. Psychiatrists are pressured into admitting them, mainly because they fear media pressure and litigation. A patient may be detained and treated in an ER for up to a week without any need of a section or court order. Because of time pressure, lack of proper assessment, this may lead to unjustified detention.

I will describe three cases which I observed over the course of a Friday night in a busy New York ER.

A Hispanic boy of 15 was brought into the ER with a diagnosis of cocaine abuse. Several months earlier he had signed himself voluntarily into a private hospital to deal with the problem. He had been in the hospital for four months and described a tough behavioural regime with an overlay of psychoanalytically oriented groups and individual psychotherapy, along with some thioridazine. He decided that he wanted to leave and gave his "3 day notice". He was told, however, that he would be put on a PC2 and so withdrew the notice. He then behaved well, got a leave pass and, once out, refused to go back. Because he was frightening his mother, pushing her around, she got a note from the family doctor requesting help from the police to return him to hospital. He was brought in by eight police. There was an emotional and angry scene with the mother as he pleaded with her not to have him sent back to the hospital. He was eventually taken to the hospital in a strait-jacket.

A white drug abuser with a known history of violence was brought in and had to be strapped to the trolley because he was threatening violence. The psychiatrist responded to pressure from the staff to get rid of him and arranged admission to the forensic unit of a psychiatric hospital. She admitted that there was no evidence of mental illness as such, although she said that even if he wasn't psychotic he was so "oppositional" that admission was appropriate.

The third case was that of a 13 year-old black child who was remanded to hospital by the courts because his mother was unable to cope with him at home. A psychologist had recommended that he be admitted to psychiatric hospital for evaluation of his mental state on the basis of auditory hallucinations: the devil telling him to harm his mother and sister. In the ER he was written up for haloperidol which was a routine procedure in case he was difficult over the weekend as he would not be seen again by a doctor until the following Monday morning. The psychiatrists on duty were surprised that he'd been admitted by a psychologist, but said that there was nothing they could do because it was a court remand. They thought that he would be an in-patient for a minimum of one month and that he'd probably go on to the State Hospital. I saw him a few hours later in the men's locked ward which had about forty disturbed or demented men of all ages. He was now in blue pyjamas, standing by the television next to a man who was showing him how to do some kung-fu type moves. He came up to the ward psychiatrist and asked how long he was going to be there. He said that on one occasion he had heard a voice inside his head telling him to steal from his mother. He denied other abnormal experiences, but admitted that he often got into a rage at his mother and at his sister for "telling on him".

Psychiatric intervention was probably necessary in this last case, although it is unlikely that he would have been admitted to hospital in most European countries. If admission were required it would be to a children's unit. This also applies to the Soviet Union. In this case the boy was admitted to a locked, adult ward because his mother could not pay for private treatment and because there were no other facilities in the public sector.

The issue of social control is particularly relevant to certain sections of the population, the ethnic minorities. There is evidence that black patients in Britain and the USA are more likely to be admitted and treated against their will and that the police are more likely to be involved in the admissions (Lipsedge, 1985; Edeh, 1987). Littlewood and Lipsedge (1988) write that West Indians in Britain are rarely offered psychotherapy and are treated with higher doses of medication in comparison to whites with equivalent conditions. There are more blacks in secure units and special hospitals.

General issues
Psychiatry and psychology are often seen as challenging certain views about the nature of man, especially concerning the issue of free will. In this context psychiatry may be perceived as a threat to individual liberty, and, consequently, is a target for the champions of individualism. Soviet psychiatry, based on a materialist philosophy of mind and set in a collectivist society, is the obvious paradigm for this. This is perhaps one of the hidden agendas in the debate on Soviet and Western psychiatry.

Within any society there is a tension arising out of the conflict between individual freedom and the broader interests of society. Structures and organizations within society are caught up in this conflict and some structures, including various public health agencies and inspectorates, are perceived as representing the interests of society above those of the individual. Psychiatry is generally perceived as representing the collective interest over that of the individual. Such structures will be opposed by individuals or groups who consider that the freedom of the individual is paramount and are repelled by any degree of social control or collectivism. In the West this opposition has come from the libertarian left and radical right, successors to the traditional opponents of collectivism, the anarchists and laissez-faire liberals. One can assume that a person's position on this issue would influence their views about the role of psychiatry, psychiatrists' responsibilities, record keeping, computerized or otherwise, the follow-up and tracing of patients, and family interventions. This chapter has perhaps shown that the differences between the Soviet and Western psychiatric systems with regards to the balance between the rights of the individual and those of society are not as profound as one might have expected. This is partly because the influence of the radical right on Western government has been more limited than is commonly supposed. There have been shifts in economic policy, but many their fundamental tenets have been left out in the cold. These include opposition to any form of censorship (with extremist elements championing the right to child pornography etc), opposition to laws which aim to control individual behaviour (including drink-driving laws and bans on narcotics) and resistance to any form of surveillance or record-keeping.

There are different kinds of pressure from society to protect its interests at the expense of particular individuals. There is public opinion, sometimes represented by the media, and there is the threat of litigation by potential victims of the individual. In the USA this results in caution in discharging patients, essentially a restriction of individual freedom. One obvious result is the fact that most admission wards in American hospitals are locked. In Britain psychiatrists are perhaps somewhat freer to implement policies which allow greater freedom for patients. Admission and discharge policies are more liberal than those in the Soviet Union or the USA. These policies, however, can only be implemented in a society which does not extract too high a price, either in terms of adverse publicity, litigation or bureaucratic censure, for possible adverse consequences. It is paradoxical that in USA, with its individualistic and anti-collectivist political philosophy, the balance has tilted away from the individual and towards the interests of society in that it is the very system of free enterprise (and individual resource to the law) which leads to restrictive practices, essentially the denial of individual freedom, towards certain patients.

There are pressures on psychiatrists which are common to all systems. Psychiatrists are expected to do something when people perceived as mentally ill behave in a socially disruptive manner. Most psychiatrists will have had experience of doctors, policemen, neighbours and relatives vehemently expressing their views that a particular patient should be admitted to hospital or should never have been allowed to "escape". There may also be pressure for patients to be maintained on drugs even when this is considered clinically inappropriate. In my experience the pressure that Soviet psychiatrists face in this respect is similar to that faced by Western psychiatrists. The fond myth that Western doctors are somehow bound in a duty to their patients is no more true than the myth that Soviet doctors are only concerned in serving the interests of the state. One obvious difference, of course, is how the balance is arrived at. In the Soviet Union it is usually determined downwards, via official policy. In the USA it seems to be determined upwards through litigation and public opinion. The law recognizes the needs of society in the sense that society is made up of many individuals who invoke the law for their protection. It may be that this system will lead to greater restrictions for the individual than a centrally planned system which might be more prepared to take risks on behalf of particular individuals.

Treatment
Some general criticisms of treatment are also discussed in chapters 3 and 6.

Do economic factors influence treatment?

The charge here is that economic rather than clinical factors influence American psychiatrists in their choice of treatment to the detriment of patients. An article in the American Journal of Psychiatry (Markowitz et al, 1987) describes the care of 74 patients with manic-depressive psychosis. They report that those given ECT immediately, rather than after a trial of antidepressants, had an average admission of 13 days less than those receiving drugs. This led to a saving of $6400 dollars per patient. The question, of course, is whether this is justified on clinical grounds when drugs would have been effective in the majority of the patients. Psychiatrists are being put under pressure to make decisions about treatment on purely economic grounds. Patients, and, more significantly, relatives, will of course be offered the choice. This is an important consideration with a treatment such as ECT which is still controversial in the eyes of many people (as indicated by the "political" restrictions on its use in some mainland European countries, for instance Holland, Switzerland and Germany, as well as in certain states in the USA).

A more alarming trend is the use of ECT in mania because it works faster (Small, 1988). This could lead to accusations that ECT is being used as a measure of control, dealing with disruptive or aggressive behaviour, either on economic grounds or because of limited resources (a difficult to manage patient requires high staff input). Thus, although the treatment is apparently justified on the basis of the diagnosis, in reality it is being used because of other factors, essentially how much of a perceived threat the patient represents and whether or not they can be contained. Often this simply comes down to the size of a patient, but it is also related to social, cultural and, possibly, racial factors. More traditional Soviet psychiatrists like Babayan (1985) are particularly concerned about the use of ECT which he refers to as a "traumatic method of treatment", claiming that in the USA it is used too widely, sometimes as a repressive measure.

The financial aspects of treatment have become an important issue in the USA. Psychiatric journals and even textbooks now carry numerous articles about payments, billing, claims, filling in forms. Langsley (1985) describes the "Professional Standards Review Organization" (PSRO) procedure which arose out of the 1972 legislation aimed at controlling expenditure on health. Peer review, the review of treatment methods by fellow professionals, has a key role and is generally carried out by a medical committee, assisted by a nurse reviewer. The trend is to move towards a standard period of admission for particular conditions..."using standards or criteria that have been established in advance according to diagnosis" with longer admissions having to be agreed locally by the medical committee. He describes the PSRO as applied to psychiatry, giving the example of a 34-year-old woman admitted to a community hospital with depression. Within a day of admission the case is reviewed by the Peer Review Nurse Coordinator. She finds that the hospital's Peer Review Committee has agreed a median stay of 18 days for this condition and so hospitalization is agreed for 18 days. There is no improvement after 10 days on imipramine and so the patient is changed to another antidepressant. By day 17 there is still no improvement and it is decided to use ECT if there is no improvement by day 24. A 12 day extension for a course of ECT is requested and approved. A further extension for recovery time requires a phone call to the chairman of the committee, but in this case the full time is not allowed. It is claimed that the system does work, both allowing time for treatment and saving money. It is also being introduced to office-based psychiatry, with periods of treatment being agreed in advance according to the DSM-III diagnosis.

It is clear that financial considerations are becoming important in determining the kind of treatment that patients receive. Insurance cover is time limited (for instance allowing 30 days in hospital), after which patients or relatives have to pay the treatment bills. Inevitably, therefore, there will be pressure on psychiatrists for quick results and those psychiatrists and hospitals that deliver the economic goods will stay in business. Physical treatments will be favoured over psychological (for those without adequate insurance or funds). At worst, patients with depression who are unwilling to have ECT will have the prospect of this hanging over them unless they "get better" within a month or so.

Soviet psychiatrists accept the importance of peer review and medical audit. What is considered a dangerous trend in the West is the way it is being related to economic rather than clinical issues, the pressure to treat patients by the quickest rather than the most appropriate methods. Ironically, perhaps, another criticism is that it will limit individual differences in practice and create excessive conformity.

The pharmaceutical industry

Collier (1989) criticizes the pharmaceutical industry for the way in which copy-cat or "me-too" drugs proliferate in search of bigger profits. He writes that doctors are under intense pressure to prescribe new drugs, not always tried, and not always in the patients' best interests. There is pressure from advertising and from various forms of indirect bribery such as post-marketing surveillance. There are reports of various forms of bribery to get leading psychiatrists to promote certain products.

The pharmaceutical industry claims that it has proved itself by giving the world a wide range of effective, safe drugs. The claim is justified in many respects, although it cannot be proved that this is because of the way the system operates. That said, however, the Soviet pharmaceutical industry has produced a much smaller range of drugs, virtually none of which are in use in the West. The Soviet response is that essential drugs rather than me-too drugs are produced and that there is also greater caution with regard to safety standards [50].

Psychotherapy

A general criticism of Soviet psychiatry has been the lack of psychotherapy. The Soviet response is that psychotherapy is widely used in all patients in the Soviet Union (although not psychoanalytic psychotherapy) and that psychotherapy is only available to a few patients in the West, essentially those in the private sector. Therefore a large section of the population are not receiving adequate overall treatment in that they are offered only hospitalization and/or physical treatments. It is true that patients in the public sector are unlikely to receive psychotherapy, but it is more widely available than might be expected in that the better insurance policies cover a limited amount of psychoanalytic psychotherapy. Chodoff (1987) discusses the concern about the future of psychotherapy. He notes that Blue Cross and Blue Shield, the main two medical insurance companies, used to pay 80% of

50. Thalidomide, for instance, failed the testing procedure and was not used in the Soviet Union.

psychotherapy fees up to a maximum of $50,000 for an individual. This has now dropped to 70% of the fees and allows a maximum of 50 visits per year. The result is a drop in the number of clients. Full psychoanalytic treatment is really only an option for the relatively well off and the seriously rich [51].

Psychiatry for profit and its impact on the doctor's allegiance
Consumer led demand in the USA has led to a growth in the number of profit-making psychiatric hospitals which specialize in dealing with difficult adolescents. Admissions of adolescents to profit-making mental hospitals rose from 6,452 in 1970 to 43,000 in 1986 (Newsweek, 28.8.89). A programme entitled "The Child Fixers" (BBC 15.3.1985) looked at the American profit-oriented hospitals for difficult adolescents, often children doing badly at school or being openly rebellious. The programme described the aggressive marketing and the advertising campaigns. It was directed mainly towards white adolescents (blacks were more likely to go to detention centres), but also some children as young as five years old. The basic treatment was a strict regime of behaviour therapy, with routine use of intramuscular drugs and patients being strapped to their beds for up to twelve hours at a time. The patients were technically voluntary because they were admitted by their parents, paying up to 400 dollars a day, but they were kept as in-patients, against their will, for periods of up to two years.

This issue raises an important question about the relationship between diagnosis and commerce. DSM-III has been criticized on a number of counts, one of which is that it is geared towards the market place, providing categories that facilitate the business of psychiatry. Perhaps the most notorious in this respect is "Oppositional Disorder". The criteria for this are that there should have been a period of at least six months of disobedient, negativistic, and provocative opposition to authority figures, as manifested by at least two of the following:

    i   violations of minor rules
    ii   temper tantrums
    iii argumentativeness
    iv   provocative behaviour
    v   stubbornness

This set of criteria could cover almost any difficult adolescent (and many older people) and can be used to justify compulsory detention and treatment [52]. Similar accusations might be made about the "Adjustment disorders", "Impulse Control disorders" and some of the personality disorder categories.

The impact of market forces upon medical ethics and the psychiatrist's allegiance is a related issue. Market forces clearly respond to the interests of those

---

51. Thus, LeBeau (1988), writing in the American Journal of Psychotherapy, describes the "silver-spoon" syndrome, a disorder of the extremely rich. She talks about narcissism, high regard for public self, low regard for private self and disturbed family patterns of relationships. To work free of the silver-spoon syndrome families should use their prosperity in healthier ways. An article entitled "Children of the Rich" by F.S. Pittman The Third (1985) covers similar ground. An article on the psychoanalytic consequences of bankruptcy (Ginsburg and Ginsburg, 1983) perhaps balances the picture.

52. A full-page advert in the American Journal of Psychiatry for St Francis (episcopal) Homes shows a picture of a smiling mother sitting at her desk writing a letter which reads: "Thank you, doctor, for helping us give Tommy the care he needed. Thanks to you and St. Francis, Tommy is a changed young man. After just a year in their therapy program and under their full-time supervision, Tommy is no longer the hostile and rebellious teenager we saw hanging around with the wrong crowd and getting deeper and deeper into trouble. Thanks to you, we found a way to help a boy who didn't want to be helped." Outside the window we see a boy, presumably Tommy, pushing a lawn-mower.

paying the bills, but in psychiatry, more than in other disciplines, this is usually not the patient himself. Is the doctor's duty to the patient or to the person who pays the bill? The more the doctor is involved in the market the sharper the issue becomes, and it is a problem not dissimilar to those concerning doctors' allegiance to the state or the individual. [53] As the world spins faster and faster to the tune of market forces perhaps the greatest danger lies in the abuse of psychiatry for profit.

---

53. This issue has come sharply into focus in Japan where psychiatry is dominated by the private sector. The potential for abuse is compounded by poor mental health legislation which allows a single family member and one doctor, often the owner of the psychiatric hospital, to admit someone to hospital for an indefinite period of time (Cohen, 1988). 87% of the psychiatric beds in Japan are private and 75% of all psychiatric admissions are involuntary, the highest rate in the world (Lancet, 1986b). The average stay for compulsorily detained patients is over 8 years. Cohen (1988) gives an even more graphic account, writing about "horrific" conditions and systematic violence. He reports that there were many scandals in the 1970s and gives example of three hospitals owned by the Juzenkai corporation where 859 out of 2100 patients died over a period of nine months. There was no improvement in the 1980s. He condemns the World Psychiatric Association for its lack of action. Harding (1987) writes: "Those who advocate competition, free enterprise and profit incentives in health care would indeed do well to take a long, hard look at Japan's private psychiatric hospitals and their 300,000 involuntary patients".

REFERENCES

(note: Kors refers to the Korsakoff Journal of Neurology and Psychiatry)

Abrahamson D. (1988) Bulletin of the Royal College of Psychiatrists 12 (9) 378-379

Abramov L.I. et al (1987) Kors 87, 1050-1059

Aksentiev S.B. et al (1987) Kors 87, 432-437

Aliev N.A. (1985) Kors 85, 1382-1385

Allen M.G. (1973) American Journal of Psychiatry 130, 1333-1337

Andreasen N.C. (1989) Schizophrenia Bulletin 15, 4, 519-531

Andriushkiavechene Ye. and Visotskas P.P. (1986) Kors 86 (9) 1405-1406

Annals of Internal Medicine (1986) 104, 405-409

Annals of Internal Medicine (1988) 108, 279-288

Anokhina (1985) In: "The Structure of Psychiatry in the Soviet Union" edited by Babayan E. International Universities Press Inc, New York.

Appelbaum P.S. (1988) American Journal of Psychiatry 145, 413-419

Aronson J. (1968) International Journal of Psychiatry 6, 363-364

Asatiani N.M. et al (1983) In: "Borderline neuropsychiatric disorders" Moscow

Auster S.L. (1967) American Journal of Psychiatry 124, 538

Avrutsky G.Ya. and Neduva A.A. (1981) "The treatment of mentally ill patients" Meditsina, Moscow

Avrutsky G.Ya et al (1987) Kors 87 (4) 573-578

Avrutsky G.Ya. et al (1988) Kors 88 (4) 100-105

Babayan E. (1985) "The Structure of Psychiatry in the Soviet Union" International Universities Press Inc, New York.

Bacherikov N.E. et al (1989) "Clinical Psychiatry" Zdarovia, Kiev

Bassuk E.L. (1984) American Journal of Psychiatry 141, 1546-1550

Baxter S. (1983) Lancet i 876

Beardshaw V. (1981) "Conscientious Objectors at Work: Mental Hospital Nurses - A Case Study" Social Audit, London

Bech P. (1987) British Journal of Psychiatry 151, 271

Beers M. et al (1988) Journal of the American Medical Association 260, 3016-3020

Bekhtereva N. (1984) Social Sciences 3, 34-40.

Bennett M.I. (1988) American Journal of Psychiatry 145, 1273

Berrios G. and Bulbena M. (1987) Acta Psychiatrica Scandinavica 76, 89-93

Bleuler E. (1911) "Dementia Praecox oder Gruppe der Schizophrenien" Deutike, Leipzig

Bloch S. and Reddaway P. (1977) "Russia's Political Hospitals" Victor Gollancz, London

Bloch S. and Reddaway P. (1984) "Soviet Psychiatric Abuse" Victor Gollancz, London

Bochkarev V.K. et al (1987) Kors 87 (4) 564-570

British Medical Journal (1985) 290, 1-2

British Medical Journal (1988) 297, 879-880

Brod J. (1984) British Medical Journal 288, 1288-1292

Brown G.W. and Harris T. (1978) Social Origins of Depression Tavistock, London

Bukovsky V. (1978) "To Build a Castle: My life as a dissenter" Andre Deutsch, London.

Bullock M.L. et al (1989) Lancet i 1435-1439

Cancro R. (1985) In: "Comprehensive Textbook of Psychiatry IV" edited by Kaplan H.I. and Sadock B.J. Williams and Wilkins, Baltimore

Casey P.R. and Tyrer P. (1990) British Journal of Psychiatry 156, 261-265

Cawley R.H. (1983) Handbook of Psychiatry, Volume 4 Cambridge University Press, Cambridge.

Chodoff P. (1987) American Journal of Psychiatry 144, 1293-1297

Churkin A.A. Gurovitch I.Ye. Kisilyev A.C. (1987) Kors 87 (11) 1725-1731

Claghorn J. et al (1987) Journal of Clinical Psychopharmacology 7, 377-384

Clare A. (1986) In: "Essentials of Postgraduate Psychiatry" edited by Hill P., Murray R. and Thorley A. Grune and Stratton, London.

Claridge (1987) British Journal of Psychiatry 151, 735-743

"Clinical Psychiatry" (1989) edited by Bacherikov N.E. Zdarovia, Kiev

Cohen D. (1988) "Forgotten Millions" Paladin, London

Cohen D. (1989) "Soviet Psychiatry" Paladin, London

Coid J.W. (1987) British Medical Journal 295, 606

Coid J.W. (1988) British Medical Journal 296, 1779-1782

Collier J. (1989) "The Health Conspiracy" Century, London

"Comprehensive Textbook of Psychiatry IV" (1985) edited by Kaplan H.I. and Sadock B.J. Williams and Wilkins, Baltimore

Cornwell R. (1989a) Independent Magazine 25.3.1989

Cornwell R. (1989b) Independent 13.3.1989

Corson S.A. (1976) Editor: "Psychiatry and Psychology in the USSR" Plenum, New York

Cooper A.M. (1985) American Journal of Psychiatry 142, 1395-1402

Cowdry R.W. and Gardner D.L. (1988) Archives of General Psychiatry 45, 111-119

Crammer J. (1988) British Journal of Psychiatry 153, 709-710

Crome L. (1973) Times 5.9.1973

Crow T.J. et al (1986) British Journal of Psychiatry 148, 120-127

Curson D.A. et al (1985) British Journal of Psychiatry 246, 464

Curson D.A. et al (1986) British Medical Journal 293, 726-728

Cutting J. (1985) "The Psychology of Schizophrenia" Churchill Livingstone

Dalton D.R. (1973) "Two disparate philosophies" Regency Press, London

David A.S. (1988) British Medical Journal 296, 1016

Davidow M. (1976) "Cities without Crisis" International Publishers, New York

Davis D.R. (1987) British Medical Journal 294, 265-266

Davis C.M. (1989) In: "Success and Crisis in National Health Systems" Edited by M.G. Field Routledge, London

Deutsch A. (1948) "The shame of the states" (Mental Illness and social policy: The American Experience Series) Ayer Company Publications

Dispatches (1989) Channel 4 11.1.89

Dodwell D. and Goldberg D. (1989) British Journal of Psychiatry 154, 635-639

Dongier M. and Wittkower E.D. (1981) Editors: "Divergent Views in Psychiatry" Harper and Row, New York

Dorway and Schlesinger (1988) American Journal of Psychiatry 145, A17

Dragunskaya L.S. (1987) Kors 87, 1387-91

Druzhinina Ye. (1989) Science in the USSR 3, 77

Dudaeva K.I. et al (1990) Kors 90 (4) 99-103

Edeh J. (1987) Lancet i 45

Edmonds R. (1965) In: "Fathers and Sons" by Ivan Turgenev Penguin, London

Eisenberg L. (1988) Psychological Medicine 18, 1-9

Endicott J. et al (1982) Archives of General Psychiatry 39, 884-889

Endicott J. et al (1985) Archives of General Psychiatry 43, 13-19

Epifanova N.M. et al (1988) Kors 88 (2) 78-81

Erlichman J. (1988) Guardian 28.7.1988

Fagin L. (1985) Bulletin of Royal College of Psychiatrists 9, 112-114

Fagin L. and Purser H. (1986) Bulletin of Royal College of Psychiatrists 10, 303-306

Farndale J. (1961) "The Day Hospital movement in Great Britain" Pergamon Press

Field M. (1967) "Soviet Socialized Medicine" Free Press, New York

Field M.G. (1989) Editor: "Success and Crisis in National Health Systems" Routledge, London

Fish F. (1967) "Clinical psychopathology" Wright and Sons, Bristol.

Fuller Torrey E. (1971) American Journal of Psychiatry 128, 153

Fuller Torrey E. (1987) British Journal of Psychiatry 150, 598-608

Futiryan Y. (1990) Medical Gazette 6.4.1990

Galachian A.G. (1968) in "Psychiatry in the Communist World" edited by Kiev A. Science House, New York.

Galanter M. (1982) American Journal of Psychiatry 139, 1539-1548

Galanter M. (1991) American Journal of Psychiatry 148, 90-95

Garrison O.V. (1974) "The Hidden Story of Scientology" Arlington books, London

Gellner E. (1985) "The Psychoanalytic Movement" Paladin, London.

Giliarovsky V.A. (1931,1935,1938,1954) "Psychiatry" Biomedgiz, Moscow and Leningrad

Gill M. (1988) British Medical Journal 297, 1426

Ginsburg L.M. and Ginsburg S.A. (1983) Journal of Psychiatry and Law 11, 19-28

Gladishev A.S. (1977) Kors 77, 1734-1739

Gluzman S. (1989) Medical Gazette 21.5.89

Goldberg S. et al (1986) Archives of General Psychiatry 43,680-686.

Goldman H.H. (1983) In "New Directions for Mental Health Services: Deinstitutionalization" edited by Bachrach L.L. Jossey-Bass, San Francisco

Gorchakova L.N. (1988) Kors 88 (5) 76-82

Gorman M. (1969) International Journal of Psychiatry 8, 841-861

Granville-Grossman K. (1983) In "Handbook of Psychiatry" Volume 2 Cambridge University Press, Cambridge

Gray J.A. (1979) "Pavlov" Fontana

Grigorieva E.A. and Nikiforov A.I. (1987) Kors 87 (4) 550-555

Grinker R. (1982) In: "Psychiatrists on Psychiatry" edited by Shepherd M. Cambridge University Press, Cambridge

Gross G. (1989) British Journal of Psychiatry 155 (suppl. 7) 21-25

Gunderson et al (1981) American Journal of Psychiatry 138, 896-903

Gurland et al (1979) Psychological Medicine 9, 781-788

Gurevitch et al (1985) Kors 85 (4) 550-556

"Handbook of Psychiatry" (1983) edited by Snezhnevsky A.V. Meditsina, Moscow

Harding T.W. (1987) Lancet i, 1264

Harding C.M. et al (1987) American Journal of Psychiatry 144, 718-735

Haslam (1987) British Journal of Clinical and Social Psychiatry 5, 43-47

Healy P. Times 22.2.83

Hein G. (1968) International Journal of Psychiatry 6, 346-362

Hoch P. and Palatin J. (1949) Psychiatric Quarterly 23, 248-276

Hoenig J. (1983) British Journal of Psychiatry 142, 547-556

Holland J. (1975) In: "The Future Role of the State Hospital" edited by Zusman J. and Bertsch E.F. Lexington Books, Toronto

Holland J. (1976) "Psychiatry and Psychology in the USSR" edited by Corson S.A. Plenum, New York

Holland J. (1977) Schizophrenia in the Soviet Union: Concepts and Treatment. In: "Annual Review of the Schizophrenia Syndrome" edited by Cancro R.

Holland J. and Shakhmatova-Pavlova I. (1977) Schizophrenia Bulletin 3, 277-287

Howard R.C. (1984) Psychological Medicine 14, 569-580

Hutton J.B. (1960) "Danger from Moscow" Neville Spearman, London

Hyde G. (1973) British Journal of Social Psychiatry and Community Health 6, 157-169

Hyde G. (1974) "The Soviet Health Service" Lawrence and Wishart, London

Hyde G. (1988) UK-USSR Medical Exchange Programme Newsletter March 1988

Isaev (1974) International Journal of Mental Health 1974, 3, 47-56

Isakoff Yu. V. et al (1987) Kors 87 (12) 1832-1835

Jablensky A. (1982) In: "Psychiatrists on Psychiatry" edited by Shepherd M. Cambridge University Press

Jablensky A. (1986) Schizophrenia Bulletin 12, 52-73

Jackson P.R. and Warr P.B. (1984) Psychological Medicine 605-614

John E.R. et al. (1988) Science 239, 162-169

Johnstone E.C. et al (1988) Lancet ii 119-125

Jones K. (1972) "A History of the Mental Health Services" Routledge and Kegan Paul, London.

Kabanov M.M. (1986) In: Current Psychiatric Therapies. Edited by Masserman J.H. Grune and Stratton, New York

Kabanov M.M. and Zachepitsky R.A. (1982) International Journal of Mental Health 11 (3) 133-147

Karvasarsky B.D. (1980) "Nevrosi" Meditsina, Moscow

Karvasarsky B.D. (1986) In: Current Psychiatric Therapies edited by Masserman J.H. Grune and Stratton, New York

Kaser M. (1976) "Health care in the Soviet Union and Eastern Europe." Westview Press, Boulder, Colorado.

Kastrup M. (1988) European Journal of Psychiatry 2, 22-31

Katz S. (1985) In: "Comprehensive Textbook of Psychiatry IV" edited by Kaplan H.I. and Sadock B.J. Williams and Wilkins, Baltimore

Kazanetz E.P. (1979) Archives of General Psychiatry 36, 740-745
Kazanetz E.P. (1989) British Journal of Psychiatry 155, 160-165
Kendell R.E. (1975) British Journal of Psychiatry 127, 305-315
Kendell R.E. (1981) In "Divergent Views in Psychiatry" edited by Dongier M.
     and Wittkower E.D. Harper and Row, New York
Kendell R.E. (1989) British Medical Journal 299, 1237-1238
Kendell R.E. and Gourlay J. (1970) British Journal of Psychiatry 117, 261-266
Kendell RE and Brockington IF (1980) British Journal of Psychiatry 137, 324 - 331
Kendell RE et al (1971) Archives of General Psychiatry 25, 123
Kendler K.S. et al (1985) Archives of General Psychiatry 42; 770-779
Kerbikov O.V. (1971) "Selected Works" Meditsina, Moscow
Kiev, Ari (1968) Editor: "Psychiatry in the Communist World" Science House,
     New York.
Kiloh L.G. et al (1962) British Medical Journal i 1225-1227
Kiloh L.G. et al (1988) British Journal of Psychiatry 153, 752-757
Klaf F.S. and Hamilton J.G. (1961) Journal of Mental Science 107, 819-827
Kleist K. (1953) Mschr. Psychiat. Neurol. 125, 526
Koniukhova E.N. (1985) Kors 85, 584-588
Kontsevoi O.V. and Kolesnikov E.S. (1987) Kors 87 (9) 1401-1403
Korkina M. Tsivilko M. Kossova E. (1980) "Lecons pratiques de psychiatrie"
     Mir, Moscow
Korkina M.V. et al (1989) Kors 89 (2) 82-87
Kornilov A.A. et al (1987) Kors 87 (11) 1694-1697
Korolev V.V. (1983) Kors 83 (11) 1695-1699
Korsakoff S.S. (1893, 1913) "A course in psychiatry" Moscow
Koryagin A. (1981) Lancet i 821-824
Koryagin A. (1988) Lancet ii 268-269
Kosenko V.G. (1989) Kors 89 (1) 117-120
Kozulin A. (1984) "Psychology in Utopia" MIT Press Cambridge, Massachusetts
Kramer M. (1989) In: "The Scope of Epidemiological Psychiatry" edited by
     Williams P. et al Routledge, London
Krasick and Logvinovitch (1977) Kors 77 1711-1715
Kronfeld A. (1928) Nervenarzt 53 (1) 46-51
Kutsenok B.M. (1988) "Residual schizophrenia" Zdarovia, Moscow
Kuzmina M.E. and Panyushkina S.V. (1975) Kors 8 1218-1222
Lader M. (1977) "Psychiatry on Trial" Penguin, London
Laing R.D. (1965) "The Divided Self" Pelican, London
Lakosina N.D. and Trunova M.M. (1983) Kors 83 (11) 1664-1670
Lancet (1984) ii 1350-1351
Lancet (1985) ii 253
Lancet (1986a) i 1014-1015
Lancet (1986b) ii 701
Lancet (1987a) ii 773-774
Lancet (1987b) i 678-679
Lancet (1988a) i 1467-1468
Lancet (1988b) ii 919
Lancet (1988c) ii 316-317

Lancet (1988d) i 134-135

Lancet (1988e) ii 1402-4

Lancet (1989a) i 1462

Lancet (1989b) i 1195

Langfeldt G. (1937) "The Prognosis in Schizophrenia and the Factors influencing the Course of the Disease" Levin and Munksgaard, Copenhagen.

Langfeldt G. (1956) Acta Psychiatrica Neurologica Scandinavica, Supplement 13

Langsley D.G. (1985) In: "Comprehensive Textbook of Psychiatry IV" edited by Kaplan H.I. and Sadock B.J. Williams and Wilkins, Baltimore

Lauterbach W. (1984) "Soviet Psychotherapy" Pergamon Press, Oxford and New York

LeBeau J. (1988) American Journal of Psychotherapy 42, 425-436

Lee A.S. and Murray R.M. (1988) British Journal of Psychiatry 153, 741-751

Lehman and Cancro (1985) In: "Comprehensive Textbook of Psychiatry IV" edited by Kaplan H.I. and Sadock B.J. Williams and Wilkins, Baltimore

Leighton D.C et al (1963) "The Character of Danger" Basic books, New York.

Leonhard K. (1961) Journal of Mental Science 107, 633-648

Levitan K. (1982) "One is not born a personality" Progress, Moscow

Levy R. (1972) Lancet ii 185

Lewis A. (1953) British Journal of Sociology 4, 109-124

Lewis D.O. et al (1986) American Journal of Psychiatry 143, 838-841

Lewis D.O. et al (1988) American Journal of Psychiatry 145, 584-589

Lezhepekova L.N. and Pervov L.G. (1977) Kors 77, 1862-1866

Lichko A.E. (1977) Kors 77, 1833- 1838

Lichko A.E. (1986) In: "Current Psychiatric Therapies" edited by Masserman J.H. Grune and Stratton, New York

Linn (1985) In: "Comprehensive Textbook of Psychiatry IV" edited by Kaplan H.I. and Sadock B.J. Williams and Wilkins, Baltimore

Linn M.W. et al (1985) Archives of general Psychiatry 42, 544-551

Lipkowitz M.H. and Idupuganti S. (1985) American Journal of Psychiatry 142, 634-637

Lipsedge M.S. (1985) British Journal of Hospital Medicine 2, 25-27

Lisitsin and Batygin (1978) "The USSR: Public Health and Social Security" Progress, Moscow

Littlewood R. and Lipsedge M. (1988) British Medical Journal 296, 950-951

Lovett L.M. and Shaw D.M. (1987) British Journal of Psychiatry 151, 113-116

Lukanitsa S.K. (1986) Kors 86 (9) 1417-1427.

Lukacher G. Ya et al (1989) Kors 89 (1) 83-87

McGlashan (1983) Archives of General Psychiatry 40, 1311-1323

McGlashan (1986) Archives of General Psychiatry 43, 20-30

McGlashan (1987) Archives of General Psychiatry 44, 143-148

Mangan G.L. (1982) "The Biology of Human Conduct" Pergamon

"Manual of Psychiatry" (1985) edited by Snezhnevsky A.V. Meditsina, Moscow

"Manual for Psychiatrists" (1990) edited by Voronkov G.L., Vidrenko A.E. and Shevchuk I.D. Zdarovia, Kiev

Mark V.H. and Ervin F.R. (1970) "Violence and the Brain" Harper and Row, New York

Markelova et al (1986) Kors 86, 1708-1712

Markovsky V.M. and Fel F.M. (1988) Kors 86 (9) 1401-1404

Markowitz J. et al (1987) American Journal of Psychiatry 144, 1025-1029

Marneros A. (1988) British Journal of Psychiatry 152, 625-68

Masserman J.H. (1986) Editor: "Current Psychiatric Therapies" Grune and Stratton, New York

Matuzas W. et al (1987) American Journal of Psychiatry 144, 493-496

Mchedlov M. (1982) "Religion in the World Today" Progress, Moscow

"Medical Preparations" (1985) Mashkovsky M.D. Meditsina, Moscow

Medvedev Z.A. and Medvedev R.A. (1971) "A Question of Madness" MacMillan, London

Melikhov D.E. (1963) "The clinical basis of assessing work capability in schizophrenia" Medgiz, Moscow

Melville D.I. et al (1985) Psychological Medicine 15, 789-793

Mersky H. and Shafran B. (1986) British Journal of Psychiatry 148, 247-256

Miasishchev V.N. (1960) "Personality and neuroses" Leningrad

Mikheeva T.V. et al (1987) Kors 87, 109-113

Mikolaisky M.V. (1988) Kors 88 (5) 102-106

Minsker et al (1977) Kors 77 (8) 1209-1214

Mombaur W.(1984) In: "Training and Education in Psychiatry" edited by Lopez Ibor Alino J.J. and Lenz G. Facultas-Verlag, Vienna.

Morozov G.V. (1985) In: "The Structure of Psychiatry in the Soviet Union" edited by Babayan E. International Universities Press Inc, New York.

Morozov G.V. and Kalashnik Ya.M. (1970) "Forensic Psychiatry" In the Soviet Law and Government series, International Arts and Sciences Press, Inc. White Plains, New York

Mosketi K.V. et al (1984) Kors 84 (4) 589-596

Mosolov S.N. and Moshchevitin S.Y. (1990) Kors 90 (4) 121-125

Mosolov S.N. et al (1989) Kors 89 (4) 87-93

Mugutdinov T.M. (1985) Kors 85 (2) 232-236

Mullan M.J. and Murray R.M. (1989) British Journal of Psychiatry 154, 591-595

Nadjarov R.A. (1972) In: "Schizophrenia: a multidisciplinary study" edited by Snezhnevsky A.V. Meditsina, Moscow

National Economy of the USSR (1987) Finance and Statistics, Moscow

National Economy of the USSR (1989) Finance and Statistics, Moscow

Nemtsov A.V. et al (1989) Kors 89 (2) 93-97

Nesse et al (1984) Archives of General Psychiatry 41, 771-776

Nevidimova T.I. et al (1988) Kors 88 (10) 81-87

New England Journal of Medicine (1988) 318, 843-847

New York State Journal Of Medicine (1986) 86, 620-621

Nuller Yu. L. (1976) Kors 76 (5) 717-723

Nuller Y.L. (1986) In: "Current Psychiatric Therapies" edited by Masserman J.H. Grune and Stratton, New York

Nuller Yu.L. and Mikhalenko I.N. (1988) "The Affective Psychoses" Meditsina, Leningrad

Nuller Yu L. et al (1986) Kors 86 (4) 547-551

Ogonyok (1984) 42, 22-23

Osipov V.P. (1931) "Handbook of Psychiatry" Gosizdat, Moscow and Leningrad
Oskolkova S.N. (1985) Kors 85, 560-565
Papadopolous T.F. and Shakhmatova-Pavlova I.V. (1983) In: "Handbook of Psychiatry" edited by Snezhnevsky A.V. Meditsina, Moscow
Pelosi A.J. (1988) British Journal of Psychiatry 153, 412
Philip P. et al (1991) Biological Psychiatry 29, 451-456
Pittman F.S. the third (1985) Family Processes 24, 461-472
Platt S. and Kreitman N. (1985) Psychological Medicine 15, 113-123
Podrabinek A. (1980) "Punitive Medicine" Karoma, Ann Arbor
Poliakov S.E. and Kokhanov V.P. (1988) Kors 88 (10) 133-137
Poliakov Yu. F. et al (1987) Kors 87 (7) 1059-1064
Polischuk Yu. I. (1989) Kors 89 (5) 148-149
Pollock G. (1988) American Journal of Psychiatry 145, 1055
Ponomareff G.L. (1986) In: "Current Psychiatric Therapies" edited by Masserman J.H. Grune and Stratton, New York
Ponomareff G.L. (1989) Guest Editor: Psychotherapy in "Soviet Neurology and Psychiatry" Winter 1988-1989 edition M.E.Sharpe, Armonk, New York
Popper K.R. and Eccles J.C. (1977) "The Self and its Brain" Springer, Berlin
Portnov A.A. et al (1987) Kors 87 (7) 1076-1086
Potapova V.A. (1985) Kors 85 (9) 1378-1381
Potapova V.A. and Trubnikov V.I. (1987) Kors 87, 727-732
Powell J.C. et al (1988) British Journal of Psychiatry 153, 689-692
Pravda (1987a) Pravda International July 1987
Pravda (1987b) Pravda International February 1987
Prokhorova I.S. (1985) Kors 85 (4) 570-574
Prokopochky A.A. et al (1988) Kors 88 (5) 82-87
Radhakrishnan et al (1983) British Journal of Psychiatry 142, 557-559
Raevsky K.S. (1985) Kors 85, 574-570
Regier D.A. et al (1988) Archives of General Psychiatry 45, 977-986
Reiser M.F. (1988) American Journal of Psychiatry 145, 158
Rich V. (1989) Nature 338, 608
Rich V. (1991a) Lancet 337, 723-724
Rich V. (1991b) Lancet 338, 1197-1198)
Robin A. and DeTissera S. (1982) British Journal of Psychiatry 141, 357-366
Robinson and Berger (1988) Bulletin of the Royal College of Psychiatrists 12, 95-97
Roemer R. (1987) American Journal of Public Health 78, 241-247
Rollin N. (1972) "Child Psychiatry in the Soviet Union: Preliminary Observations" Harvard University Press Cambridge Massachusetts
Rosenhan D.L. (1973) Science 179, 250
Rosenshtein L.M. (1933) "Mild forms of schizophrenia" In: "Current problems in schizophrenia" Moscow and Leningrad
Ross D.R. et al (1988) American Journal of Psychiatry 1988 145, 242-245
Roth M. (1986) In: "Contemporary Issues in Schizophrenia" edited by Kerr A. and Snaith P. Gaskell, 1986
Roth L.R. (1989) American Journal of Psychiatry 146 135-137
Rotstein V.G. (1977) Kors 77 569-574
Rotstein V.G. et al (1987) Kors 87, 931-936

Rozhnov V.E. (1985) In: "The Structure of Psychiatry in the Soviet Union" edited by Babayan. International Universities Press Inc, New York.

Rozhnov V.E. (1989) Kors 89 (1) 58-62

Rubinstein S.L. (1942 and 1946) "Foundations of General Psychology" Moscow

Rudy L.H. (1985) In: "Comprehensive Textbook of Psychiatry IV" edited by Kaplan H.I. and Sadock B.J. Williams and Wilkins, Baltimore

Rutter M. (1987) British Journal of Psychiatry 150, 443-458

Ryan M. (1982) British Medical Journal 285, 496-497

Ryan M. (1985) British Medical Journal 290, 1414-1416

Ryan M. (1989) British Medical Journal 299, 383-384

Ryan M. and Prentice R. (1983) British Medical Journal 286, 1494-1495

Sackeim H.A. et al (1987) American Journal of Psychiatry 144, 1449-1455

Salzman L. (1963) Comprehensive Psychiatry 4 (4) 237-245

Sartorius N. (1988) British Journal of Psychiatry 152, supplement 1, 9-14

Saugstadt L. and Odegard O. (1985) Psychological Medicine 15, 1-2

Scadding J.G. (1967) Lancet ii 877-882

Sedgewick P. (1982) "Psychopolitics" Pluto Press, London

Segal B.N. (1975) American Journal of Psychotherapy 29, 503-523

Segal S.P. (1989) American Journal of Psychiatry 146 187-193

Sekirina T.P. et al (1988) Kors 88 (7) 90-95

Sekerina T.P. et al (1989) Kors 89 (5) 95-97

Semenov S.F. et al (1988) Kors 88 (1) 100-107

Serbsky V.P. (1906, 1912) "Psychiatry: a handbook of mental disorders" Moscow

Shakhmatova-Pavlova I.V. et al (1975) In: "New Dimensions in Psychiatry: World View" edited by Arieti S. and Chrzanowski G. John Wiley and Sons, New York

Shmaunova L.M. (1985) In "Manual of Psychiatry" edited by Snezhnevsky A.V. Meditsina, Moscow

Shmaunova L.M. and Lieberman Ye. I. (1979) Kors 79 (6) 770-780

Shmaunova L.M. et al (1988) Kors 88 (5) 66-71

Shore D. et al (1985) American Journal of Psychiatry 142, 308-312

Shumsky N.G. (1985) In: "Manual of Psychiatry" edited by Snezhnevsky A.V. Meditsina, Moscow

Sidorenko G.V. and Soroko S.I. (1989) Kors 89 (6) 92-98

Sigerist H.E. (1937) "Socialized Medicine in the Soviet Union" Victor Gollancz, London

Signer S.F. (1988) British Journal of Psychiatry 152, 296-297

Silver G.A. (1989) Lancet ii 95

Simms A. (1988) "Symptoms in the Mind" Bailliere Tindall, London

Simpson and May (1985) In: "Comprehensive Textbook of Psychiatry IV" edited by Kaplan H.I. and Sadock B.J. Williams and Wilkins, Baltimore

Sinitsky V.N. et al (1988) Kors 88 (9) 84-95

Sirotkin P. (1968) American Journal of Psychiatry 125, 656-660Slater and Shields (1969) "Studies of Anxiety" edited by Lader M.H. British Journal of Psychiatry Special Publication Number 3

Sluchevsky F.I. and Petsevitch M.E. (1988) Kors 88 (3) 93-97

Small J.G. (1988) Archives of General Psychiatry 45, 727-732

Smith R. (1985) British Medical Journal 291, 1191-1195 and 1492-1495 and 1263-1266 and 1563-1566

Smulevitch A.B. (1983) In "Handbook of Psychiatry" edited by Snezhnevsky A.V. Meditsina, Moscow

Smulevitch A.B. (1985) In "Manual of Psychiatry" edited by Snezhnevsky A.V. Meditsina, Moscow

Smulevitch A.B. (1987) "Slow-flow schizophrenia and borderline conditions" Meditsina, Moscow

Smulevitch A.V. and Panteleeva G.P. (1983) Kors 83 (9) 1345-1351

Snaith R.P. (1987) British Journal of Hospital Medicine 38, 147

Snezhnevsky A.V. (1968) In: "Modern Perspectives in World Psychiatry" edited by Howells J.G. Oliver and Boyd, London and Edinburgh.

Snezhnevsky A.V. (1972) "Schizophrenia: multidisciplinary research" Meditsina, Moscow.

Snezhnevsky A.V. (1983) Editor: "Handbook of Psychiatry" Meditsina, Moscow

Snezhnevsky A.V. (1985) Editor: "Manual of Psychiatry" Meditsina, Moscow

Snezhnevsky A.V. (1987) In "Slow-flow schizophrenia and borderline conditions" Smulevitch A.B. Meditsina, Moscow

Sochneva (1985) In: "The Structure of Psychiatry in the Soviet Union" edited by Babayan E. International Universities Press Inc, New York

Sonnick G.T. (1984) Vrachebnoe delo 3, 99-101

Spencer J. (1975) British Journal of Psychiatry 126, 556-559

Spitzer R.L. (1976) Archives of General Psychiatry 33, 459-470

Srole L. et al (1962) "Mental Health in the Metropolis" McGraw-Hill, New York

Steaman H. (1983) International Journal of Law and Psychiatry , 381-390

Steele D.W. (1985) British Medical Journal 290, 561-562

Sternberg E.Ya. (1983) In "Handbook of Psychiatry" edited by Snezhnevsky A.V. Meditsina, Moscow

Stone A. (1984) In: "Law, Psychiatry and Morality" pages 3-39 American Psychiatric Press Inc, Washington

Sturt J. and Waters H. (1985) Lancet i 507-508

Szasz T. (1961) "The Myth of Mental Illness" Secker and Warburg, London

Szasz T. (1988) Lancet ii 573

Szasz T. (1989) British Journal of Psychiatry 154, 864-869

Tarsis V. (1965) "Ward 7" Collins and Harvill, London

Taube C.A. et al (1988) American Journal of Psychiatry 145, 210-213

Thompson J.W. and Blaire J.D. (1987) American Journal of Psychiatry 144, 557-562

Thornicroft G. (1988) Bulletin of the Royal College of Psychiatrists 12 (7) 286-288

Tsaritsinsky V.I. (1984) Kors 84 (4) 92-98

Tselmz G. (1989) Literaturnaya Gazeta 31.5.89

Tyrer P. (1985) Lancet i, 685-688

Tyrer P. (1986) Journal of Affective Disorders 11, 99-104

Tyrer and Murphy (1987) British Journal of Psychiatry 151, 719-723

Umansky K. (1989) "Everyday neuropathology" Mir, Moscow

Vaillant and Perry (1985) In: "Comprehensive Textbook of Psychiatry IV" edited by Kaplan H.I. and Sadock B.J. Williams and Wilkins, Baltimore

Valenstein E.S. (1986) "Great and Desperate Cures" Basic Books, New York

Vartanian M. (1983) In "Handbook of Psychiatry" edited by Snezhnevsky A.V. Meditsina, Moscow

Vasiljeva O.A. et al (1989) American Journal of Psychiatry 146, 284-285

Vein A.M. and Rodshtat I.V. (1974) "Neurological and neurophysiological aspects of the approach to the problem of neuroses" Meditsina, Moscow

Vetlugina T.P. et al (1989) Kors 89 (5) 102-105

Vilkov G.A. et al (1987) Kors 87 (8) 1241-1243

Vishnevsky V.A. (1984) Kors 84 (4) 563-567

Vishnevsky V.A. (1988) Kors 88 (12) 73-78

Visotsky H.M. (1968) American Journal of Psychiatry 125, 650-655

Vovin R.Y. (1986) In: "Current Psychiatric Therapies" edited by Masserman J.H. Grune and Stratton, New York

Vovin R.Y. (1987) Kors 87, 1396-1400

Vovin R.Y. and Aksenova I.O. (1982) "Prolonged Depressive Disorders" Meditsina, Leningrad

Volovik V.M. (1986) In: "Current Psychiatric Therapies" edited by Masserman J.H. Grune and Stratton, New York

Voronkov G.L., Vidrenko A.E. and Shevchuk I.D. (1990) "Manual for psychiatrists" Zdarovia, Kiev

Vrono M. (1988) Kors 88 (10) 1514-1517

Vul F.R. et al (1988) Kors 88 (10) 111-116

Wallace E.R. (1988) American Journal of Psychiatry 145, 137

Warner R. (1985) "Recovery from Schizophrenia: psychiatry and political economy" Routledge and Kegan Paul, London.

Weller M. et al (1988) British Medical Journal 297, 559-560

West D.J. (1989) British Journal of Psychiatry 154, 870-871

Wilkinson G. (1986) British Medical Journal 293, 641-642.

Wing J.K. (1974) British Medical Journal 1, 433-436

Wing J.K. (1987) British Medical Journal 291, 1219-1220

Winn R. (1962) "Psychotherapy in the Soviet Union" Peter Owen, London

Winslade et al (1984) American Journal of Psychiatry 141, 1349

WHO (1973) "Report of the International Pilot Study of Schizophrenia" WHO, Geneva

Wolpert L. (1987) Journal of the Royal College of Physicians of London 21, 159-165

Wortis J. (1950) "Soviet Psychiatry" Williams and Wilkins, Baltimore

Wortis J. (1979) Psychiatric News 14 (4): 2, 14

Wylie H.W. and Wylie M.L. (1987) American Journal of Psychiatry 144, 489-492

Wynn A. (1987) "Notes of a non-conspirator" Andre Deutsch, London

Yenikeyev et al (1989) Science in the USSR 5, 124-127

Youssef H.A. (1973) Lancet i 595-596

Zachepitsky R.A. (1986) In: "Current Psychiatric Therapies" edited by Masserman J.H. Grune and Stratton, New York

Zagalsky L. (1989) Literaturnaya Gazeta 28.6.89

Zavilianskaya L.I. (1987) "The psychotherapy of the neurosis-like disorders" Zdarovia, Kiev

Zenevich G.V. (1986) In: "Current Psychiatric Therapies" edited by Masserman J.H. Grune and Stratton, New York

Zharikov N.M. (1983) In "Handbook of Psychiatry" edited by Snezhnevsky A.V.
   Meditsina, Moscow
Zharikov N.M. and Sokolova E.D. (1989) Kors 89 (5) 63-66
Ziferstein I. (1966) American Journal of Psychiatry 123, 440
Ziferstein I. (1968) International Journal of Psychiatry 6, 366-370
Zilboorg G. (1944) American Review of Soviet Medicine 562-575

INDEX

Page numbers given in **bold type** indicate where the definition
or main description of a term is given.